Age-Related Macular Degeneration

Age-Related Macular Degeneration

Weiye Li

Professor emeritus of Ophthalmology
Drexel University College of Medicine
Philadelphia, Pennsylvania
United States

ELSEVIER

Elsevier
Radarweg 29, PO Box 211, 1000 AE Amsterdam, Netherlands
The Boulevard, Langford Lane, Kidlington, Oxford OX5 1GB, United Kingdom
50 Hampshire Street, 5th Floor, Cambridge, MA 02139, United States

Notices
Knowledge and best practice in this field are constantly changing. As new research and
experience broaden our understanding, changes in research methods, professional
practices, or medical treatment may become necessary.

Practitioners and researchers must always rely on their own experience and knowledge in
evaluating and using any information, methods, compounds, or experiments described
herein. In using such information or methods they should be mindful of their own safety
and the safety of others, including parties for whom they have a professional
responsibility.

To the fullest extent of the law, neither the Publisher nor the authors, contributors, or
editors, assume any liability for any injury and/or damage to persons or property as a
matter of products liability, negligence or otherwise, or from any use or operation of any
methods, products, instructions, or ideas contained in the material herein.

Library of Congress Cataloging-in-Publication Data
A catalog record for this book is available from the Library of Congress

British Library Cataloguing-in-Publication Data
A catalogue record for this book is available from the British Library

ISBN: 978-0-12-822061-0

For information on all Elsevier publications visit our website at
https://www.elsevier.com/books-and-journals

Publisher: Cathleen Sether
Acquisitions Editor: Kayla Wolfe
Editorial Project Manager: Mona Zahir
Production Project Manager: Niranjan Bhaskaran
Cover Designer: Matthew Limbert

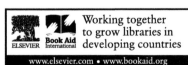

Working together
to grow libraries in
developing countries

www.elsevier.com • www.bookaid.org

Typeset by TNQ Technologies

To my wife, Xinru, for her encouragement, support, and love. To my family who understands the hard and meaningful work writing this book. To my mentors, Dr. Katherine Yuen-Tsieu Lao, Dr. Tennyson Tiansheng Hu, and Dr. John H. Rockey who inspired me and guided my path to be a physician-scientist.

Contents

About the author

Weiye Li, MD, PhD

Dr. Weiye Li, Professor Emeritus, is a retinal surgeon and researcher of Drexel University, College of Medicine. In this book, Dr. Li shares his experience and insight as an internationally renowned expert in the study of diabetic retinopathy and age-related macular degeneration.

Preface

Age-related macular degeneration (AMD) is a leading cause of blindness of the elderly worldwide. AMD is a macular disease with heterogeneous disease manifestations and with complex genetic heritability. In the recent two decades, substantial progress has been made in both basic and clinical research of this devastating disease.

This book tries to update the basic understanding of AMD genetics and the interplay between genetic and environmental factors in the pathogenesis of AMD. In the early 21st century, the Human Genome Project was completed. It provided a necessary map of the human genome, onto which polymorphism data had been collected over years. Genome-wide single-nucleotide polymorphic association studies with AMD case-control cohorts discovered the association of a variant (Y402H) in the complement factor H (*CFH*) gene with late-stage AMD in 2005.[1] This discovery opened the gate of AMD molecular genetics and pointed out the association between genetic risk factor, that is, tyrosine-histidine polymorphism, and underlying mechanisms of AMD, such as drusen formation, alternative complement pathway activation, and complement-mediated inflammation. In recent years, the molecular mechanistic link between complement dysregulation and AMD pathobiology has been investigated in great depth.[2] Meanwhile epidemiological studies from AREDS1 to AREDS2 have revealed that age and smoking are important environmental risk factors for AMD. Expectedly, the interaction between environmental factors such as dietary supplements in AREDS2 and genotype of patients with AMD is complex. Future studies in larger populations that include different stages of AMD, focusing on the identification of rare and potentially highly penetrant variants in the genes that already have been implicated from common loci, are essential. Studies in molecular genetics and molecular pathobiology have elucidated key pathogenic events of AMD, which include oxidative stress, radical oxygen species generation, inflammation, complement/inflammasome activation, dysfunctional autophagy, programmed cell death, and pathological angiogenesis.

The aim of this book is to discuss how these research achievements can be translated into clinical application from a physician's perspective. Again, in less than two decades, multimodal imaging technology, especially optical coherence tomography (OCT), has become the most frequent and powerful ancillary test in clinical retinal practice. OCT has started a new era on clinical AMD and other retinal diseases. To date, OCT is able to analyze retina at the cellular level in vivo and to have validated and revised both dry and wet AMD classification.[3] Based on the consensus on classification and nomenclatures, heterogeneous phenotypes of AMD can be accurately stratified for better searching geno-phenotype interaction and possible therapeutic targets. Based on a better understanding of pathogenic events, numerous approaches are under development in the AMD treatment pipeline. In 2005, the field celebrated the success of intravitreal anti-VEGF therapy, translated and adapted from clinical oncology for neovascular AMD.[4] This therapy has revolutionized the treatment of neovascular AMD, because the anti-VEGF not only can prevent vision loss but also lead to vision improvement. Notably, the success of anti-VEGF therapy is incomplete in the clinical setting, which has prompted us to search for targets beyond VEGF-driven angiogenesis. For instance, regulation of complement/inflammasome, neuroprotection, gene-therapy, and cell-based stem cell therapy will help us surmount obstacles in AMD treatment. Although we are facing a challenging future, more advances in basic and clinical AMD studies may lead us to eventually control this blinding disease.

The topic of AMD studies is far-ranging, which is beyond my ability to comprehensively describe. I humbly present this book to readers, to make some introductory remarks to set the ball rolling for future breakthroughs.

References

1. Klein RJ. Complement factor H polymorphism in age-related macular degeneration. *Science*. 2005;308(5720):385−389. https://doi.org/10.1126/science.1109557.
2. Calippe B, Augustin S, Beguier F, et al. Complement factor H inhibits CD47-mediated resolution of inflammation. *Immunity*. 2017;46(2):261−272. https://doi.org/10.1016/j.immuni.2017.01.006.
3. Drexler W. Cellular and functional optical coherence tomography of the human retina: the Cogan lecture. *Invest Ophthalmol Vis Sci*. 2007;48(12):5339−5351. https://doi.org/10.1167/iovs.07-0895.
4. Rosenfeld PJ, Moshfeghi AA, Puliafito CA. Optical coherence tomography findings after an intravitreal injection of bevacizumab (avastin) for neovascular age-related macular degeneration. *Ophthalmic Surg Lasers Imaging*. 2005;36(4):331−335.

Acknowledgments

Writing a monograph on age-related macular degeneration (AMD), a leading cause of irreversible blindness in the elderly, is an enormous undertaking. During my three decades at the Drexel University at Philadelphia, my research and clinical work allowed me to continuously build on my understanding of the complexities of AMD. I am very grateful to Dr. Samuel Zigler for his critical comments and careful editing of the manuscript. I also appreciate the critiques and editing efforts of Dr. Aparna Ramasubramanian, Dr. Guotong Xu, and Dr. Jingfa Zhang. Thanks also go out to the production team at Elsevier whose delicate and hard work made publishing this book possible.

Overview and definition of age-related macular degeneration

1

Age-related macular degeneration as a leading cause of blindness among the elderly population

Age-related macular degeneration (AMD) is the leading cause of irreversible blindness of the elderly worldwide.[1] Based on the Global Vision Database, among the global population, the cause for blindness due to AMD in 1990 and 2010 was 5% and 7%, respectively.[2] In the United States, the number of persons having AMD will increase by 50% to 2.95 million in 2020.[3] AMD is a central-retina disease from early to late stage, with various severities (Fig. 1.1).[4] Earlier, it had been believed that this kind of blindness is predominantly from a rapidly progressing form, that is, neovascular or wet AMD. Currently, it is understood that the etiologies of visual impairment in AMD patients consist of both wet AMD and an advanced form of dry AMD, that is, geographic atrophy (GA). Vision loss by GA is characterized by a gradual progression, due to the subtle nature of GA growth and its poor association with vision impairment. In real life, enlarging GA lesions could be

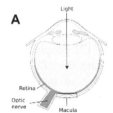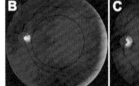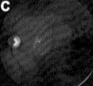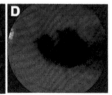

FIGURE 1.1

A spectrum of clinical presentation of AMD. The macula is the central part of the retina (A). Clinical photographs of posterior retina demonstrate the different features of AMD: (B) soft drusen at the posterior pole of fundus, the black circle indicates the macula; (C) geographic atrophy, advanced stage of dry AMD; (D) neovascular AMD with subretinal hemorrhage.

Modified from McHarg S, Clark SJ, Day AJ, Bishop PN. Age-related macular degeneration and the role of the complement system. Mol Immunol. 2015;67(1):43–50. doi: 10.1016/j.molimm.2015.02.032.

Age-Related Macular Degeneration. https://doi.org/10.1016/B978-0-12-822061-0.00004-9

harbored for years before encroaching on the fovea, the center of the macula. Therefore, a large portion of GA progression is not easily discerned or quantified and the annual rate of vision impairment due to GA may be underestimated.

AMD is a serious gerontologic disease. Although the pathogenesis underlying this human age-related disease is not completely understood, advanced age appears to be the strongest risk factor.[5] The evidence from epidemiological studies shows that the prevalence of AMD increases with age. In the United States, approximately one in eight people (12.5%) over the age of 60 has some degree of macular degeneration. For seniors over age 80, one in three (33%) has AMD. The number of people living with macular degeneration is expected to reach 196 million worldwide by 2020 and increase to 288 million by 2040.[6] As a whole, the rapidly rising incidence of AMD is caused by the aging of the population worldwide. The social and economic impact of AMD is enormous.

AMD and its negative impact on quality of life

AMD involves the progressive dysfunction and degeneration of the macula's photoreceptors that eventually lead to loss of central vision. With the increase in the aging population, AMD will become an even more common problem. As AMD incidence increases, it is important to understand how it affects the visual function and quality of life (QoL) of patients. The test of QoL is a subjective measure, using patient-reported outcome measures, normally via a questionnaire.[7] When central scotomas extend beyond 20 degrees of diameter at the advanced stage of AMD, usually in both eyes, the profound loss of central vision leads to visual disability, including inability to drive, to read, or to recognize human faces. This severe consequence has a negative impact on the patients' autonomy and QoL.[8] Among central visual functions, face recognition is an important daily activity. It is agreed that peoples spend more time looking at faces than any other complex visual stimuli. Face recognition is essential to social interactions.[9] Difficulties with face recognition can lead to embarrassment and anxiety in social situations, which in turn can lead to social isolation and depression.[10] Based on studies from 1988 to 2002, 171 people with AMD from five cohort studies received the QoL test to evaluate the effect of AMD on face recognition.[11–15] These studies collected a range of outcomes including familiar face recognition, facial expression discrimination, and eye movements when viewing an image of a face. AMD patients performed worse on categorizing facial expressions than on yes-no questions. Familiar face recognition and facial expression detection performance worsened with reduced luminance. One study reported significant differences in eye movements with AMD compared to the controls.[14] The profound visual impairment of AMD patients such as the inability of face recognition may lead to depression.[16] Depression is the most frequent psychiatric disorder in AMD patients (33.7%). Meanwhile, a significant association also was found between AMD and anxiety, adjustment disorders, and somatoform disorders.[16]

AMD may also trigger the development of multiple psychiatric conditions. It has been found that patients with AMD are at greater risk for cognitive impairment than the non-AMD controls,[17] suggesting that this ophthalmological disease is not just associated with depression and anxiety. The relationship between depression, anxiety, and AMD is complex and involves several possibilities. One hypothesis is that valued activities are impaired among AMD patients with major visual function loss, indirectly increasing the risk of developing affective suffering and distress.[18] It is noteworthy that elderly patients with AMD are often affected by other chronic conditions. As a result, it is possible that individuals with AMD are depressed not only because of the impairment of their visual acuity but also because of the impact of their other medical conditions on their daily lives. This fact highlights the importance of interdisciplinary management of patients with AMD to prevent the development of depression and anxiety.

In the retinal clinic, wet AMD patients receiving intravitreal antivascular endothelial growth factor (VEGF) therapy often describe a physical and psychological stress. Most studies on depression associated with AMD are earlier reports, before the era of intravitreal anti-VEGF therapy, now the mainstay of treatment for wet AMD. This revolutionized therapy has significantly reduced the risk of central vision loss caused by wet AMD. This is a positive impact on vision outcomes. On the other hand, the patients need repeated intravitreal injections often for many years to maintain the anti-VEGF efficacy. This is a stressful event with anticipatory anxiety for many patients. It has been reported that the prevalence of depression and anxiety in the wet AMD patients with anti-VEGF treatment is still significantly higher than in the general population.[19] A recent study utilizing qualitative data and validated questionnaires showed that anxiety is associated with intravitreal anti-VEGF injections. The source of anxiety is related not only to the fear of the injection, but also to concern over effectiveness of the treatment. The levels of clinical depression, not anxiety levels, are significantly higher in association with the initial three injections than with subsequent injections.

AMD and its socioeconomic burden for the healthcare system

AMD accounts for 8.7% of all blindness worldwide based on data published in 2014.[6] The Global Burden of Disease Study 2010 reported an increase of 160% in vision-related years lived with disability due to AMD from 1990 to 2010.[20] Because of increased aging population and an increasingly negative impact of environmental risk factors for AMD, specifically smoking and obesity, its incidence is expected to be higher in the next decade.[6] For instance, AMD will affect almost 200 million people globally in 2020. Substantial AMD patients in those aged 55–85 years (3.5%–17.6%) will develop late-stage AMD.[21] Among populations in the US and UK, the proportion with GA and neovascular AMD is about equal among late AMD patients.[22] Since patients with neovascular AMD require multiple anti-VEGF treatments, the demands of anti-VEGF therapy will be surged continuously.

Currently aflibercept, ranibizumab and bevacizumab are intravitreal anti-VEGF agents used in the United States. The surge in demand for these anti-VEGF agents makes AMD treatment cost a serious medical and economic challenge. In 2000, only 3000 Medicare-covered intravitreal injections were documented. In 2008, the number of injections increased to 1 million. In 2013, 2.5 million intravitreal injections were covered by Medicare at a cost of more than $300 million. The American Academy of Ophthalmology estimated more than 6 million injections would be given in 2016.[23]

AMD as a disease of the macular neurovascular complex

AMD affects the central region of the retina, that is, the macula. The characteristic visual impairment for both advanced forms of AMD is the loss of central vision (Fig. 1.1A). The central region of the fundus comprises photoreceptors (PRs), retinal pigment epithelium (RPE), Bruch's membrane (BrM), and choroid, specifically choriocapillaris (CC) (Fig. 1.2). These cell types interdependently and reciprocally link to form a multicellular entity that has been called the PR/RPE/BrM/CC complex.[24] In this book, we will call it the macular neurovascular complex (MNC), which is adapted from the concept of the neurovascular unit of the central nerve system (CNS). Our focus will be on the coupling between photoreceptor degeneration and RPE-BrM/CC dysfunction at the macular region in AMD.[25] The term neurovascular unit has been successfully used to illustrate pathogenesis in diabetic retinopathy, in which the coupling between neurosensory retina and retinal vasculature is studied.[26] Based on the concept of neurovascular unit, there must be an interface between the CNS and the peripheral circulatory system. The physical and functional barrier is located at the level of cerebral vascular endothelial cells with tight junctions. RPE constitutes a monolayer of cells with tight junctions located between PRs and CC. The neurosensory retina is a part of the central nervous system due to its embryological origins.[27] The CC, a porous capillary system, is the peripheral vascular bed that supplies the avascular outer retina.[28,29] Among PRs, RPE, and CC of the proposed neurovascular complex, RPE coupling of photoreceptor activity to the choroidal blood flow serves as the structural and functional outer blood-retinal barrier.[30] Geographic atrophy (GA), a subtype of AMD, is an example demonstrating how AMD is considered to be a disease of the MNC. GA is characterized by the presence of sharply demarcated atrophic lesions of PRs, RPE, and underlying CC. Furthermore, a recent study using Swept-Source OCT angiography demonstrated a correlation between choriocapillaris flow deficits around GA and enlargement rates of the photoreceptor degeneration and RPE atrophic lesion.[31,32]

The intimate anatomic relationship between PRs and RPE starts from early embryonic development through the process of organogenesis of the eye, which begins at embryonic day 25. As the neural tube closes, the optic vesicles remain attached to the neural tube by optic stalks composed of neuroectodermal cells. As the optic vesicle approaches the outer wall of the embryo, the cell populations of the optic

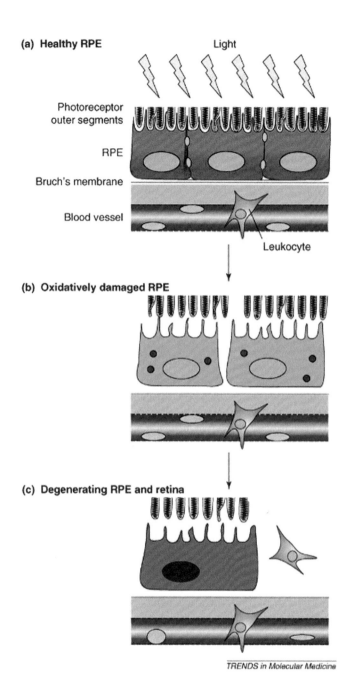

(a) Healthy RPE

Light

Photoreceptor
outer segments

RPE

Bruch's membrane

Blood vessel

Leukocyte

(b) Oxidatively damaged RPE

(c) Degenerating RPE and retina

TRENDS in Molecular Medicine

FIGURE 1.2

AMD affects a histologic complex of posterior pole of fundus, comprising photoreceptors (PRs), retinal pigment epithelium (RPE), Bruch membrane (BrM), and choroid, especially choriocapillaris. This tissue entity is called PR/RPE/BrM/CC complex.[33]

Modified from Kang KH, Lemke G, Kim JW. The PI3K-PTEN tug-of-war, oxidative stress and retinal degeneration.
Trends Mol Med. *2009;15(5):191–198. doi: 10.1016/j.molmed.2009.03.005.*

vesicle differentiate and extend, resulting in the invagination of its temporal and lower walls and the formation of the optic cup. Neuroectodermal cells of the inner layer of the optic cup evolve as the neurosensory retina. Differentiation of the neurosensory retina begins at the center of the optic cup and gradually expands peripherally. PRs are neurons located at the outermost layer of the neurosensory retina (Fig. 1.3). Differentiation of the PRs and glial cells in the fovea occurs simultaneously. In the different cell types, synapses as well as intercellular junctions, are established by 15 weeks of gestation. The fovea becomes the focal point of the retina. The highest concentration of PRs is in the central retina, which facilitates the central vision and permits high-resolution visual acuity. On the other hand, the RPE is derived from the outer layer of the optic cup. By 8 weeks of gestation, the RPE is organized as a single layer of hexagonal columnar cells adjacent to the developing neurosensory retina. RPE cells are polarized epithelial cells. They have long, microvillous processes on their apical surfaces interdigitating with the outer segments of PRs. The basement membrane of the RPE becomes the inner portion of BrM. The outer layer of BrM is also a basement membrane, which is laid down by the CC layer. In fact, the embryonic pigment epithelial cells have a profound impact on the development of both choroid and neurosensory retina. For instance, in the process of eye development, RPE is one of key endogenous stem/progenitor cells, which is able to differentiate into overlying retinal neurons.[34,35] Increasing evidence shows that, in AMD, the death and dysfunction of PRs appear to be secondary to the loss of RPE cells (also see Chapter 7).

RPE exists primarily as a selective diffusion barrier, but in contrast to the classic concept of the neurovascular unit, not at the level of endothelium. This is the reason that this book uses the term of neurovascular complex instead of the neurovascular unit. However, RPE acts as the outer blood-retinal barrier with the presence of tight cell—cell junctions, which is similar to the retinal endothelial cells acting as the inner blood-retinal barrier. The functions of the RPE include protection of the retina from oxidative stress, facilitation of nutrient delivery and waste disposal, ionic homeostasis, phagocytosis of photoreceptor outer segments, synthesis and reisomerization of all-trans-retinal during the visual cycle, and establishment of ocular immune privilege. In addition, RPE cells interact with other cellular components of the neurovascular complex such as neural glial cells, that is, Muller cells. Although these two types of cells do not directly contact each other, they are the major contributors to the pool of secreted molecules, that is, secretome, in the retinal milieu.[36] Secreted trophic factors are key to maintaining the structural and functional integrity of the retina, as they regulate cellular pathways responsible for survival, function, and response to injury. Nevertheless, these same factors can also be involved in retinal pathologies, as a consequence of the impairment of the secretory function of cells. RPE cells are polarized, differentially synthesizing and releasing molecules either through the apical or basolateral membrane. This is demonstrated by the secretion of molecules that regulate angiogenesis in the retina. Pigment epithelial-derived factor (PEDF) is secreted from the apical membrane of RPE with antiangiogenetic function, whereas vascular endothelial growth factor A (VEGF-A), a potent

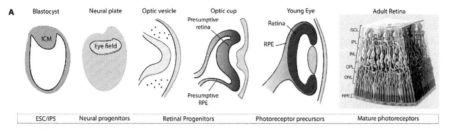

FIGURE 1.3

A schematic demonstration of the various stages of eye development, from the blastocyst stage through to the mature adult retina. At very early stages, the eye field domain is specified from a region of the neural plate. This region extends laterally to form the optic vesicle, and then invaginates to form the optic cup. Further specification of this region gives rise to the young eye, which contains a two-layered optic cup; at this stage, the developing neural retina (red) is situated in the inner region of this structure, whereas the RPE forms the outer RPE layer (orange). Further differentiation gives rise to the mature retina containing all retinal cell types.

Modified from Jayakody SA, Gonzalez-Cordero A, Ali RR, Pearson RA. Cellular strategies for retinal repair by photoreceptor replacement. Prog Retin Eye Res. 2015;46:31–66. doi: 10.1016/j.preteyeres.2015.01.003.

proangiogenic factor, is secreted through the basolateral membrane of RPE. In hypoxic retinal vascular diseases, Muller cells decrease PEDF secretion and increase VEGF-A secretion, thus shifting the angiogenetic balance.[24] In wet AMD, the RPE secretes excessive amounts of VEGF-A from its basolateral membrane, and this contributes to the breakdown of the blood-retinal barrier and sprouting of underlying CC through BrM into the RPE level thus forming macular neovascularization. Shifting levels of VEGF and PEDF documented in surgical specimens of choroidal neovascularization membranes obtained from patients with wet AMD provide evidence of these mechanisms.[37]

In the neurovascular complex, neuron–glia interaction is essential. Müller cells are specialized macroglial cells of the retina, which span the entire thickness of the neurosensory retina. In addition to their supportive and homeostatic functions for the retina in general, Müller cells closely interact with photoreceptors at the macula. First, Muller cells form a structure of "Müller cell cone shape" at the central retina, which means that the PRs are surrounded by the outer processes of Müller cells at the fovea wall to maintain photoreceptor configuration. This structure guides image formation. Second, Müller cells crucially support the function and viability of photoreceptors, particularly the cones. The local cone-to-Müller ratio roughly equals one.[38] Müller cells and photoreceptors linking other transition retinal neurons represent the smallest functional unit for the processing of visual information.[39] Third, recent studies identify two different visual cycles that regenerate chromophores of photopigments, that is, the rods and the cones.[40,41] Rod-derived all-trans retinal is recycled to 11-cis-retinal in RPE, while cone-derived all-trans retinal is processed by Müller cells. Although its physiological function remains to be established, the rapid supply of the cone chromophore through Müller cells may be critical for extending the dynamic range of cones to light and dark adaptation after light exposure.[42] Dysfunction of MNC has been associated with the pathogenesis of AMD in relation to increased oxidative stress, mitochondrial destabilization, complement dysregulation-related inflammation, and proangiogenetic state (see Chapters 7 and 8). Therefore, the MNC, which is involved in AMD, is not only a disease-mechanistic unit but also as a therapeutic target for the coupling of both neural degeneration and vascular dysfunction.[43]

AMD as an inflammatory disease

AMD is a chronic low-grade inflammatory disease.[44,45] The existence of retinal drusen is clinical evidence of the inflammation process. In the early phases of AMD, accumulation of intracellular lipofuscin in the RPE and its extracellular deposit between RPE cells and BrM can be clinically detected (see Chapters 3 and 4). Because of the high content of polyunsaturated fatty acids in photoreceptor outer segments (POS), which are constantly ingested by RPE, and substantial exposure to light, RPE is susceptible to excessive oxidative stress. When continuous ingestion of POS exceeds the capability of nondividing and aging RPE cells, the accumulation of an undegradable metabolite, that is, lipofuscin, along with the suppressed function of lysosomal enzymes leads to oxidative stress and inflammation.[46] Although the sub-RPE deposits are heterogeneous in nature,[47] the compositional analysis of drusen is able to reveal their origin. Drusen consists of (oxidatively modified) lipids, proteins, and minerals, particularly inflammation-related proteins.[48] Various inflammation-related factors are detected in retinal drusen, such as complement components, immunoglobulins, HLA molecules, and acute-phase proteins like vitronectin, fibrinogen, al-antichymotrypsin, and pentraxins.[49] Therefore, components of drusen likely induce a complement cascade and sustain a low-grade inflammation, resulting in local cellular damage at the very early onset of AMD.

The inflammatory response in AMD occurs in the absence of infection, and thus is a so-called sterile inflammation of low-grade and chronic nature. This kind of inflammation responds to host-derived elements ranging from oxidized lipids or lipoproteins to deposits of protein/lipid aggregates.[50] These host-derived stimuli trigger activation of pattern recognition receptors (PRRs) of the innate immune system (Chapters 7 and 9). Toll-like receptors (TLRs), a family of PRRs, are exemplified for explaining the relationship between activation of an innate immune system and AMD pathogenesis. TLRs are located either on the cell surface or in endosomal compartments. The activation of TLRs initiates signal transduction pathways that determine the type and duration of the inflammatory response.[44] When TLRs recognize host products that are mis-localized or appear to be "nonself," a change in lipid constitution of the RPE plasma membrane can force TLRs into lipid rafts allowing for proximity-enabled activation.[51] Alternatively, carboxyethyl-pyrrole, an oxidative-stress modifier, plays a role as an endogenous ligand activating TLR2 in AMD.[52] Activation of TLRs results in recruitment of downstream signaling proteins to orchestrate a proinflammatory response.

Association of AMD with variants in complement system genes serves as an inflammatory node in the pathogenesis of AMD. The complement pathway, as the host inflammatory response, is an essential part of the innate immune system, responsible for eliminating foreign antigens and pathogens. Variants of several genes encoding proteins in the complement system are of particular interest: complement factor H (CFH),[53] complement factor B (CFB), complement component 2 (C2),[54] complement component 3 (C3),[55] and C5.[56] CFH inhibits activation of the alternative complement pathway.[53] The CFH polymorphism resulting in tyrosine to histidine at position 402 (Y402H) may be associated with up to 50% of all AMD cases,[57] suggesting a critical role for this polymorphism in the inflammatory process in AMD. C3, the central molecule of the complement cascade that includes the classical, alternative, and lectin pathways, is activated by numerous inciting factors. In the alternative complement pathway, C3 activation is under the control of CFB, and CFH.[58] Genetic evidence implicates both C3 and CHH as contributory factors to AMD etiology (see Chapter 9).[59]

Other inflammatory factors, for example, chemokines and their receptors as well as inflammatory cytokines, have been found to be upregulated systemically in the serum or locally in the ocular tissue of patients with AMD. Chemokine receptors are expressed on immune cells and other cell types, such as endothelial cells in response to ligation by their cognate chemokine. Genetic variants of the chemokine receptor CX3CR1 have been associated with AMD.[60,61] A correlation of systemic levels of IL-6, IL-18, and TNF-α with CFH haplotypes has been found in AMD patients.[62] Systemic IL-6 levels also have been found to correlate with both the incidence and progression of AMD.[63,64] However, the underlying mechanisms by which systemically or locally elevated cytokines mediate inflammation in AMD have not been established. A recent clinical study showed that among 41 tested cytokines in aqueous humor, only growth-regulated oncogene, macrophage-derived chemokine, and macrophage inflammatory protein-1α are significantly higher in AMD patients than controls. In this report, the aqueous humor VEGF of AMD patients is not significantly different from the control group.[65] The authors suggest that wet AMD has more localized pathology, because the upregulation of VEGF was documented previously by immunohistochemical methods in choroidal neovascularization membrane.[37] Nonetheless, AMD has been associated with genetic variants of various inflammatory molecules, suggesting that several inflammatory pathways can lead to the same clinical disease (see Chapter 7).

Genetics of AMD

The importance of heritability of AMD was revealed by twin studies. The fundus features and vision loss are strikingly similar in monozygotic twins with AMD but not in dizygotic twins.[66] The breakthrough in the molecular genetics of AMD is the result of the Human Genome Project. Then, the novel and replicated loci such as chromosome 1q31, in affected individuals, were found by genome-wide family-based linkage studies.[67] Moving forward, four genome-wide single-nucleotide polymorphic (SNP) association studies with AMD case-control cohorts discovered the association of a variant (Y402H) in the CFH gene with AMD in 2005.[53,59,68,69]

The variant observed is an SNP where thymine substitutes for cytosine at nucleotide 1277 in exon 9, with a resulting tyrosine to histidine change in amino acid position 402, that is, Y402H of the protein. The CHF gene, located at chromosome 1q25-31, regulates a protein that inhibits the activation of the alternative complement pathway. The genetic association of CFH with AMD indicates the critical role of activation of the alternative complement pathways in outer-retina tissue-specific inflammation. It has been proposed that external and intrinsic tissue-specific inflammatory molecules target proteins with genetic variants and modify the function of the alternative complement pathway in the macular milieu. This process theoretically could contribute to the inflammatory pathogenesis in AMD. Meanwhile, more complex mechanisms for variants other than CHF have emerged from rapidly growing studies. Other complement pathway genes and other inflammation/immune-related genes have been evaluated for possible association with AMD. In addition, one of the ultimate goals of genetic studies is to identify individuals at high risk for AMD by using genetic variation and environmental risk factor data. More detailed genetic studies on AMD pathogenesis and on clinical management will be discussed in Chapter 9.

Translation of the advances in research on AMD into better clinical management for patients

Visual impairment due to AMD affects patients, caregivers, and society in multiple ways. In addition to the cost of anti-VEGF treatment, the economic consequences of vision impairment are enormous, including the direct costs, indirect costs, and intangible effects related to visual impairment.[70] Hospitalization of AMD patients who are vulnerable to other chronic conditions, contributes the most to direct medical costs. Assistive devices/aids, and home services take the major proportion of direct nonmedical costs. The indirect costs arising from patients and caregivers include productivity losses, employment changes, income loss, premature mortality, etc.[23] Therefore, the burden of AMD has turned into a challenge in the daily patient care.

AMD is the leading blinding disease among the elderly. However, it is fortunate that because of the advances from studies on AMD pathogenesis, anti-VEGF therapy has been successfully integrated into clinical practice for wet AMD patients. This therapy improves or stabilizes the vision of most patients with wet AMD, although the long-term outcome needs to be further investigated. Recent mechanistic studies of AMD have widened the therapeutic view beyond anti-VEGF therapy. Targeting inflammation-based mechanisms, complement modulating agents such as multiple complement C5 inhibitors are in the pipeline, which block the terminal complement activity-induced inflammation (Chapter 11). Focusing on cell-death based mechanisms, inhibitors of cell-death related pathways, that is, neuro-protectants, have shown protection from cell death of photoreceptors and RPE cells.[71] Studying on angiogenesis-based mechanisms in wet AMD, inhibition of the angiopoietin-Tie signaling pathway leads to suppression of vascular permeability by tightening endothelial cell junctions, thereby inhibiting the recruitment of angiogenetic macrophages to the inflammatory lesions.[72]

In addition to therapies for AMD, there are still numerous challenges in prevention and management of AMD. Fortunately, the key modifiable environmental risk factors such as smoking, obesity, and diet have been identified. Among these factors, smoking is the most consistently implicated as a risk factor of AMD development by the published studies. A larger portion of the epidemiologic and cohort studies showed significant causative association between smoking and AMD with an increased risk of AMD of two- to three-fold in current-smokers compared with never-smokers.[73] These data are convincing because the association between smoking and AMD shows a dose-response effect, a temporal relationship, and reversibility of effect. A mandate of tobacco control and smoking cessation may have beneficial effects in minimizing the risk of AMD.

Rapidly emerging innovations in diagnostic technologies in the field of AMD allow unprecedented high-resolution visualization of disease morphology. For instance, a variety of optical coherence tomography provides a promising horizon for early disease detection and efficient therapeutic follow-up. Based on growing genetic and proteomic data, valid biomarkers have been studied to provide a practical base for disease management. It is fortunate that AMD-related basic and clinical science is one of the most active and promising fields, which encompass the essence of the achievements in neuroscience, particularly brain research, oncology, angiogenesis, immunology, gerontology, and medical imaging. Advances in regenerative research will guide improvements in gene-therapy and cell-based therapy of this disease.

Taken together, a comprehensive scientific definition of AMD may be summarized as follows:

Definition

AMD is a spectrum central-retina disease ranging from early to late stage, with various severities, involving photoreceptor/retinal pigment epithelium/Bruch's membrane/choriocapillaris, a neurovascular complex. AMD is pathogenically characterized as a chronic progressive degenerative and inflammatory disease. AMD is genetically characterized as having polygenic and multifactorial inheritance. The strongest risk factor of AMD is advanced age. The aged individuals whose retinas are modified by environmental and genetic factors have a higher incidence than the normal aging population for developing clinical phenotypes of macular degeneration.

References

1. Bressler NM. Age-related macular degeneration is the leading cause of blindness. *JAMA.* 2004;291(15):1900−1901. https://doi.org/10.1001/jama.291.15.1900.

2. Bourne RRA, Stevens GA, White RA, et al. Causes of vision loss worldwide, 1990−2010: a systematic analysis. *Lancet Glob Health.* 2013;1(6):e339−349. https://doi.org/10.1016/S2214-109X(13)70113-X.

3. Friedman DS, O'Colmain BJ, Muñoz B, et al. Prevalence of age-related macular degeneration in the United States. *Arch Ophthalmol.* 2004;122(4):564−572. https://doi.org/10.1001/archopht.122.4.564.

4. McHarg S, Clark SJ, Day AJ, Bishop PN. Age-related macular degeneration and the role of the complement system. *Mol Immunol.* 2015;67(1):43−50. https://doi.org/10.1016/j.molimm.2015.02.032.

5. Luu J, Palczewski K. Human aging and disease: lessons from age-related macular degeneration. *Proc Natl Acad Sci USA.* 2018;115(12):2866−2872. https://doi.org/10.1073/pnas.1721033115.

6. Wong WL, Su X, Li X, et al. Global prevalence of age-related macular degeneration and disease burden projection for 2020 and 2040: a systematic review and meta-analysis. *Lancet Glob Health.* 2014;2(2):e106−116. https://doi.org/10.1016/S2214-109X(13)70145-1.

7. Clemons TE, Chew EY, Bressler SB, McBee W, Age-Related Eye Disease Study Research Group. National eye institute visual function questionnaire in the age-related eye disease study (AREDS): AREDS report no. 10. *Arch Ophthalmol.* 2003;121(2):211−217. https://doi.org/10.1001/archopht.121.2.211.

8. Maniglia M, Cottereau BR, Soler V, Trotter Y. Rehabilitation approaches in macular degeneration patients. *Front Syst Neurosci.* 2016;10:107. https://doi.org/10.3389/fnsys.2016.00107.

9. Pascalis O, Kelly DJ. The origins of face processing in humans: phylogeny and ontogeny. *Perspect Psychol Sci.* 2009;4(2):200−209. https://doi.org/10.1111/j.1745-6924.2009.01119.x.

10. Yardley L, McDermott L, Pisarski S, Duchaine B, Nakayama K. Psychosocial consequences of developmental prosopagnosia: a problem of recognition. *J Psychosom Res.* 2008;65(5):445−451. https://doi.org/10.1016/j.jpsychores.2008.03.013.

11. Alexander MF, Maguire MG, Lietman TM, Snyder JR, Elman MJ, Fine SL. Assessment of visual function in patients with age-related macular degeneration and low visual acuity. *Arch Ophthalmol.* 1988;106(11):1543−1547. https://doi.org/10.1001/archopht.1988.01060140711040.

12. Boucart M, Dinon J-F, Despretz P, Desmettre T, Hladiuk K, Oliva A. Recognition of facial emotion in low vision: a flexible usage of facial features. *Vis Neurosci.* 2008;25(4):603−609. https://doi.org/10.1017/S0952523808080656.

13. Tejeria L, Harper RA, Artes PH, Dickinson CM. Face recognition in age related macular degeneration: perceived disability, measured disability, and performance with a bioptic device. *Br J Ophthalmol.* 2002;86(9):1019−1026. https://doi.org/10.1136/bjo.86.9.1019.

14. Seiple W, Rosen RB, Garcia PMT. Abnormal fixation in individuals with age-related macular degeneration when viewing an image of a face. *Optom Vis Sci.* 2013;90(1):45−56. https://doi.org/10.1097/OPX.0b013e3182794775.

15. Bullimore MA, Bailey IL, Wacker RT. Face recognition in age-related maculopathy. *Invest Ophthalmol Vis Sci.* 1991;32(7):2020−2029.

16. Jacob L, Spiess A, Kostev K. Prevalence of depression, anxiety, adjustment disorders, and somatoform disorders in patients with age-related macular degeneration in Germany. *Ger Med Sci.* 2017;15:Doc04. https://doi.org/10.3205/000245.

17. Woo SJ, Park KH, Ahn J, et al. Cognitive impairment in age-related macular degeneration and geographic atrophy. *Ophthalmology.* 2012;119(10):2094−2101. https://doi.org/10.1016/j.ophtha.2012.04.026.

18. Rovner BW, Casten RJ. Activity loss and depression in age-related macular degeneration. *Am J Geriatr Psychiatr.* 2002;10(3):305−310.

19. Senra H, Balaskas K, Mahmoodi N, Aslam T. Experience of anti-vegf treatment and clinical levels of depression and anxiety in patients with wet age-related macular degeneration. *Am J Ophthalmol.* 2017;177:213−224. https://doi.org/10.1016/j.ajo.2017.03.005.

20. Pascolini D, Mariotti SP. Global estimates of visual impairment: 2010. *Br J Ophthalmol.* 2012;96(5):614−618. https://doi.org/10.1136/bjophthalmol-2011-300539.

21. Colijn JM, Buitendijk GHS, Prokofyeva E, et al. Prevalence of age-related macular degeneration in Europe: the past and the future. *Ophthalmology.* 2017;124(12):1753−1763. https://doi.org/10.1016/j.ophtha.2017.05.035.

22. Danis RP, Lavine JA, Domalpally A. Geographic atrophy in patients with advanced dry age-related macular degeneration: current challenges and future prospects. *Clin Ophthalmol.* 2015;9:2159−2174. https://doi.org/10.2147/OPTH.S92359.

23. Cannon E. Managed care opportunities and approaches to supporting appropriate selection of treatment for sight preservation. *Am J Manag Care.* 2019;25(10 Suppl):S182−S187.

24. Bhutto I, Lutty G. Understanding age-related macular degeneration (AMD): relationships between the photoreceptor/retinal pigment epithelium/Bruch's membrane/choriocapillaris complex. *Mol Aspects Med.* 2012;33(4):295−317. https://doi.org/10.1016/j.mam.2012.04.005.

25. Iadecola C. The neurovascular unit coming of age: a journey through neurovascular coupling in health and disease. *Neuron.* 2017;96(1):17−42. https://doi.org/10.1016/j.neuron.2017.07.030.

26. Gardner TW, Davila JR. The neurovascular unit and the pathophysiologic basis of diabetic retinopathy. *Graefes Arch Clin Exp Ophthalmol.* 2017;255(1):1−6. https://doi.org/10.1007/s00417-016-3548-y.

27. Hoon M, Okawa H, Della Santina L, Wong ROL. Functional architecture of the retina: development and disease. *Prog Retinal Eye Res.* 2014;42:44−84. https://doi.org/10.1016/j.preteyeres.2014.06.003.

28. Saint-Geniez M, D'Amore PA. Development and pathology of the hyaloid, choroidal and retinal vasculature. *Int J Dev Biol.* 2004;48(8-9):1045−1058. https://doi.org/10.1387/ijdb.041895ms.

29. Törnquist P, Alm A. Retinal and choroidal contribution to retinal metabolism in vivo. A study in pigs. *Acta Physiol Scand.* 1979;106(3):351−357. https://doi.org/10.1111/j.1748-1716.1979.tb06409.x.

30. Buxton RB, Frank LR. A model for the coupling between cerebral blood flow and oxygen metabolism during neural stimulation. *J Cerebr Blood Flow Metabol.* 1997;17(1):64−72. https://doi.org/10.1097/00004647-199701000-00009.

31. Thulliez M, Zhang Q, Shi Y, et al. Correlations between choriocapillaris flow deficits around geographic atrophy and enlargement rates based on swept-source oct imaging. *Ophthalmol Retina*. 2019;3(6):478−488. https://doi.org/10.1016/j.oret.2019.01.024.

32. Sohn EH, Flamme-Wiese MJ, Whitmore SS, et al. Choriocapillaris degeneration in geographic atrophy. *Am J Pathol*. 2019;189(7):1473−1480. https://doi.org/10.1016/j.ajpath.2019.04.005.

33. Kang KH, Lemke G, Kim JW. The PI3K-PTEN tug-of-war, oxidative stress and retinal degeneration. *Trends Mol Med*. 2009;15(5):191−198. https://doi.org/10.1016/j.molmed.2009.03.005.

34. Jayakody SA, Gonzalez-Cordero A, Ali RR, Pearson RA. Cellular strategies for retinal repair by photoreceptor replacement. *Prog Retin Eye Res*. 2015;46:31−66. https://doi.org/10.1016/j.preteyeres.2015.01.003.

35. Opas M, Davies JR, Zhou Y, Dziak E. Formation of retinal pigment epithelium in vitro by transdifferentiation of neural retina cells. *Int J Dev Biol*. 2001;45(4):633−642.

36. Araújo RS, Santos DF, Silva GA. The role of the retinal pigment epithelium and Müller cells secretome in neovascular retinal pathologies. *Biochimie*. 2018;155:104−108. https://doi.org/10.1016/j.biochi.2018.06.019.

37. Tatar O, Adam A, Shinoda K, et al. Expression of VEGF and PEDF in choroidal neovascular membranes following verteporfin photodynamic therapy. *Am J Ophthalmol*. 2006;142(1):95−104. https://doi.org/10.1016/j.ajo.2006.01.085.

38. Lindenau W, Kuhrt H, Ulbricht E, Körner K, Bringmann A, Reichenbach A. Cone-to-Müller cell ratio in the mammalian retina: A survey of seven mammals with different lifestyle. *Exp Eye Res*. 2019;181:38−48. https://doi.org/10.1016/j.exer.2019.01.012.

39. Reichenbach A, Siegel A, Rickmann M, Wolff JR, Noone D, Robinson SR. Distribution of Bergmann glial somata and processes: implications for function. *J Hirnforsch*. 1995;36(4):509−517.

40. Reichenbach A, Bringmann A. New functions of Müller cells. *Glia*. 2013;61(5):651−678. https://doi.org/10.1002/glia.22477.

41. Wang J-S, Kefalov VJ. The cone-specific visual cycle. *Prog Retin Eye Res*. 2011;30(2):115−128. https://doi.org/10.1016/j.preteyeres.2010.11.001.

42. Wang J-S, Estevez ME, Cornwall MC, Kefalov VJ. Intra-retinal visual cycle required for rapid and complete cone dark adaptation. *Nat Neurosci*. 2009;12(3):295−302. https://doi.org/10.1038/nn.2258.

43. Neuwelt EA. Mechanisms of disease: the blood-brain barrier. *Neurosurgery*. 2004;54(1):131−140. https://doi.org/10.1227/01.neu.0000097715.11966.8e. discussion 141-142.

44. Mulfaul K, Rhatigan M, Doyle S. Toll-like receptors and age-related macular degeneration. *Adv Exp Med Biol*. 2018;1074:19−28. https://doi.org/10.1007/978-3-319-75402-4_3.

45. Wilhelm I, Nyúl-Tóth Á, Kozma M, Farkas AE, Krizbai IA. Role of pattern recognition receptors of the neurovascular unit in inflamm-aging. *Am J Physiol Heart Circ Physiol*. 2017;313(5):H1000−H1012. https://doi.org/10.1152/ajpheart.00106.2017.

46. Ferrington DA, Sinha D, Kaarniranta K. Defects in retinal pigment epithelial cell proteolysis and the pathology associated with age-related macular degeneration. *Prog Retin Eye Res*. 2016;51:69−89. https://doi.org/10.1016/j.preteyeres.2015.09.002.

47. Thompson RB, Reffatto V, Bundy JG, et al. Identification of hydroxyapatite spherules provides new insight into subretinal pigment epithelial deposit formation in the aging eye. *Proc Natl Acad Sci USA*. 2015;112(5):1565−1570. https://doi.org/10.1073/pnas.1413347112.

48. Bergen AA, Arya S, Koster C, et al. On the origin of proteins in human drusen: The meet, greet and stick hypothesis. *Prog Retin Eye Res.* 2019;70:55—84. https://doi.org/10.1016/j.preteyeres.2018.12.003.

49. Kauppinen A, Paterno JJ, Blasiak J, Salminen A, Kaarniranta K. Inflammation and its role in age-related macular degeneration. *Cell Mol Life Sci.* 2016;73(9):1765—1786. https://doi.org/10.1007/s00018-016-2147-8.

50. Rock KL, Latz E, Ontiveros F, Kono H. The sterile inflammatory response. *Annu Rev Immunol.* 2010;28:321—342. https://doi.org/10.1146/annurev-immunol-030409-101311.

51. Levy O, Calippe B, Lavalette S, et al. Apolipoprotein E promotes subretinal mononuclear phagocyte survival and chronic inflammation in age-related macular degeneration. *EMBO Mol Med.* 2015;7(2):211—226. https://doi.org/10.15252/emmm.201404524.

52. West XZ, Malinin NL, Merkulova AA, et al. Oxidative stress induces angiogenesis by activating TLR2 with novel endogenous ligands. *Nature.* 2010;467(7318):972—976. https://doi.org/10.1038/nature09421.

53. Klein RJ, Zeiss C, Chew EY, et al. Complement factor H polymorphism in age-related macular degeneration. *Science.* 2005;308(5720):385—389. https://doi.org/10.1126/science.1109557.

54. Gold B, Merriam JE, Zernant J, et al. Variation in factor B (BF) and complement component 2 (C2) genes is associated with age-related macular degeneration. *Nat Genet.* 2006;38(4):458—462. https://doi.org/10.1038/ng1750.

55. Yates JRW, Sepp T, Matharu BK, et al. Complement C3 variant and the risk of age-related macular degeneration. *N Engl J Med.* 2007;357(6):553—561. https://doi.org/10.1056/NEJMoa072618.

56. Baas DC, Ho L, Ennis S, et al. The complement component 5 gene and age-related macular degeneration. *Ophthalmology.* 2010;117(3):500—511. https://doi.org/10.1016/j.ophtha.2009.08.032.

57. Thakkinstian A, Han P, McEvoy M, et al. Systematic review and meta-analysis of the association between complement factor H Y402H polymorphisms and age-related macular degeneration. *Hum Mol Genet.* 2006;15(18):2784—2790. https://doi.org/10.1093/hmg/ddl220.

58. Pickering MC, Cook HT, Warren J, et al. Uncontrolled C3 activation causes membranoproliferative glomerulonephritis in mice deficient in complement factor H. *Nat Genet.* 2002;31(4):424—428. https://doi.org/10.1038/ng912.

59. Edwards AO, Ritter R, Abel KJ, Manning A, Panhuysen C, Farrer LA. Complement factor H polymorphism and age-related macular degeneration. *Science.* 2005;308(5720):421—424. https://doi.org/10.1126/science.1110189.

60. Tuo J, Smith BC, Bojanowski CM, et al. The involvement of sequence variation and expression of CX3CR1 in the pathogenesis of age-related macular degeneration. *FASEB J.* 2004;18(11):1297—1299. https://doi.org/10.1096/fj.04-1862fje.

61. Yang X, Hu J, Zhang J, Guan H. Polymorphisms in CFH, HTRA1 and CX3CR1 confer risk to exudative age-related macular degeneration in Han Chinese. *Br J Ophthalmol.* 2010;94(9):1211—1214. https://doi.org/10.1136/bjo.2009.165811.

62. Cao S, Ko A, Partanen M, et al. Relationship between systemic cytokines and complement factor H Y402H polymorphism in patients with dry age-related macular degeneration. *Am J Ophthalmol.* 2013;156(6):1176—1183. https://doi.org/10.1016/j.ajo.2013.08.003.

63. Klein R, Myers CE, Cruickshanks KJ, et al. Markers of inflammation, oxidative stress, and endothelial dysfunction and the 20-year cumulative incidence of early age-related macular degeneration: the Beaver Dam eye study. *JAMA Ophthalmol*. 2014;132(4): 446−455. https://doi.org/10.1001/jamaophthalmol.2013.7671.

64. Seddon JM, George S, Rosner B, Rifai N. Progression of age-related macular degeneration: prospective assessment of C-reactive protein, interleukin 6, and other cardiovascular biomarkers. *Arch Ophthalmol*. 2005;123(6):774−782. https://doi.org/10.1001/archopht.123.6.774.

65. Agrawal R, Balne PK, Wei X, et al. Cytokine profiling in patients with exudative age-related macular degeneration and polypoidal choroidal vasculopathy. *Invest Ophthalmol Vis Sci*. 2019;60(1):376. https://doi.org/10.1167/iovs.18-24387.

66. Meyers SM, Greene T, Gutman FA. A twin study of age-related macular degeneration. *Am J Ophthalmol*. 1995;120(6):757−766. https://doi.org/10.1016/s0002-9394(14)72729-1.

67. Barral S, Francis PJ, Schultz DW, et al. Expanded genome scan in extended families with age-related macular degeneration. *Invest Ophthalmol Vis Sci*. 2006;47(12):5453−5459. https://doi.org/10.1167/iovs.06-0655.

68. Hageman GS, Anderson DH, Johnson LV, et al. A common haplotype in the complement regulatory gene factor H (HF1/CFH) predisposes individuals to age-related macular degeneration. *Proc Natl Acad Sci USA*. 2005;102(20):7227−7232. https://doi.org/10.1073/pnas.0501536102.

69. Haines JL, Hauser MA, Schmidt S, et al. Complement factor H variant increases the risk of age-related macular degeneration. *Science*. 2005;308(5720):419−421. https://doi.org/10.1126/science.1110359.

70. Köberlein J, Beifus K, Schaffert C, Finger RP. The economic burden of visual impairment and blindness: a systematic review. *BMJ Open*. 2013;3(11):e003471. https://doi.org/10.1136/bmjopen-2013-003471.

71. Miller JW. Beyond VEGF-The Weisenfeld lecture. *Invest Ophthalmol Vis Sci*. 2016; 57(15):6911−6918. https://doi.org/10.1167/iovs.16-21201.

72. Saharinen P, Eklund L, Alitalo K. Therapeutic targeting of the angiopoietin-TIE pathway. *Nat Rev Drug Discov*. 2017;16(9):635−661. https://doi.org/10.1038/nrd.2016.278.

73. Thornton J, Edwards R, Mitchell P, Harrison RA, Buchan I, Kelly SP. Smoking and age-related macular degeneration: a review of association. *Eye*. 2005;19(9):935−944. https://doi.org/10.1038/sj.eye.6701978.

Epidemiology of age-related macular degeneration

Prevalence and incidence

Numerous population-based studies of age-related macular degeneration (AMD) have been reported around the world. AMD is the leading cause of irreversible blindness of the elderly worldwide.[1] The reported prevalence of AMD, which varies regions, populations, and disease definitions, is constantly updating. In 2014, a systemic review and meta-analysis established worldwide prevalence and projected the number of people with AMD from 2020 to 2040.[2] The pooled global prevalence of early and late-stage disease in adult populations was 8.01% (3.95%−15.49%) and 0.37% (0.18%−0.77%), respectively. The overall prevalence of any AMD was 8.69% (4.26%−17.40%). It has been realized that the prevalence of AMD varies in different ethnicities. Any AMD was more prevalent in populations of European ancestry than Asian (12.3% vs. 7.4%; Bayes factor 4.3, suggesting moderate evidence); and European ancestry had a higher prevalence than African ancestry for early, late, or any AMD. Particularly, the comparison of prevalence of late AMD between the people with European and African ancestry was 12.3% versus 7.5%; Bayes factor 31.3, suggesting very strong evidence. Subgroup analysis (8 of the 39 studies with information on geographic atrophy (GA) and neovascular subtypes) showed that Europeans had a higher prevalence of GA (1.11%, 0.53%−2.08%) than Africans (0.14%, 0.04%−0.45%), Asians (0.21%, 0.04%−0.87%), and Hispanics (0.16%, 0.05%−0.46%). There was no significant difference in the prevalence of neovascular AMD between ethnicities.[2] In 2013, Bourne et al. reported that the proportion of blindness caused by AMD worldwide was higher in women than in men.[3] Contrary to this previous report, the recent meta-analysis did not show evidence of gender difference in both early and late AMD prevalence.[2] This finding is consistent with other reviews in people of European ancestry, where no significant gender difference was found in the prevalence of neovascular AMD and GA.[4] Wong et al. by using UN World Population Prospects, assessed differences by ethnicity, region, and sex, and projected the individuals affected worldwide by the condition in 2020 and 2040. The projected number of people with AMD is around 196 million in 2020, and increasing to 288 million in 2040 (Fig. 2.1).[2] The prevalence of AMD

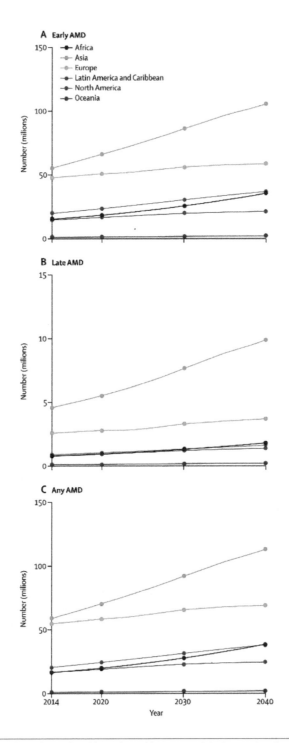

FIGURE 2.1

Projection of number of people with early and late age-related macular degeneration (AMD) by regions, that is, Africa, Asia, Europe, Latin America and Carrabin, North America and Oceania in 2014, 2020, 2030, and 2040.

Reprinted with permission from Elsevier (Wong WL, Su X, Li X, et al. Global prevalence of age-related macular degeneration and disease burden projection for 2020 and 2040: a systematic review and meta-analysis. The Lancet Global Health. 2014;2(2):e106-e116. doi:10.1016/S2214-109X(13)70145-1).

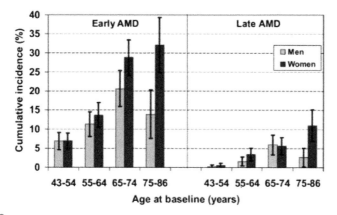

FIGURE 2.2

Fifteen-year cumulative incidence and 95% confidence intervals of early and late age-related macular degeneration (AMD) by age and gender in the beaver dam eye study. The overall age-adjusted differences between men and women and the incidence of early ($P = .16$) and late ($P = .16$) AMD were not statistically significantly different.

Modified from Klein R, Klein BEK, Knudtson MD, Meuer SM, Swift M, Gangnon RE. Fifteen-year cumulative incidence of age-related macular degeneration. Ophthalmology. *2007;114(2):253–262. doi:10.1016/j.ophtha.2006.10.040.*

at these given time points helps assess the socioeconomic burden and distribute the resource for management.

On the other hand, the incidence of AMD at a certain period helps examine risk factors for AMD and genetic and environmental interactions in the etiology of AMD. It may be exemplified by the Beaver Dam Eye Study,[5] which is a population-based longitudinal cohort study of residents of Beaver Dam, Wisconsin, aged 43–84 years in 1987–1988. A 15-year cumulative incidence of both early and late AMD was reported in the Beaver Dam Eye Study population with different age groups. The high incidence of early AMD (24%) and late AMD (8%), respectively, was observed in those who were >75 years age at baseline, indicating advanced age is a key risk factor for both early and late AMD (Fig. 2.2).[6]

Based on the data from the longitudinal cohort Beaver Dam Eye Study, the change of incidence of every 5-year interval was studied. This cohort study was designed to have four examination visits, 5 years apart in 1988–90, 1993–95, 1998–2000, and 2003–05. While controlling for age, smoking, blood pressure, and other related factors, the 5-year incidence of AMD was 60% declined for each successive generation.[7] The decline in the incidence across three generations suggests that environmental and/or behavioral factors are significant risk factors in the etiology of AMD because rapid genetic changes are unlikely.

Risk factors of AMD by various epidemiologic studies

AMD is a complex multifactorial disease with numerous genetic and environmental risk factors. The genetics of AMD is introduced in Chapter 9. It is critical that identification of potentially modifiable risk factors, that is, environmental factors, is required because it may provide mechanistic evidence for developing an effective therapy for AMD. Both Blue Mountains Eye Study (BMES) and Rotterdam Study are the classical epidemiology studies of AMD, in which a detailed grading system and similar definitions for grading of AMD are used.[8,9] In the BMES, participants were measured based on their smoking history. Current smoking was significantly associated with late AMD (odds ratio [OR], 3.92), including neovascular AMD (OR, 3.20) and GA (OR, 4.54), and early AMD (OR, 1.75). The significant association of past smokers with late AMD (OR, 1.83) but not early AMD. Passive smoking, defined as the spouse of smokers, was associated with an increased but insignificant odds ratio for late AMD. These findings show a causal association between smoking and AMD exists. The strongest risk was found for current smokers, suggesting potential benefits of targeting education to older people who are current smokers and have signs of early AMD.

The findings by Rotterdam Study are essentially similar to that of BMES.[8] Current smokers younger than 85 years, had a 6.6-fold increased risk of neovascular AMD compared with those who had never smoked. Past smokers had a 3.2-fold increased risk of neovascular AMD compared with never smokers in this age group. A strongly increased risk of neovascular AMD was present in those who had smoked more than 10 pack-years (relative risk, 6.5). Persons who had quitted smoking 20 or more years before the eye examination had no increased risk. The distinct findings by Rotterdam Study are that the above associations were not observed in participants 85 years or older and no association of smoking with atrophic AMD was found, although the underlying mechanisms are currently unclear.[9]

In summary, the dose-dependent association between smoking and AMD found in both BMES and Rotterdam study indicates a causative relationship of smoking in the development of AMD. This causative relationship had been confirmed by a 5-year follow-up study of survivals from BMES. The participants were divided into subgroups based on their status of smoking. The 5-year incidence rates of AMD of survivals in different subgroups were measured. The incidence rates for late AMD based on the smoking status, that is, current, past, and never smokers were 3.1%, 1.2%, and 1.4%, respectively. The incidence rates for early AMD corresponding to smoking status were 10.6%, 8.2%, and 9.3%, respectively. The 5-year follow-up data also showed that current smokers developed late AMD at a significantly earlier age than never or past smokers.[8] A recent cohort study showed that current smokers developed neovascular AMD at an average 5.5 years younger age than never smokers and 4.4 years younger age than past smokers, respectively. Most importantly, this study pointed out that the smoking status influences the treatment outcome of neovascular AMD patients by anti-VEGF agent.[10] Current smokers compared with never smokers had greater odds of presence of subretinal fluid at 12-

month anti-VEGF treatment. It is worthy to note that the smoking status was not significantly associated with visual acuity over 12 months.[10]

In addition to cigarette smoking, other environmental and behavioral risk factors for AMD have been recognized as follows: obesity, low dietary intake of vitamins A, C, and E, and zinc, low dietary intake of lutein and omega-3 fatty acids, and unhealthy lifestyle related to the cardiovascular risk factor.[11,12] Several epidemiologic studies suggest a possible role of antioxidants in reducing the risk of AMD.[13] The National Eye Institute initiated the Age-Related Eye Disease Study (AREDS) in 1990. It was a double-masked AMD clinical trial that enrolled participants with criteria of early, intermediate, and late AMD. In this study, the progression of AMD and loss of visual acuity were compared between groups receiving antioxidant supplementation or placebo, and those receiving zinc treatment or placebo. The mean follow-up of the participants was 6.3 years.[14] AREDS was designed to evaluate the clinical course of AMD, including rates of progression and risk factors.[15] To fulfill this purpose, a simplified severity scale for AMD was crucial in the AREDS for evaluating fundus photographs from clinical studies worldwide.[16] In this study, drusen were categorized by size as small (<63 µm), intermediate ($63-124$ µm), or large (>125 µm) (Fig. 2.3).

Persons with no visible drusen or pigmentary abnormalities are considered to have no signs of AMD, that is, stage 0. In AREDS, persons with few small drusen (stage 1), with many small drusen or few intermediate drusen, that is, stage 2, and many intermediate drusen or even single large drusen, that is, stage 3 were classified. The participants with neovascular AMD or geographic atrophy are referred to have late AMD, that is, stage 4. Based on additional analyses from AREDS, the classification scheme presented by the Beckman Initiative for Macular Research Classification Committee is introduced.[17,18] By this clinical classification, in addition to drusen, pigmented abnormality, an indication of retinal pigment epithelium (RPE) changes, was included.[18] The grading systems, severity scales, and classification scheme used in AREDS have obtained large consensus. In 2016, a simplified but more comprehensive 4-point grading scale based on AREDS for classifying the severity of AMD and predicting the disease course was further evolved in Table 2.1.[17,18] The application of this classification system is further discussed in Chapter 3.

When risk factor points are totaled across both eyes to reach a number between 0 and 4 as described in Table 2.1, they can be used to estimate patients' 5-year and 10-year risk of developing advanced AMD in one eye (Table 2.2).[19]

AREDS demonstrated a beneficial relationship between certain micronutrients and decreased risk of AMD. After 5 years of follow-up, the estimated probability of progression to advanced AMD was 28% of participants in the placebo group, 23% and 22% for those receiving antioxidants and zinc, respectively, and 20% for those receiving antioxidants plus zinc.[21] A single-arm comparison of treatment groups with placebo found statistically significant risk reductions for the antioxidants plus zinc arm ($P < .05$) and borderline significance in the zinc arm ($P = .05$), but not in the antioxidants arm alone.[14]

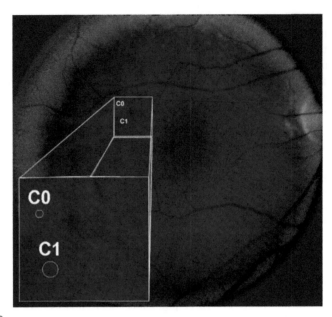

FIGURE 2.3

In an eye with multiple types of drusen, the age-related eye disease study drusen grading circles C0 (63 μm diameter) and C1 (125 μm diameter) are superimposed for size comparison. Small drusen are smaller than the C0 circle (drupelets). Lesions larger than C0 but less than C1 are considered intermedium drusen, and lesions larger than C1 are large drusen. Within the inset, drupelets and medium drusen are seen. Faint reticular drusen also may be seen in the superior macular region.

Modified from Ferris FL, Wilkinson CP, Bird A, et al. Clinical classification of age-related macular degeneration. Ophthalmology. *2013;120(4):844–851. doi:10.1016/j.ophtha.2012.10.036.*

A follow-up study, AREDS2, was initiated in 2006 to evaluate the effect of the inclusion of lutein, zeaxanthin, and omega-3 fatty acids into the original AREDS formula on progression to advanced AMD over a period of 5 years.[14] The data of AREDS2 confirmed the overall risk reduction found in the original AREDS. The data showed that lutein and zeaxanthin had similar effects to β-carotene. Unlike β-carotene, the intake of lutein and zeaxanthin did not increase the risk for lung cancer in current and past smokers. Although AREDS2 confirmed that 80 mg of zinc is an appropriate dose for AMD prophylaxis, a lower dose of zinc (from 80 to 25 mg daily) has been used in the clinic to minimize the side effect of high zine intake. Currently, patients with stage 3 or 4 AMD are advised to take the AREDS2 supplement.[12,20]

In previous epidemiologic studies such as the Rotterdam Study, homozygous carriers for the CFH rs1061170 risk allele seemed to benefit from daily dietary intake of zinc, lutein, and zeaxanthin, and omega-3 fatty acids. The carrier status was able to reduce the risk for early AMD almost to the level of a noncarrier, that is, without

Table 2.1 Definitions of the age-related eye diseases study simplified severity scale.

Age-related eye diseases study simplified severity scale	Definition
0	No large drusen (>125 μm) or pigment changes in either eye
1[a]	Large drusen or pigment changes in one eye only, or bilateral medium-sized drusen in both eyes
2[b]	Large drusen and pigment changes in one eye only, or large drusen or pigment changes in both eyes, or late AMD in one eye, and no large drusen or pigment changes in the fellow eye
3	Large drusen and pigment changes in one eye and large drusen or pigment changes in the fellow eye, or late AMD in one eye and large drusen or pigment changes in the fellow eye
4	Large drusen and pigment changes in both eyes, or late AMD in one eye and both large drusen and pigment changes in the fellow eye

AMD, *age-related macular degeneration.*
[a] *In the absence of large drusen in either eye, the presence of bilateral medium drusen (half the diameter of large drusen or more) constitutes a score of 1.*
[b] *An eye that has late AMD (choroidal neovascularization or center geographic atrophy) is assigned a score of 2. The presence of large drusen or pigment changes in the other eye will increase this score to a maximum of 4.*

Table 2.2 Five-year and ten-year risks of advanced AMD in one eye.

AREDS simplified		
Risk factor points	5-year risk, %	10-year risk, %
0	0.4	1
1	3.1	7
2	11.8	22
3	25.9	50
4	47.3	67

Modified from AAO Retina and Vitreous 2019–20 BCSC; Ferris FL, Davis MD, Clemons TE, et al. A simplified severity scale for age-related macular degeneration: AREDS Report No. 18. Arch Ophthalmol. 2005;123(11):1570–1574. doi:10.1001/archopht.123.11.1570; Ferris FL, Wilkinson CP, Bird A, et al. Clinical classification of age-related macular degeneration. Ophthalmology. 2013;120(4): 844–851. doi:10.1016/j.ophtha.2012.10.036; Liew G, Joachim N, Mitchell P, Burlutsky G, Wang JJ. Validating the AREDS simplified severity scale of age-related macular degeneration with 5- and 10-year incident data in a population-based sample. Ophthalmology. 2016;123(9):1874–1878. doi:10.1016/ j.ophtha.2016.05.043; Chew EY, Clemons TE, Agrón E, et al. Ten-year follow-up of age-related macular degeneration in the age-related eye disease study: AREDS report No. 36. JAMA Ophthalmol. 2014;132(3):272. doi:10.1001/jamaophthalmol.2013.6636; American Academy of Ophthalmology. Retina and Vitreous.; 2019.

CFH risk variant.[22] However, AREDS2 was conducted to assess whether lutein and zeaxanthin, omega-3 fatty acids, β-carotene, or zinc could negate the effects of deleterious genotypes at two major loci associated with AMD, that is, CFH and ARMS2. There was no significant interaction between these dietary supplements and CFH rs1061170 or ARMS2 rs10490924 genotype with regard to the progression to late AMD. Based on these data, no changes to the current AREDS2 formula were recommended for any genetic subgroup.[23] The possible reason for the absence of a genotype interaction effect with dietary supplements in AREDS2 is complex. First, the previous epidemiology study was a population-based study, which had different population characteristics as compared to that of AREDS2. In other words, the AREDS2 participants were peoples who already had intermediate AMD or high risk of AMD progression. Second, the dose of micronutrients investigated in AREDS2 was much higher than the daily intake through food, but the study duration of AREDS2 was much shorter than the course in the epidemiology studies. In fact, the epidemiologic studies showing gene–diet interactions, not just AREDS2 formula, were in a population-based setting and evaluated the progression from no AMD to early AMD.[23] Third, it is possible that gene–diet interactions played a role only earlier on in disease development. Future studies in larger populations, focusing on other AMD-related genetic factors as well, are essential.

Subretinal drusenoid deposits/reticular pseudodrusen and AMD

In the epidemiology studies, conventional drusen, deposits of extracellular matrix below RPE, have been recognized as the hallmark of AMD, because drusen formation and development are the courses of AMD progression. In the aging and AMD eyes, a peculiar yellowish network pattern in the retina was identified, named as reticular pseudodrusen (RPD), in 1990 by Mimoun et al.[24] Both histopathologic studies and clinical optical coherence tomography (OCT) images have confirmed that RPD is located in the subretinal space above RPE (Fig. 2.5).[25,26] These deposits contain overlapping protein compositions of drusen. Because of the location and composition, the material was also called subretinal drusenoid deposits (SDD).[27] It is not easy to distinguish SDD/RPD with soft indistinct drusen (SID) by viewing with color photographs alone[28] (Fig. 2.4B). The prevalence of SDD/RPD was <1% in the earlier population-based epidemiology studies by using stereoscopic color photographs.[29] Nowadays, by using multimodal imaging techniques, particularly autofluorescence imaging, SDD/RPD was defined as clusters of discrete round or oval lesions of hypo-autofluorescence that are usually similar in size or confluent ribbon-like patterns with intervening areas of normal or increased autofluorescence (Fig. 2.4A).[30]

Clinically, SDD/RPD is frequently associated with late AMD.[31] Most interestingly, it has been reported that outer retinal atrophy develops in the eyes with regression of RPD. Therefore, RPD associated AMD was hypothesized as a newly

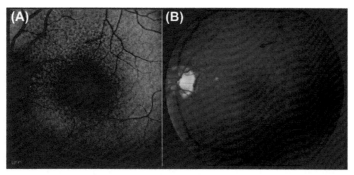

FIGURE 2.4

(A) Fundus autofluorescence (FAF) image and (B), color photograph showing reticular pseudodrusen (RPD) (*arrow*). By using autofluorescence imaging, RPD was defined as clusters of discrete round or oval lesions of hypoautofluorescence that are usually similar in size or confluent ribbon-like patterns with intervening areas of normal or increased autofluorescence.

Modified from Domalpally A, Agrón E, Pak JW, et al. Prevalence, risk, and genetic association of reticular pseudodrusen in age-related macular degeneration. Ophthalmology. *2019;126(12):1659–1666. doi: 10.1016/j.ophtha.2019.07.022.*

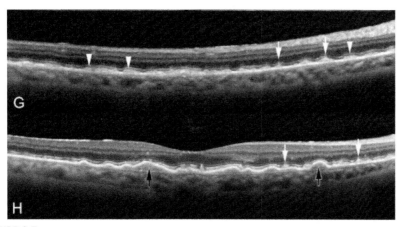

FIGURE 2.5

(G), an OCT through the superior macula shows a nearly confluent accumulation of material in the subretinal space. (H), an OCT through the fovea shows cross-sections of the soft drusen (black *arrows*) and a subretinal deposition of material that is clearly differentiable from the underlying RPE (white *arrows*).

Modified from Zweifel SA, Spaide RF, Curcio CA, Malek G, Imamura Y. Reticular pseudodrusen are subretinal drusenoid deposits. Ophthalmology. *2010;117(2):303–312.e1. doi:10.1016/j.ophtha.2009.07.014.*

recognized form of late AMD.[26] The study of RPD composition revealed that RPD shared major tissue markers of conventional soft drusen, but had no by-products of photoreceptors. It indicates that RPD and conventional drusen undergo different formation mechanisms. In the process of RPD formation, RPE lost normally polarized vectorial functions for both apical and basolateral secretion.[27] Therefore, RPD is an independent risk marker of AMD progression beyond conventional drusen. Its epidemiological feature has been extensively studied.

Based on the data of the Rotterdam Study follow-up in 2016, the epidemiology of SDD/RPD was studied in a large population-based setting.[28] The Rotterdam classification consists of five grades of AMD as described earlier. Both the near-infrared (NIR) imaging and color fundus photographs (CFP) were used to identify RPD. RPD was detected in 4.9% of study participants. 92.7% RPD was detected with NIR imaging and 38% on CFP. Most eyes with RPD showed coexistence of SID, whereas other drusen types coincided less frequently. RPD was significantly associated with age and female gender.[28] In another multimodal imaging study, the relationship between RPD and the severity of AMD was reported. The prevalence of SDD/RPD increases to 25% in eyes with intermediate AMD, 36%−54% in eyes with neovascular AMD, and 29%−92% in eyes with GA.[32,27] These data indicate that SDD/RPD has distinct association with AMD because the presence of SDD/RPD in AMD eyes is different from other types of conventional drusen. Most importantly, SDD/RPD is strongly associated with late AMD, as a significant marker of both neovascular AMD and GA. It has been documented that major AMD risk variants were significantly associated with SDD/RPD and SID; however, *ARMS2, C3,* and *VEGFA* variants were more associated with RPD (RPD vs. SID $P < .05$). Although the genetic risk profile of RPD and SID was different, the total genetic risk score did not differ significantly ($P = .88$) in this report.[28] In a recent post hoc analysis of cross-sectional data from US participants in the Comparison of AMD Treatments Trials, among patients with neovascular AMD, the AMD risk alleles *ARMS2* and *HTRA1* were associated with an increased risk of RPD, while the risk allele *CFH* Y402H was associated with a lower risk of SDD/RPD.[33]

Based on epidemiology studies on AMD worldwide, it is clear that AMD is the most common cause of blindness in the elderly. Therefore, the demand for new effective treatments and socioeconomic burden is enormous. For neovascular AMD, although the utilization of anti-VEGF agents has revolutionized the treatment, it is only effective for suppression of pathologic angiogenesis. Not to mention, no therapy is successful for dry AMD. Learning from epidemiology study on AMD has led to further identification of risk factors, understanding of their modifiable mechanisms, and investigation of the interplay between genetic and environmental factors, resulting in new therapeutic achievement in both early and late AMD.

References

1. Bressler NM. Age-related macular degeneration is the leading cause of blindness. *J Am Med Assoc.* 2004;291(15):1900. https://doi.org/10.1001/jama.291.15.1900.
2. Wong WL, Su X, Li X, et al. Global prevalence of age-related macular degeneration and disease burden projection for 2020 and 2040: a systematic review and meta-analysis. *Lancet Global Health.* 2014;2(2):e106−e116. https://doi.org/10.1016/S2214-109X(13) 70145-1.
3. Bourne RRA, Stevens GA, White RA, et al. Causes of vision loss worldwide, 1990−2010: a systematic analysis. *Lancet Global Health.* 2013;1(6):e339−e349. https://doi.org/10.1016/S2214-109X(13)70113-X.
4. Smith W, Assink J, Klein R, et al. Risk factors for age-related macular degeneration: pooled findings from three continents. *Ophthalmology.* 2001;108(4):697−704. https://doi.org/10.1016/s0161-6420(00)00580-7.
5. Klein R, Knudtson MD, Lee KE, Gangnon RE, Klein BEK. Age-period-cohort effect on the incidence of age-related macular degeneration: the beaver dam eye study. *Ophthalmology.* 2008;115(9):1460−1467. https://doi.org/10.1016/j.ophtha.2008.01.026.
6. Klein R, Klein BEK, Knudtson MD, Meuer SM, Swift M, Gangnon RE. Fifteen-year cumulative incidence of age-related macular degeneration. *Ophthalmology.* 2007;114(2): 253−262. https://doi.org/10.1016/j.ophtha.2006.10.040.
7. Cruickshanks KJ, Nondahl DM, Johnson LJ, et al. Generational differences in the 5-year incidence of age-related macular degeneration. *JAMA Ophthalmol.* 2017;135(12): 1417−1423. https://doi.org/10.1001/jamaophthalmol.2017.5001.
8. Mitchell P, Wang JJ, Smith W, Leeder SR. Smoking and the 5-year incidence of age-related maculopathy: the blue mountains eye study. *Arch Ophthalmol.* 2002;120(10): 1357−1363. https://doi.org/10.1001/archopht.120.10.1357.
9. Smith W, Mitchell P, Leeder SR. Smoking and age-related maculopathy. The blue mountains eye study. *Arch Ophthalmol.* 1996;114(12):1518−1523. https://doi.org/10.1001/ archopht.1996.01100140716016.
10. Detaram HD, Joachim N, Liew G, et al. Smoking and treatment outcomes of neovascular age-related macular degeneration over 12 months. *Br J Ophthalmol.* 2019;26. https:// doi.org/10.1136/bjophthalmol-2019-314849. Published online September bjophthalmol-2019-314849.
11. Lim LS, Mitchell P, Seddon JM, Holz FG, Wong TY. Age-related macular degeneration. *Lancet.* 2012;379(9827):1728−1738. https://doi.org/10.1016/S0140-6736(12)60282-7.
12. Age-Related Eye Disease Study 2 Research Group. Lutein + zeaxanthin and omega-3 fatty acids for age-related macular degeneration: the age-related eye disease study 2 (AREDS2) randomized clinical trial. *J Am Med Assoc.* 2013;309(19):2005−2015. https://doi.org/10.1001/jama.2013.4997.
13. Sperduto RD, Ferris FL, Kurinij N. Do we have a nutritional treatment for age-related cataract or macular degeneration? *Arch Ophthalmol.* 1990;108(10):1403−1405. https://doi.org/10.1001/archopht.1990.01070120051026.
14. Gorusupudi A, Nelson K, Bernstein PS. The age-related eye disease 2 study: micronutrients in the treatment of macular degeneration. *Adv Nutr.* 2017;8(1):40−53. https:// doi.org/10.3945/an.116.013177.

15. Age-Related Eye Disease Study Research Group. The age-related eye disease study (AREDS): design implications. AREDS report no. 1. *Control Clin Trials*. 1999;20(6): 573−600. https://doi.org/10.1016/s0197-2456(99)00031-8.

16. Ferris FL, Davis MD, Clemons TE, et al. A simplified severity scale for age-related macular degeneration: AREDS Report No. 18. *Arch Ophthalmol*. 2005;123(11):1570−1574. https://doi.org/10.1001/archopht.123.11.1570.

17. Ferris FL, Wilkinson CP, Bird A, et al. Clinical classification of age-related macular degeneration. *Ophthalmology*. 2013;120(4):844−851. https://doi.org/10.1016/j.ophtha. 2012.10.036.

18. Liew G, Joachim N, Mitchell P, Burlutsky G, Wang JJ. Validating the AREDS simplified severity scale of age-related macular degeneration with 5- and 10-year incident data in a population-based sample. *Ophthalmology*. 2016;123(9):1874−1878. https://doi.org/ 10.1016/j.ophtha.2016.05.043.

19. Chew EY, Clemons TE, Agrón E, et al. Ten-year follow-up of age-related macular degeneration in the age-related eye disease study: AREDS report No. 36. *JAMA Ophthalmol*. 2014;132(3):272. https://doi.org/10.1001/jamaophthalmol.2013.6636.

20. American Academy of Ophthalmology. *Retina and Vitreous*. 2019.

21. Age-Related Eye Disease Study Research Group. A randomized, placebo-controlled, clinical trial of high-dose supplementation with vitamins C and E, beta carotene, and zinc for age-related macular degeneration and vision loss: AREDS report no. 8. *Arch Ophthalmol*. 2001;119(10):1417−1436. https://doi.org/10.1001/archopht.119.10.1417.

22. Ho L, van Leeuwen R, Witteman JCM, et al. Reducing the genetic risk of age-related macular degeneration with dietary antioxidants, zinc, and ω-3 fatty acids: the Rotterdam study. *Arch Ophthalmol*. 2011;129(6):758−766. https://doi.org/10.1001/archophthalmol. 2011.141.

23. van Asten F, Chiu C-Y, Agrón E, et al. No CFH or ARMS2 interaction with omega-3 fatty acids, low versus high zinc, or β-carotene versus lutein and zeaxanthin on progression of age-related macular degeneration in the age-related eye disease study 2: age-related eye disease study 2 report No. 18. *Ophthalmology*. 2019;126(11):1541−1548. https://doi.org/10.1016/j.ophtha.2019.06.004.

24. Mimoun G, Soubrane G, Coscas G. Macular drusen. *J Fr Ophtalmol*. 1990;13(10): 511−530.

25. Zweifel SA, Spaide RF, Curcio CA, Malek G, Imamura Y. Reticular pseudodrusen are subretinal drusenoid deposits. *Ophthalmology*. 2010;117(2):303−312.e1. https:// doi.org/10.1016/j.ophtha.2009.07.014.

26. Spaide RF, Ooto S, Curcio CA. Subretinal drusenoid deposits AKA pseudodrusen. *Surv Ophthalmol*. 2018;63(6):782−815. https://doi.org/10.1016/j.survophthal.2018.05.005.

27. Rudolf M, Malek G, Messinger JD, Clark ME, Wang L, Curcio CA. Sub-retinal drusenoid deposits in human retina: organization and composition. *Exp Eye Res*. 2008;87(5): 402−408. https://doi.org/10.1016/j.exer.2008.07.010.

28. Buitendijk GHS, Hooghart AJ, Brussee C, et al. Epidemiology of reticular pseudodrusen in age-related macular degeneration: the rotterdam study. *Invest Ophthalmol Vis Sci*. 2016;57(13):5593−5601. https://doi.org/10.1167/iovs.15-18816.

29. Klein R, Meuer SM, Knudtson MD, Iyengar SK, Klein BEK. The epidemiology of retinal reticular drusen. *Am J Ophthalmol*. 2008;145(2):317−326.e1. https://doi.org/ 10.1016/j.ajo.2007.09.008.

30. Domalpally A, Agrón E, Pak JW, et al. Prevalence, risk, and genetic association of reticular pseudodrusen in age-related macular degeneration. *Ophthalmology*. 2019;126(12): 1659−1666. https://doi.org/10.1016/j.ophtha.2019.07.022.

31. Arnold JJ, Sarks SH, Killingsworth MC, Sarks JP. Reticular pseudodrusen. A risk factor in age-related maculopathy. *Retina*. 1995;15(3):183−191.
32. Wang JJ, Rochtchina E, Lee AJ, et al. Ten-year incidence and progression of age-related maculopathy: the blue mountains eye study. *Ophthalmology*. 2007;114(1):92−98. https://doi.org/10.1016/j.ophtha.2006.07.017.
33. Lin LY, Zhou Q, Hagstrom S, et al. Association of single-nucleotide polymorphisms in age-related macular degeneration with pseudodrusen: necondary analysis of data from the comparison of AMD treatments trials. *JAMA Ophthalmol*. 2018;136(6):682. https://doi.org/10.1001/jamaophthalmol.2018.1231.

Classification of age-related macular degeneration

AMD classification based on drusen and pigmentary changes before OCT era

Understanding the nature and developing effective treatments for age-related macular degeneration (AMD), a consensus classification for defining this leading cause of blindness in the elderly is imperative. First, AMD is a spectrum macular disorder covering both the early and late stages of the disease with a wide range of clinical signs and symptoms. Before optical coherence tomography (OCT) era, as the early AMD is usually asymptomatic, the classification is mainly based on the presence of drusen and pigmentary changes within two disc-diameters of the fovea. Therefore, various criteria including the size of drusen (e.g., small vs. large), the type of drusen (e.g., hard vs. soft), the anatomic position (subretinal vs. sub-RPE), the number, and the area of drusen as well as the location, size, and area of pigmentary changes had been used to classify different stages of AMD among ophthalmologists in clinical practice.[1−4] Based on these features of drusen and pigmentary changes in the literature, AMD classification and the severity scale in terms of evaluation from early to late AMD are summarized in this section.[1] In addition, the severity scales of 5-year and 10-year risks of advanced AMD in one eye are shown in Tables 2.1 and 2.2 in Chapter 2. In Chapters 2 and 4 of this book, the morphologic and clinical characteristics of drusen including cuticular drusen and reticular pseudodrusen have been introduced by multimodal imaging techniques.

Conventionally, AMD has been divided into two main types. Dry AMD is the most common type, consisting of 90% of diagnosed cases. Geographic atrophy (GA) is the advanced stage of dry AMD. Wet (neovascular) AMD is less common than dry, but is associated with more rapid loss of sight. The main manifestations are choroidal neovascularization (CNV), subretinal fluid, and pigment epithelial detachment (PED). In recent years, two additional conditions, retinal angiomatous proliferation and polypoidal choroidal vasculopathy (PCV) have been included under the term neovascular AMD, which is collectively characterized as macular neovascularization (MNV).

Based on the age-related eye disease study (AREDS) data by using color fundus photography (CFP), an expert consensus committee pointed out that identification of clinical risks at the early stage that leading to late AMD development is the most

Age-Related Macular Degeneration. https://doi.org/10.1016/B978-0-12-822061-0.00013-X

important goal for the consensus of classification system.[5] This system unifies vocabulary of practice into a common nomenclature for all clinical providers and researchers. According to this guideline, patients at early stages with the potential loss of vision could be identified. For these patients, additional and/or specific therapy might be discovered and utilized to prevent blindness. The consensus of the classification system is a guideline of all clinical providers and researchers for the communication with their patients and among themselves. In this classification, the size of the drusen and the presence of pigmentary alterations are the most important factors. When the size of drusen is smaller than 63 μm, the term "drupelet" is used as a distinct type of drusen, because drusen of this size contribute no risk of subsequent late AMD. Therefore, the presence of drupelets is considered a normal aging change. The presence of medium drusen (63−125 μm) is a risk factor for the development of large drusen. By calculation of the 5-year rate of progression to large drusen, >50% for patients with medium drusen in both eyes and ∼25% for patients with medium drusen in one eye may develop large drusen. In contrast, the 5-year risk for the development of large drusen in eyes with small or no drusen is less than 5%. The overall 10-year risk for the development of late AMD in patients with bilateral medium drusen is ∼13% and those with unilateral medium drusen is ∼5%, respectively.[5] Based on a post hoc analysis of fundus images taken during the AREDS trial, the risk factors for CNV development correlated with the presence of large drusen (>125 m) within the 2-disc diameter of the fovea were statistically significant.[6]

The pigmentary changes at the macula were analyzed in nine subfields inside the circle with a 2-disc diameter of the fovea.[7] The pigmentary changes were categorized as (1) retinal pigment epithelial degeneration defined as the percentage area of each subfield; (2) increased retinal pigment defined as the presence of granules or clumps of gray or black pigment in or beneath the retina; (3) pigmentary abnormality defined as the presence of either retinal pigment epithelium (RPE) degeneration or increased retinal pigment in the central macular subfield.[7] By using these three criteria, the prevalence of various signs of maculopathy including these three pigmentary changes was estimated by using the Beaver Dam Eye Study (1988−90) data. Retinal pigment epithelial degeneration was present in 20.7%, increased retinal pigment in 24.5%, and pigmentary abnormalities of the RPE in 26.6% of the persons aged 75 years or older, as compared to 3.7%, 6.9%, and 7.3% of persons with age ranging 43−54, respectively.[7] The post hoc analyses of the AREDS trial support these findings that the presence of pigment at the macula is the risk factor for CNV development.[6] The clinical classification of AMD is provided in Table 3.1.[5]

The classification of AMD and the disease severity scale based on the consensus of experts' opinions have provided a guideline for follow-up of the disease course from early and intermediate to late AMD. As both large drusen and pigmentary changes in one or both eyes are individually proved to be risk factors for late AMD development, it is reasonable to deduce that patients with an increasing combination of these risk factors are at increased risk. If a risk score of 1 for each risk factor in each eye is assigned, the maximum risk score of 2 can be obtained per eye or 4 per patient. For example, a person who has large drusen and pigmentary abnormalities in both eyes

Table 3.1 Clinical classification of AMD.

Classification of AMD	Definition (Lesions assessed within two disc diameters of fovea in either eye)
No apparent aging changes	No drusen and No AMD pigmentary abnormalities[a]
Normal aging changes	Only drupelets (small drusen ≤ 63 μm) and No AMD pigmentary abnormalities[a]
Early AMD	Medium drusen >63 μm and ≤125 μm and No AMD pigmentary abnormalities[a]
Intermediate AMD	Large drusen > 125 μm and/or Any AMD pigmentary abnormalities[a]
Late AMD	Neovascular AMD and/or Any geographic atrophy

AMD, age-related macular degeneration.
[a] AMD pigmentary abnormalities = any definite hyper- or hypopigmentary abnormalities associated with medium or large drusen but not associated with known disease entities.
Modified from Ferris FL, Wilkinson CP, Bird A, et al. Clinical classification of age-related macular degeneration. Ophthalmology. 2013;120(4):844–851. https://doi.org/10.1016/j.ophtha.2012.10.036.

receives a score of 4. Therefore, a 5-step severity scale of 0 (no risk factor) to 4 (both risk factors in both eyes) can be established. For instance, the 5-year risk of late AMD development increases from a score of 0 to a score of 4 (see Table 2.1 in Chapter 2 and Fig. 3.1).[5] Most importantly, the prediction of late AMD development according to the severity scale can be understood by both providers and patients. During the follow-up, the modifiable risk factors and dietary/nutritional regimen

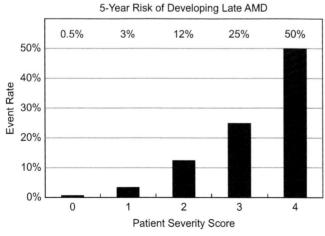

FIGURE 3.1

Graph showing AREDS clinical severity scale for AMD, demonstrating the 5-year risk of developing late AMD for different risk groups. For instance, the risk rate of the group with scale 3 is 25.9% and that with scale 4 is 47.3%, respectively.
AREDS, Age-related eye disease study.
Modified from Ferris FL, Wilkinson CP, Bird A, et al. Clinical classification of age-related macular degeneration. Ophthalmology. 2013;120(4):844–851. https://doi.org/10.1016/j.ophtha.2012.10.036.

could be discussed with the patients. The necessary genetic tests and possible future treatment can be conducted based on accurate classification of AMD.

Validation and revision of the AREDS classification of AMD in OCT era

It is clear that the AREDS classification of AMD was established by data mainly obtained by CFP and fluorescein angiography (FA) in a semiquantitative manner known as "a study in FA era." For more than a decade, the AREDS classification system has been the gold standard for AMD grading and risk stratification. However, this classification system of AMD and treatment algorithms for late AMD has been revised with OCT imaging. In fact, some studies have described confounding errors in the CFP classification of intermediate AMD. In a comparative study, druse areas identified by CFP were compared to those measured by SD-OCT. There was general agreement between CFP and SD-OCT in identifying the presence and absence of drusen. While, the disagreement of these two methods occurred mainly at how to determine druse margins. As CFP-measured drusen may be influenced by the bias of graders, the calculated drusen burden was underestimated particularly in larger drusen with pigmentation.[8–10] Nowadays, it is achievable to quantify RPE and RPE drusen complex (RPEDC) in eyes of intermediate AMD with semi- or automated OCT. By delineating the inner aspect of the RPE plus drusen material and the outer aspect of Bruch's membrane, the RPEDC volume containing drusen materials (including subretinal drusenoid deposits) can be measured (Fig. 3.2).[10,11] Although

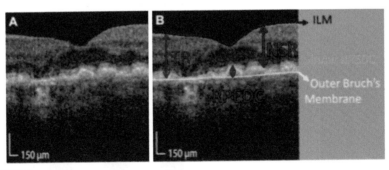

FIGURE 3.2

Definition of the target segmented layers and layer boundaries by SD-OCT. (A) Magnified foveal SD-OCT image with 6.70 μm lateral resolution and 3.24 μm axial resolution. (B) Delineation of the target layer boundaries: the inner aspect of the inner limiting membrane (ILM) in blue, the inner aspect of the retinal pigment epithelium drusen complex (RPEDC) in green, and the outer aspect of Bruch's membrane in yellow. (A) and (B), These boundaries isolate the total retina (TR) (orange *arrow* from blue to yellow), neurosensory retinal (NSR) (purple *arrow* from blue to green), and RPEDC (red *arrow* from green to yellow).

Modified from Farsiu S, Chiu SJ, O'Connell RV, et al. Quantitative classification of eyes with and without intermediate age-related macular degeneration using optical coherence tomography. Ophthalmology. 2014; 121(1):162–172. https://doi.org/10.1016/j.ophtha.2013.07.013.

during the measurement process, the thickness of RPEDC in AMD and the control are largely overlapping, the SD-OCT images successfully distinguished RPEDC thickness of patients with intermediate AMD from the control eyes. Therefore, practically OCT-measured RPEDC thickness became the single most discriminative biomarker of intermediate AMD.[11] In addition, based on OCT measurement, the modified new nomenclature of atrophic AMD is described (see Chapter 5, Table 5.1).

Classification of drusen and pigmentary changes by polarization-sensitive OCT

The increase of drusen size and the development of pigmentary changes are considered as indicators for the progression of AMD. Intensity-based SD-OCT measures the intensity of the backscattered light of the retina. Generally, polarization-sensitive SD-OCT (PS-OCT) is based on the same technology and sharing the same high-resolution images as SD-OCT. In addition, PS-OCT identifies the light in a polarization state within most cellular parts of the retina except for melanin. Melanin is found mostly in RPE cell organelles and is observed in other structures including pigmentary changes in the retina and inside of the drusen.[12] Schlanitz et al. in 2015 reported additional features of drusen and pigmentary changes in early and intermediate AMD by using PS-OCT, than by using conventional SD-OCT. Drusen were classified using three internal druse SD-OCT characteristics such as shape, reflectivity, and homogeneity, and two PS-OCT characteristics including foci and content (Fig. 3.3). Note that individual foci could be both hyperreflective and depolarizing, content could be patchy, non- or depolarizing.[13] Then, the central slice of each single druse was selected and its position on the retina was analyzed statistically and used as parameters for drusen classification (Fig. 3.3).[13]

Melanin is identified as the main cause for the depolarization signal of PS-OCT. As a result, melanin-loaded RPE cells generate a depolarization signal, which is indicated as red in Figs. 3.3 and 3.4. Meanwhile depolarizing signals may also occur in other locations within the retina, especially in a disease-affected eye.[14] In PS-OCT analysis, depolarization signals, an indicator of metabolism level, were observed within drusen and drusenoid pigment epithelial detachments, which may highlight the intensity of metabolic activity of RPE in drusen formation.[13] In parallel, a heterogeneous internal reflectivity observed by conventional SD-OCT may be associated with progression to local RPE atrophy.[15] Thus, the high intensity of polarization signal detected by PS-OCT and heterogeneous internal reflectivity by SD-OCT within drusen can be used as prognostic indicators for AMD progression. These techniques relied on two different principles of optical physics. By using SD-OCT, the presence of overlying hyperreflective foci of drusen, a phenomenon of intraretinal RPE migration, is another biomarker of AMD progression.[16] In Fig. 3.4 (bottom left), a colocalized, both hyperreflective and depolarizing material,

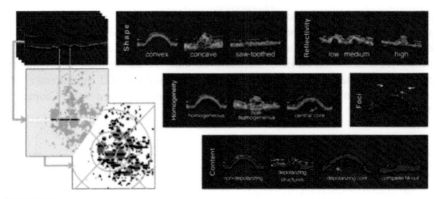

FIGURE 3.3

Classification of macular drusen by both SD-OCT and PS-OCT. Every elevation of the retinal pigment epithelium detectable in the single B-scans (Top left image) was delineated. In the next step, drusen were classified using three internal druse characteristics based on the spectral-domain optical coherence tomography classification (shape, reflectivity, and homogeneity, center and right area) and for specific depolarizing characteristics (foci and content, right and bottom area—the red color in the B-scans represents depolarizing structures segmented based on the degree of polarization uniformity calculation). Note that foci could be hyperreflective and/or depolarizing (foci, blue vs. yellow *arrow*, respectively). Finally, the central slice of each single druse was selected (Bottom left images) and its position on the retina was noted for further statistical calculations.

Modified from Schlanitz FG, Sacu S, Baumann B, et al. Identification of drusen characteristics in age-related macular degeneration by polarization-sensitive optical coherence tomography. Am J Ophthalmol. 2015;160(2): 335–344.e1. https://doi.org/10.1016/j.ajo.2015.05.008.

above the drusen suggests the origin of signals from the RPE layer. In Fig. 3.4 (bottom center and bottom right), depolarization signal is expending from RPEDC into the choroidal space, indicating PS-OCT can detect more pigment-loaded RPE activity in RPEDC than those by SD-OCT.[13] Therefore, the novel classification of PS-OCT characteristics of RPEDC has provided additional prognostic information for monitoring the progression of dry AMD.

Classification analysis of junctional zone of GA by OCT

AMD is a disease of photoreceptor/RPE/Bruch's membrane/choriocapillaris (PR/RPE/BrM/CC) complex. Segmentation technique by OCT has provided the opportunity to analyze the cross-section pathology of individual layers of this complex. Particularly, characterization of the junctional zone at the demarcation of GA by OCT could construct a three-dimensional configuration of PR/RPE/BrM/CC complex at junctional zone. For the study of the junctional zone of GA, a classification

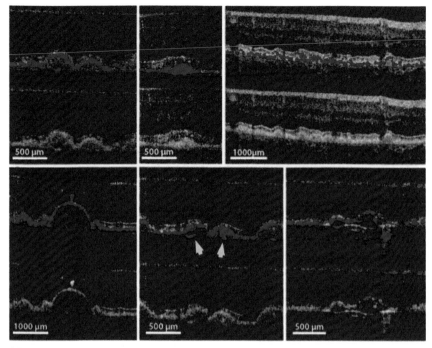

FIGURE 3.4

Macular drusen and pigmentary changes of intermediate AMD. Each image consists of two parts, showing the depolarization signal in the upper part (red) and the sole intensity image, as in SD-OCT, in the lower part. (Top left) Two neighboring drusen, of which only the left one displays depolarizing contents. (Top center) Hyperreflective druse completely filled out with depolarizing material. (Top right) Example of a saw-toothed druse formation spreading throughout the scan, with intermittent convex drusen and an irregular RPE layer. (Bottom left) Foci emanating from the RPE layer. (Bottom center and Bottom right) Depolarizing internal cores located at the base of the druse (center) or within the druse volume (right).

Modified from Schlanitz FG, Sacu S, Baumann B, et al. Identification of drusen characteristics in age-related macular degeneration by polarization-sensitive optical coherence tomography. Am J Ophthalmol. 2015;160(2): 335–344.e1. https://doi.org/10.1016/j.ajo.2015.05.008

analysis by OCT is required, because this could provide a guideline in deciding progressive, prognostic, and future therapeutic endpoints of GA enlargement. The following SD-OCT image shows a typical segmentation of the junctional zone of a patient with GA (Fig. 3.5).[17] This graded OCT image points out the start and the end of PR loss and the margin of RPE atrophy. Based on the grading data, the phenomena of PR loss are categorized as entirely inside the GA margin or as bridging across the GA margin, which is exemplified in this figure.[17]

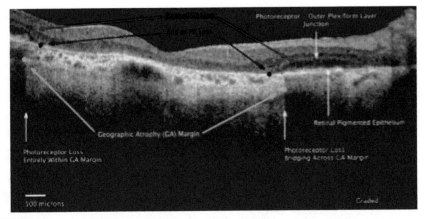

FIGURE 3.5

Graded SD-OCT image of GA margin and declining PR layer at the margin. The PR nuclear layer is the hyporeflective (darker) layer between the hyperreflective outer plexiform layer (OPL) and RPE; between the white arrows. In the normal eye, the PR inner segment to outer segment junction is visible as a separate hyperreflective band above the RPE. In this eye, that band is not clearly seen. These graded features include (1) Start of PR loss (red *dots*), (2) GA margins (green *dots*), and (3) end of PR loss (blue *dots*). The PR layer progressively thins starting at the red dot at each border of the GA until absent at the blue dot. The PR loss is categorized as entirely inside the GA margin on the left, and as bridging across the GA margin on the right. The PR layer is absent between the blue *dots*, thus the OPL is located over Bruch's membrane. The SD-OCT signal is particularly bright in the choroid and extends deeper into the choroid between the green *dots* where there is no RPE pigment to shadow.

Modified from Bearelly S, Chau FY, Koreishi A, Stinnett SS, Izatt JA, Toth CA. Spectral domain optical coherence tomography imaging of geographic atrophy margins. Ophthalmology. 2009;116(9):1762–1769. https://doi.org/10.1016/j.ophtha.2009.04.015.

In a recent cohort study, the junctional zone at GA margin was classified based on the areas of RPE defect and PR defect on OCT-measurable images. Three types of junctional configurations were classified: Type 0, exact correspondence between the edge of the RPE defect and PR defect; Type 1, loss of photoreceptors outside and beyond the edge of the RPE defect; Type 2, preservation of photoreceptors beyond the edge of the RPE defect. The overall RPE defect area was measured significantly smaller than that of PR defect in this cohort.[18] After the advent of OCT angiography (OCTA), the CC architecture and blood flow at the junctional zone have been investigated. Evidence exists that CC loss is happening outside of the atrophic margins, suggesting a compromised CC may precede outer retina and RPE atrophy in GA development.[19,20] This evidence supports that GA is a disorder of macular neurovascular complex as discussed in Chapter 1. The significance of this finding for the pathogenesis of dry AMD will be discussed in Chapter 7.

Consensus classification analyses of GA in OCT era

With advances of the OCT technique, GA can be studied in three dimensions, and the involvement of specific retinal layers can be quantified. Furthermore, OCT B-scan combined with *en face* viewing of the volumetric OCT scans for analyzing borders of atrophy can be identified. However, there had been no consensus of GA classification after entering the OCT era because the conventional classification of AMD was established based on CFP about 1 decade ago. So that there was a demand by providers who need communicate with each other and consult their patients by using the same classification of dry AMD on OCT. For this purpose, an international consensus group of experts in AMD, so-called the classification of atrophy meetings (CAM), reviewed existing data and proposed a consensus definition and nomenclature for OCT-defined atrophic AMD.[21] SD-OCT data were used because the technique possesses the following capabilities: (1) visualization of specific layers affected by the disease, (2) wide availability of this technology, and (3) patient comfort. The CAM group Report 3 recommended four terms describing atrophic AMD: (1) complete RPE and outer retinal atrophy (cRORA), (2) incomplete RPE and outer retinal atrophy (iRORA), (3) complete outer retinal atrophy, and (4) incomplete outer retinal atrophy. The representative OCT image of cRORA is illustrated in Fig. 3.6.[21]

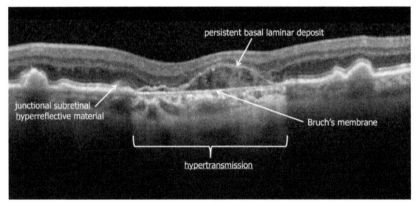

FIGURE 3.6

An OCT B-scan showing complete RPE and outer retinal atrophy (cRORA). *Bracket* indicating a zone of homogeneous choroidal hypertransmission and absence of the RPE band measuring >250 μm (hypertransmission); *Arrow* indicating the bare Bruch's membrane with the absence of RPE and overlying outer retinal thinning (Bruch's membrane) and loss of photoreceptor bands; No signs of an RPE tear; The sequela of atrophy such as junctional subretinal hyperreflective material and persistent basal laminar deposit are indicated.

Modified from Sadda SR, Guymer R, Holz FG, et al. Consensus definition for atrophy associated with age-related macular degeneration on OCT: classification of atrophy report 3. Ophthalmology. 2018;125(4):537–548. https://doi.org/10.1016/j.ophtha.2017.09.028.

The third CAM report defined cRORA as the endpoint of atrophic AMD. In the fourth CAM report in 2020, iRORA and longitudinal progression from this earlier stage to cRORA were defined. The OCT characteristics of iRORA include (1) a region of hypertransmission into the choroid, (2) a corresponding zone of attenuation or disruption of the RPE, with or without the persistence of basal laminar deposits, and (3) overlying photoreceptor degeneration such as subsidence of the INL and OPL, presence of a hyporeflective wedge in the Henle fiber layer, thinning of the outer nuclear layer, disruption of external limiting membrane, or loss of integrity of the ellipsoid zone. Overall, these features do not meet the criteria of cRORA. An example of iRORA studied by multimodal imaging is shown in Fig. 3.7.[22]

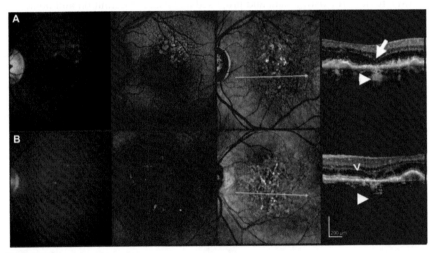

FIGURE 3.7

Examples of multimodal imaging features of incomplete retinal pigment epithelium and outer retinal atrophy (iRORA); color fundus photography (CFP; first column), fundus autofluorescence (FAF; second column), near-infrared reflectance (NIR; third column), and OCT B-scan (fourth column). (A), (B), Left maculae of two individual cases with large drusen. The first column shows CFP demonstrating drusen and pigmentary changes without evidence of geographic atrophy. The second column shows FAF imaging demonstrating only small areas of hypoautofluorescence. The third column shows NIR images illustrating no evidence of atrophy. The fourth column shows OCT B-scans demonstrating subsidence of the inner nuclear layer (large *arrow*) and outer plexiform layer. Note the hyporeflective wedge-shaped band within the limits of the Henle fiber layer (B, ar). Note the loss of photoreceptors as evidenced by outer nuclear layer thinning and loss of external limiting membrane, ellipsoid zone, and interdigitation zone. Subjacent to the area of photoreceptor loss is a zone of attenuation and disruption of the retinal pigment epithelium (<250 μm). A region of signal hypertransmission into the choroid (solid ar) is less than 250 μm in continuity. This fulfills the criteria for iRORA.

Modified from Guymer RH, Rosenfeld PJ, Curcio CA, et al. Incomplete retinal pigment epithelial and outer retinal atrophy in age-related macular degeneration: classification of atrophy meeting report 4. Ophthalmology. Published online September 30, 2019. https://doi.org/10.1016/j.ophtha.2019.09.035.

The CAM reports have defined iRORA and cRORA by using OCT. In addition to the new classification criteria and new nomenclature established in these studies, several other important points have been addressed. First, the CAM reports provided evidences that the features of iRORA predict the development of cRORA. Therefore, future clinical trial endpoint needs focusing on the prevention of GA onset, rather than the progression of preexisting atrophic lesions.[23] Second, the CAM group pointed out that the term nascent GA should be used more broadly when iRORA is present in the absence of current or prior macular neovascularization, indicating that progression toward GA has begun.[24] The rest of the detailed classification of atrophic AMD by the CAM groups are further discussed in Chapter 5.

GA growth rate dependent on lesion location

At the early stage, the GA lesion encroaches to form a parafoveal ring surrounding the fovea. During this stage of foveal sparing, patients usually have a decent central vision. As GA continues to progress, the lesion will reach the fovea and result in a dramatic loss in central vision. Therefore, by using both OCT and visual acuity, the classification of GA according to whether it is fovea spared or fovea involved has been conducted in numerous studies. In a recent literature review and meta-analysis, GA radius growth rates are defined in four location groups: macular center point involved (CPI) or spared (CPS), and foveal zone involved (FZI) or spared (FZS). GA radius enlarges linearly over time in each GA location group. Based on the GA location classification, the GA growth rate in the CPS group is $(0.203 \pm 0.013$ mm/year) 30.1% higher than that in the CPI group $((0.156 \pm 0.011$ mm/year). In comparison, the GA growth rate in the FZS group $(0.215 \pm 0.012$ mm/year) is 61.7% higher than that in the FZI group $(0.133 \pm 0.009$ mm/year). The natural GA growth can be used for the evaluation and prediction of central vision outcome of patients with GA.[25] The natural history of GA progression can be predicted based on three linear models (Fig. 3.8).[26]

Choroidal neovascularization associated AMD classification in OCT era

More than 5 decades since Gass's description of clinical features related to neovascular AMD,[27] the new nomenclature for studying wet AMD with the agreement of scientific bases had just been achieved by the Consensus on Neovascular AMD Nomenclature (CONAN) group recently.[28] With greater precision of OCT, OCTA, and other multimodal imaging, the majority of abnormalities that previously were

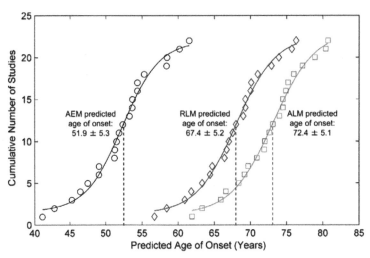

FIGURE 3.8

Natural history of GA progression based on three models. Graph showing the predicted age of geographic atrophy (GA) onset based on the area linear model (ALM), radius linear model (RLM), and area exponential model (AEM). The points were generated by subtracting the optimized translation factor in each model from the reported average age in each study. The ages of onset of GA estimated from the ALM (72.45.1 years) and RLM (67.45.2 years) are consistent with clinical observations and the literature. However, the prediction by the AEM (51.95.3 years) is outside of the observed range of age of onset reported in the literature. For all three models, the histogram of the number of studies as a function of the predicted age of onset fits a sigmoid curve, suggesting a normal distribution.

Modified from Shen L, Liu F, Grossetta Nardini H, Del Priore LV. Natural history of geographic atrophy in untreated eyes with nonexudative age-related macular degeneration: a systematic review and meta-analysis. Ophthalmol Retina. 2018;2(9):914–921. https://doi.org/10.1016/j.oret.2018.01.019.

identified by CFP and FA can be validated by OCT and OCTA. However, it is not necessary to replace the classification determined by old techniques, because the established nAMD classification can be applied to both previous data and new findings. Meanwhile, using multimodal imaging has provided additional information for modifying the classification of nAMD. The new and the old classification terms are listed in Table 3.2.[28]

Table 3.2 New versus old terminology correlates.[28]

New term	Multimodal imaging correlate	Old term	Color fundus and fluorescein imaging findings
Type 1 MNV	Type 1 MNV represents areas of neovascular complexes arising from the choroid and imaged with OCT as an elevation of the RPE by material with heterogeneous reflectivity; vascular elements may be seen. OCT angiography shows vessels below the level of the RPE	Occult CNV	Stippled hyperfluorescence over an area of elevated RPE, which expands to coalesce in the later phases of the angiography
Polypoidal choroidal vasculopathy	OCT findings similar to type 1 MNV; however, in some patients, dilated vascular elements at the outer border of the lesion are apparent. Stippled hyperfluorescence over an area of elevated RPE, which expands to coalesce in the later phases of the angiography. The pattern of the RPE elevation may suggest nodules. Indocyanine green angiography shows a branching vascular network with aneurysmal dilations	Polypoidal choroidal vasculopathy	Stippled hyperfluorescence over an area of elevated RPE that expands to coalesce in the later phases of the angiography. The pattern of the RPE elevation may suggest nodules. Indocyanine green angiography shows a branching vascular network with aneurysmal dilations
Type 2 MNV	Neovascular complex located in the subretinal space, above Ac level of the RPE May be associated with subretinal hyperreflective material and separation of the neurosensory retina from the RPE. OCT angiography demonstrates vascular elements above the level of the RPE	Classic CNV	Early hyperfluorescence and late leakage that pools in the subretinal space. Neovascular elements may be detected in the very early phase of the angiogram
Mixed type 1 and type 2 MNV	OCT findings of both type 1 and type 2 MNV together. OCT angiography demonstrates neovascularization in die subretinal pigment epithelial and subretinal compartments	Minimally classic CNV	Early hyperfluorescence with late leakage and a larger surround of stippled hyperfluorescence that also shows leakage late in the fluorescein angiogram. Difficult to differentiate from type 3 neovascularization
Type 3 MNV	Extension of hyperreflectivity from the middle retina toward to level of the RPE associated with intraretinal edema, hemorrhage, and telangiectasis. OCT angiography shows the down growth of new vessels toward or even penetrating the level of the RPE	Retinal angiomatous proliferation	Focal hyperfluorescence associated with intraretinal staining. Often shows fluorescence from deeper layers suggestive of occult CNV. The neovascularization is not necessarily CNV

Continued

Table 3.2 New versus old terminology correlates.[28]—cont'd

New term	Multimodal imaging correlate	Old term	Color fundus and fluorescein imaging findings
Retinal-choroidal anastomosis	Aberrant connection from the retinal to the choroidal circulation. Course of vessel can be seen occasionally with OCT or OCT angiography. Although visible on fluorescein angiography, indocyanine green angiography often is better at demonstrating the anastomosis	Retinal-choroidal anastomosis	Aberrant connection from the retinal to the choroidal circulation. Although visible on fluorescein angiography, indocyanine green angiography often is better at demonstrating the anastomosis
Leakage	Breakdown of the blood–retinal barrier, typically demonstrated by fluorescein angiography	Leakage	Breakdown of the blood–retinal barrier, typically demonstrated by fluorescein angiography
Intraretinal fluid	Cystoid spaces in the retina typically associated with increased retinal thickening. Readily detected using OCT	Cystoid edema	Thickening of the retina that may be difficult to detect and cystoid spaces that also may be difficult to detect by color photography. Fluorescein angiography shows the pooling of dye in some of the cystoid spaces
Subretinal fluid	Separation of the neurosensory retina from the RPE by fluid. Readily detected using OCT	Subretinal fluid	Exaggerated accumulations in the macula may be detected with stereo color photography and also may be suggested by a loss of transparency of the detached retina
Lipid (hard exudates)	Yellow-white globular material in or under the retina. OCT shows hyperreflective foci in the retina, some of which are not visible by ophthalmoscopy	Lipid (hard exudates)	Yellow-white globular material in or under the retina
Subretinal hyperreflective material	Exudation in the subretinal space of material that is hyperreflective as compared with fluid	Not named before OCT era	In extreme cases, the material is seen on color photography that is difficult to differentiate from fibrosis
Retinal PED	Several forms of elevation of the RPE monolayer from the underlying Bruch's membrane. This includes drusenoid, serous, and fibrovascular. Some forms of early type 1 neovascularization produce a relatively flat elevation. Many cases of serous PED show evidence of MNV. OCT angiography is particularly useful in detecting the presence of neovascularization	Retinal PED	Several forms of elevation of the RPE monolayer from the underlying Bruch's membrane. These include drusenoid, serous, and fibrovascular. Accurately delineating serous and fibrovascular PEDs can be difficult. Early type 1 MNV with RPE elevation may not be detectable

New Term	New Term description	Old Term	Old Term description
Hemorrhage	Blood in the retina, subretinal, or sub-RPE compartments. Exact location of blood apparent in OCT examination	Hemorrhage	Blood in the retina, subretinal, or sub-RPE compartments. Location of blood can be inferred
Fibrosis	White or yellow-white accumulation of material, usually in the subretinal or sub-RPE space. On OCT, the material is hyperreflective and may have a multilaminar appearance	Fibrosis	White or yellow-white accumulation of material, in the subretinal or sub-RPE space
Rip (or tear) of the RPE	Area of increased pigmentation from the scrolled RPE adjacent to a zone of decreased pigmentation. During fluorescein angiography, the increased pigmentation blocks the underlying fluorescence, whereas the area denuded of RPE is hyperfluorescent. OCT shows the anatomic configuration of the scrolled RPE and hypertransmission in the denuded zone	Rip (or tear) of the RPE	Area of increased pigmentation from the scrolled RPE adjacent to a zone of decreased pigmentation. During fluorescein angiography, the increased pigmentation blocks the underlying fluorescence, whereas the area denuded of RPE is hyperfluorescent
Outer retinal atrophy	On OCT imaging, loss of the ellipsoid and interdigitation zones associated with thinning of the outer nuclear layer	Not named before OCT era	No color photograph or fluorescein angiography correlates
RPE and outer retinal atrophy	OCT features of outer retinal atrophy and signs of RPE loss to include decrease or absence of the RPE monolayer and hypertransmission into the underlying neovascular lesion and choroid	Roughly correlates to geographic atrophy	The color photographic definition of geographic atrophy includes a round or oval well-defined area in which the underlying choroidal vessel are seen more easily. in neovascular cases, there is no reason the RPE loss must be round or oval and well defined. The presence of underlying neovascular lesion may block visualization of the choroidal vessels in any case

Abbreviations: CNV, choroidal neovascularization; MNV, macular neovascularization; PED, pigment epithelial detachment; RPE, retinal pigment epithelium; New Term ("Old Term" used in original table, which should be New Term).

Modified from Spaide RF, Jaffe GJ, Sarraf D, et al. Consensus nomenclature for reporting neovascular age-related macular degeneration data: consensus on neovascular age-related macular degeneration nomenclature study group. Ophthalmology. Published online November 14, 2019. doi:10.1016/j.ophtha.2019.11.004.

Based on the information of Table 3.2, CONAN group defined and subdefined the components of neovascular AMD in OCT era including neovascularization subtypes: type 1, 2, and 3 MNV (Figs. 3.9–3.11).[28] The MNV comprises the variants such as PCV; exudative features related to MNV such as leakage, subretinal fluid, lipid, and subretinal hyperreflective exudative material; lesions in addition to MNV such as RPE detachment, hemorrhage, fibrosis and RPE tear (rip); and the macular atrophy in the context of neovascular AMD. As the disease components related to neovascular AMD are also discussed in Chapters 4 and 5 in depth, this section is only focusing on MNV showed by cartoons in order to be clear at a glance.

In summary, AREDS AMD classification at FA era, based on CFP and FA data, elucidated the nature of AMD, that is, a spectrum macular disorders, provided guidelines for epidemiologic studies and clinical trials, and established the gold standard

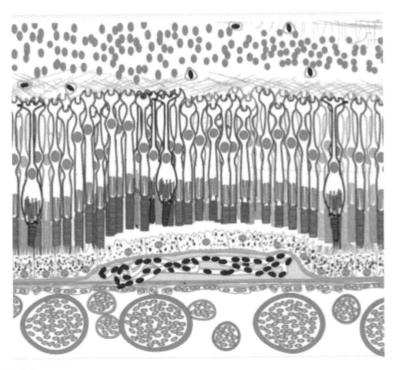

FIGURE 3.9

Cartoon diagram showing type 1 macular neovascularization. The ingrowth of vessels arises from the choriocapillaris and extends up to and under the retinal pigment epithelium.

Modified from Spaide RF, Jaffe GJ, Sarraf D, et al. Consensus nomenclature for reporting neovascular age-related macular degeneration data: consensus on neovascular age-related macular degeneration nomenclature study group. Ophthalmology. Published online November 14, 2019. https://doi.org/10.1016/j.ophtha.2019.11.004.

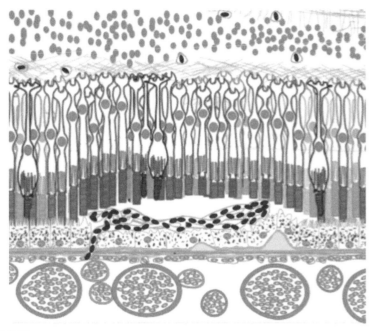

FIGURE 3.10

Cartoon diagram showing type 2 macular neovascularization. The ingrowth of vessels arises from the choriocapillaris and extends up through the retinal pigment epithelium (RPE) monolayer to proliferate in the subretinal space. To arrive in the subretinal space, the blood flow must traverse the sub-RPE space to reach the plane of neovascularization.

Modified from Spaide RF, Jaffe GJ, Sarraf D, et al. Consensus nomenclature for reporting neovascular age-related macular degeneration data: consensus on neovascular age-related macular degeneration nomenclature study group. Ophthalmology. *Published online November 14, 2019. https://doi.org/10.1016/j.ophtha.2019.11.004.*

in classification and diagnosis of AMD. AREDS AMD classification has been validated and revised by using multimodal imaging techniques, that is, those at OCT era. AMD, a spectrum disorder of macula, has been further analyzed as a disease of the photoreceptor/RPE/Bruch's membrane/choriocapillaris complex in three-dimensional approach in OCT era. As a result, novel quantitative biometry of the drusen, pigmentary changes, RPE, macula, and macular neovascularization represents a paradigm shift in the diagnosis and classification of early and late AMD. However, the AREDS AMD classification should not be replaced by the new AMD classification. The two systems share the common essential nomenclatures for the created datasets exchangeable and communicable. The data of previous epidemiologic studies and clinical trials can be longitudinally studied.

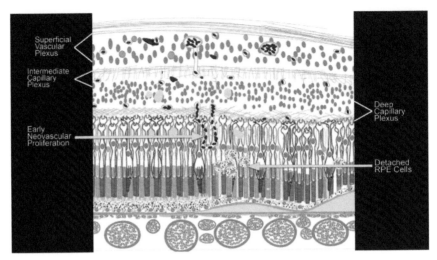

FIGURE 3.11

Type 3 neovascularization formation. When the regional proangiogenic and antiangiogenic balances shift in favor of neovascularization, new vessels occur along a proangiogenic concentration gradient. The new vessels originate from and invade into tissues below the plane of the deep capillary plexus. Elevated cytokines, particularly VEGF levels, can induce vascular leakage and intraretinal hemorrhage in addition to stimulating angiogenesis. *RPE*, retinal pigment epithelium.

Modified from Spaide RF, Jaffe GJ, Sarraf D, et al. Consensus nomenclature for reporting neovascular age-related macular degeneration data: consensus on neovascular age-related macular degeneration nomenclature study group. Ophthalmology. Published online November 14, 2019. https://doi.org/10.1016/j.ophtha.2019.11.004.

References

1. Ferris FL, Davis MD, Clemons TE, et al. A simplified severity scale for age-related macular degeneration: AREDS Report No. 18. *Arch Ophthalmol.* 2005;123(11):1570—1574. https://doi.org/10.1001/archopht.123.11.1570.
2. Bird AC, Bressler NM, Bressler SB, et al. An international classification and grading system for age-related maculopathy and age-related macular degeneration. The International ARM Epidemiological Study Group. *Surv Ophthalmol.* 1995;39(5):367—374. https://doi.org/10.1016/s0039-6257(05)80092-x.
3. Seddon JM, Sharma S, Adelman RA. Evaluation of the clinical age-related maculopathy staging system. *Ophthalmology.* 2006;113(2):260—266. https://doi.org/10.1016/j.ophtha.2005.11.001.
4. Davis MD, Gangnon RE, Lee L-Y, et al. The Age-Related Eye Disease Study severity scale for age-related macular degeneration: AREDS Report No. 17. *Arch Ophthalmol.* 2005;123(11):1484—1498. https://doi.org/10.1001/archopht.123.11.1484.
5. Ferris FL, Wilkinson CP, Bird A, et al. Clinical classification of age-related macular degeneration. *Ophthalmology.* 2013;120(4):844—851. https://doi.org/10.1016/j.ophtha.2012.10.036.

6. Friberg TR, Bilonick RA, Brennen P. Is drusen area really so important? An assessment of risk of conversion to neovascular AMD based on computerized measurements of drusen. *Invest Ophthalmol Vis Sci.* 2012;53(4):1742−1751. https://doi.org/10.1167/iovs.11-9338.

7. Klein R, Klein BEK, Linton KLP. Prevalence of age-related maculopathy: the beaver Dam eye study. *Ophthalmology.* 2020;127(4S):S122−S132. https://doi.org/10.1016/j.ophtha.2020.01.033.

8. Jain N, Farsiu S, Khanifar AA, et al. Quantitative comparison of drusen segmented on SD-OCT versus drusen delineated on color fundus photographs. *Invest Ophthalmol Vis Sci.* 2010;51(10):4875−4883. https://doi.org/10.1167/iovs.09-4962.

9. Leuschen JN, Schuman SG, Winter KP, et al. Spectral-domain optical coherence tomography characteristics of intermediate age-related macular degeneration. *Ophthalmology.* 2013;120(1):140−150. https://doi.org/10.1016/j.ophtha.2012.07.004.

10. Nittala MG, Ruiz-Garcia H, Sadda SR. Accuracy and reproducibility of automated drusen segmentation in eyes with non-neovascular age-related macular degeneration. *Invest Ophthalmol Vis Sci.* 2012;53(13):8319−8324. https://doi.org/10.1167/iovs.12-10582.

11. Farsiu S, Chiu SJ, O'Connell RV, et al. Quantitative classification of eyes with and without intermediate age-related macular degeneration using optical coherence tomography. *Ophthalmology.* 2014;121(1):162−172. https://doi.org/10.1016/j.ophtha.2013.07.013.

12. Pircher M, Götzinger E, Leitgeb R, Sattmann H, Findl O, ChristophK H. Imaging of polarization properties of human retina in vivo with phase resolved transversal PS-OCT. *Optic Express.* 2004;12(24):5940. https://doi.org/10.1364/OPEX.12.005940.

13. Schlanitz FG, Sacu S, Baumann B, et al. Identification of drusen characteristics in age-related macular degeneration by polarization-sensitive optical coherence tomography. *Am J Ophthalmol.* 2015;160(2):335−344.e1. https://doi.org/10.1016/j.ajo.2015.05.008.

14. Lammer J, Bolz M, Baumann B, et al. Detection and analysis of hard exudates by polarization-sensitive optical coherence tomography in patients with diabetic maculopathy. *Invest Ophthalmol Vis Sci.* 2014;55(3):1564−1571. https://doi.org/10.1167/iovs.13-13539.

15. Ouyang Y, Heussen FM, Hariri A, Keane PA, Sadda SR. Optical coherence tomography-based observation of the natural history of drusenoid lesion in eyes with dry age-related macular degeneration. *Ophthalmology.* 2013;120(12):2656−2665. https://doi.org/10.1016/j.ophtha.2013.05.029.

16. Ho J, Witkin AJ, Liu J, et al. Documentation of intraretinal retinal pigment epithelium migration via high-speed ultrahigh-resolution optical coherence tomography. *Ophthalmology.* 2011;118(4):687−693. https://doi.org/10.1016/j.ophtha.2010.08.010.

17. Bearelly S, Chau FY, Koreishi A, Stinnett SS, Izatt JA, Toth CA. Spectral domain optical coherence tomography imaging of geographic atrophy margins. *Ophthalmology.* 2009;116(9):1762−1769. https://doi.org/10.1016/j.ophtha.2009.04.015.

18. Qu J, Velaga SB, Hariri AH, Nittala MG, Sadda S. Classification and quantitative analysis OF geographic atrophy junctional zone using spectral domain optical coherence tomography. *Retina.* 2018;38(8):1456−1463. https://doi.org/10.1097/IAE.0000000000001824.

19. Kvanta A, Casselholm de Salles M, Amrén U, Bartuma H. Optical coherence tomography angiography OF the foveal microvasculature in geographic atrophy. *Retina.* 2017;37(5):936−942. https://doi.org/10.1097/IAE.0000000000001248.

20. Cicinelli MV, Rabiolo A, Sacconi R, et al. Optical coherence tomography angiography in dry age-related macular degeneration. *Surv Ophthalmol.* 2018;63(2):236–244. https://doi.org/10.1016/j.survophthal.2017.06.005.

21. Sadda SR, Guymer R, Holz FG, et al. Consensus definition for atrophy associated with age-related macular degeneration on OCT: classification of atrophy report 3. *Ophthalmology.* 2018;125(4):537–548. https://doi.org/10.1016/j.ophtha.2017.09.028.

22. Guymer RH, Rosenfeld PJ, Curcio CA, et al. Incomplete retinal pigment epithelial and outer retinal atrophy in age-related macular degeneration: classification of atrophy meeting report 4. *Ophthalmology.* 2019. https://doi.org/10.1016/j.ophtha.2019.09.035. Published online September 30.

23. Guymer RH. Geographic atrophy trials: turning the ship around may not Be that easy. *Ophthalmol Retina.* 2018;2(6):515–517. https://doi.org/10.1016/j.oret.2018.03.004.

24. Guymer RH, Wu Z, Hodgson LAB, et al. Subthreshold nanosecond laser intervention in age-related macular degeneration: the LEAD randomized controlled clinical trial. *Ophthalmology.* 2019;126(6):829–838. https://doi.org/10.1016/j.ophtha.2018.09.015.

25. Shen LL, Sun M, Khetpal S, Grossetta Nardini HK, Del Priore LV. Topographic variation of the growth rate of geographic atrophy in nonexudative age-related macular degeneration: a systematic review and meta-analysis. *Invest Ophthalmol Vis Sci.* 2020;61(1):2. https://doi.org/10.1167/iovs.61.1.2.

26. Shen L, Liu F, Grossetta Nardini H, Del Priore LV. Natural history of geographic atrophy in untreated eyes with nonexudative age-related macular degeneration: a systematic review and meta-analysis. *Ophthalmol Retina.* 2018;2(9):914–921. https://doi.org/10.1016/j.oret.2018.01.019.

27. Gass JD. Pathogenesis of disciform detachment of the neuroepithelium. *Am J Ophthalmol.* 1967;63(3):1–139. Suppl.

28. Spaide RF, Jaffe GJ, Sarraf D, et al. Consensus nomenclature for reporting neovascular age-related macular degeneration data: consensus on neovascular age-related macular degeneration nomenclature study group. *Ophthalmology.* 2019. https://doi.org/10.1016/j.ophtha.2019.11.004. Published online November 14.

Signs and symptoms of age-related macular degeneration

Undetectable and detectable signs of early AMD

Age-related macular degeneration (AMD) encompasses a spectrum of clinical signs ranging from undetectable to overly manifested macular disorder. The funduscopically undetected signs may overlap with the aging changes of macula. The aging changes of macula were not systemically studied in vivo until the advent of optical coherence tomography (OCT) in recent decades. The availability of a new generation of OCT such as spectral-domain OCT (SD-OCT) enables a powerful optical imaging technique to provide high-resolution optical slides in vivo of the human retina. Nowadays, SD-OCT and other newer OCT techniques can obtain multiple scans over retinal areas and generate quantitative maps of retinal thickness with high spatial resolution. By using OCT, the retinal layers at macula and the volume of macula and the architecture of macula at different locations of the posterior pole can be visualized and quantified. The OCT study on macula creates an opportunity of distinguishing the age-related macular diseases from the aging macula. The following representative SD-OCT slide shows the segmentation of retinal layers, which is compatible with histologic slides (Fig. 4.1)[1,2].

Normal aging changes of macula can be identified by both histologic and OCT approaches. Previous histologic studies showed the dynamic changes of human retinal photoreceptors and retinal pigment epithelium (RPE) cells throughout the life span (ranging from the second to the ninth decade).[2] At the foveal center, no significant differences were found in cone or RPE cell densities from the second to ninth decade. It suggests that the densities of foveal cones and RPE cells are kept stable throughout this age period. These histologic findings support the OCT findings. Specifically, the OCT measurement of center point foveal thickness on RPE, fovea cones, and their synapses with inner nuclear layers seems unchanged with age.[1] In addition, OCT measurements also showed that aging does not significantly change central subfield thickness.[1]

However, histologically measured rod density decreases by 30%, beginning from inferior to the fovea in midlife and continuously losing in an annulus between 0.5 and 3 mm eccentricity by the ninth decade.[3] Being equivalent to OCT parafoveal and perifoveal regions by early treatment diabetic retinopathy study (ETDRS)

Age-Related Macular Degeneration. https://doi.org/10.1016/B978-0-12-822061-0.00009-8

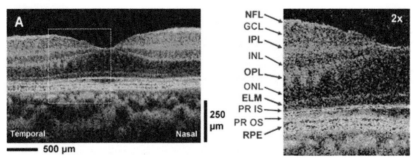

FIGURE 4.1

Definition of the normal macular layers on spectral-domain optical coherence tomography (SD-OCT). This is an SD-OCT of the central macula with layer segmentation. Inner layers are constituted by the retinal nerve fiber layer (RNFL), the ganglion cell layer (GCL), the inner plexiform layer (IPL), the inner nuclear layer (INL), and the outer plexiform layer (OPL). RNFL contains ganglion cell axons that run into the optical nerve. The ganglion cell bodies lie in the GCL. IPL is formed by the dendrites of cells in the GCL and axons of bipolar cells in the INL. Outer layers are constituted by the OPL, the outer nuclear layer (ONL), the inner segments (IS), the outer segments (OS), and the retinal pigment epithelium (RPE). The OPL is a network of synapses from cells in the INL and the photoreceptors. The photoreceptors—rods and cones—extend throughout the next three layers: ONL, which contains cell bodies of the photoreceptors; IS, which is the location for structures responsible of intracellular metabolism and transport; and OS, which contains the discs of the photoreceptors that contain photopigment. The RPE is a layer of pigmented cells that nourish and support the photoreceptors.

Modified from Ko TH, Fujimoto JG, Schuman JS, Paunescu LA, Kowalevicz AM, Hartl I,
Drexler W, Wollstein G, Ishikawa H, Duker JS. Comparison of ultrahigh- and standard-resolution
optical coherence tomography for imaging macular pathology. Ophthalmology. 2005;112(11):1922.e1-15.
https://doi.org/10.1016/j.ophtha.2005.05.027.

macular mapping, the inner and outer macula were defined as the circular zones around the macula. In fact, OCT measurements of macular regional thickness were in agreement with an age-related decrease in both inner and outer macula-subfield thickness in histology slides.[1] A recent study on the drusen evolution of intermediate AMD patients showed that the emergence and regression of drusen are associated with RPE thickness changes. Therefore, longitudinal measurement of RPE thickness may be a potential marker for predicting drusen emergence/regression and for AMD prognostic development.[4]

A decrease in the inner retina thickness of the aging retina is observed by OCT studies, specifically in the retinal nerve fiber layer (RNFL) and the retinal ganglion cell layer (GCL). Because RNFL and GCL constitute a relatively smaller proportion of the overall thickness at the fovea, the fovea is largely spared from thickness reduction due to loss of GCL and RNFL in the aging retina (Fig. 4.1).[1,5,6] Recent OCT findings reveal the significant changes of GCL thickness within the macula of intermediate AMD eyes.[7] Both age-dependent and AMD disease-dependent GCL loss were found in a location-dependent fashion.[2,7] The GCL cell loss was faster between the second and fourth decades than between the fourth and ninth decades. Meanwhile, the rod and GCL cell densities at the temporal equator maintained a constant ratio during aging, which suggests an interplay relationship between outer retinal photoreceptor loss and inner retinal neuron death,[2] although they only have trans-synaptic connections.

Both histologic and in vivo OCT findings pointed out that the early AMD signs overlap with naturally aged retina, although the aging retina does not necessarily develop into early AMD. The overlapping could be clinically undetectable in the past, but it now should be explored in the OCT era. If some OCT findings can be used as biomarkers for early AMD study, a key question is that whether the aging changes and AMD changes of chorioretinal layers can be differentiated based on location-specificity? Inferentially, when OCT measurements were used as bio-markers for the study of Alzheimers disease (AD) and other neurodegenerative diseases, distinct OCT features have been found among these diseases.[8] Because β-amyloid plaques in the retina of AD patients were located within sites of GCL degeneration and occurring in clusters in the mid- and far-periphery of the superior and inferior quadrants,[9,10] OCT findings of decreased GCL at these disease-specific regions other than generalized aging changes of GCL are very informative for helping AD diagnosis.[8] In fact, the distinct pattern of GCL thickness in intermediate AMD patients has been found that the GLC thickness alters in macula spatial clusters, with thinning toward the fovea and thickening toward the peripheral macula.[7] Whether these OCT findings of GCL are AMD-specific, and could be used as disease-specific biomarkers in clinic, merits further study.[7]

AMD is considered as a disease of macular neurovascular complex (MNC), because there is intimate anatomic relationship among PRs, RPE, and CC from early embryonic development. The choroid is a vascular tissue comprising three distinct layers, that is, choriocapillaris, Sattler's layer, and Haller's layer. The three layers of choroidal vessels begin to be identified at 21-week gestation, which coincides with the beginning of photoreceptor cell differentiation. As the choroidal vascular system is the only blood supply for oxygen and nutrient demanded by MNC, the diminishing choroidal layers, namely a decrease in choroidal blood flow observed in aging and diseases, will result in damage of this complex.[11] The observation of aging changes of CC in vivo has become accessible because of the emerging of OCT and OCT angiography (OCTA).[12,13] OCTA utilizes motion contrast technology that can detect the movement of red blood cells in consecutive scans. When OCTA is combined with OCT B-scans, both blood flow and chorioretinal structure can be simultaneously obtained.[13] When swept-source OCT was utilized, choroidal thickness at superior, inferior, nasal, and temporal sites to the fovea could be determined. The choroidal thickness was anatomically thinnest at the nasal site, followed by the order of temporal, inferior, superior, and foveal sites. The choroidal thickness overall decreased with age ranging from 21 up to 85 years.[14]

In a large cohort study measuring multiple chorioretinal segmentation parameters in elderly peoples, only a reduction of subfoveal choroidal thickness was found to be significantly associated with *CFH* risk genotype (rs1061170), a high-risk genotype of AMD development.[6,15] In a same-aged group, ranging from 21 to 82 years, choriocapillaris flow density was determined by OCTA. The choriocapillaris flow density was found to be negatively associated with advancing age.[16] Therefore, OCTA-measured choroidal signs are promising to become applicable for early AMD detection.

After teasing out aging chorioretinal changes, the location-dependent and chororetinal-layer-specific imaging markers may find detectable signs in early AMD.[11]

Drusen and pigmentary changes

Drusen [singular: druse] are the hallmark of AMD and the most common early sign of nonexudative AMD. They are visible yellowish deposits under the retina. Generally speaking, the typical location of drusen is along the basal surface of the RPE and corresponds to the thickening of the inner layer of Bruch's membrane in the posterior pole.

This clinical classification of AMD heavily depends on drusen characteristics (see Table 3.1 in Chapter 3).[17,18] Drusen are characterized by their size; their location related to the cellular structure of RPE cells, for example, subplasma membrane, and above or below basement membrane; type of drusen based on the distinct or ill-defined margin, that is, hard or soft drusen, position of predilection for macula,[19] and association with pigmentary changes.

The impact of druse size on the integrity of the overlying RPE layer and photoreceptor changes is clearly demonstrated. In a cohort study, 5933 drusen of 25 patients with early or intermedium AMD along with their adjacent RPE and photoreceptors were analyzed by polarization-sensitive OCT. In general, when the mean of druse size was 97 μm, the overlying RPE layer was still intact. If the mean druse size increased to 134 μm, the irregular RPE band appeared. It is also notable that a gradually loss of RPE integrity was correlated with the increased size of adjacent drusen. When the mean druse size reached 196 μm, up to one-third of the overlying RPE signal was missing. In this study, although the sample size of drusen with a discontinuous ellipsoid zone (EZ) was too small for statistical analysis, there was a trend with disrupted EZ more often with larger drusen. These data support the guideline of druse-size dependent AMD classification because the size of drusen can determine the degree of photoreceptor-RPE integrity.[20] In addition to the drusen size, the location of drusen related to cellular structures of RPE is illustrated in Fig. 4.2. The druse location can be precisely identified by histological and ultrastructural studies. The clinical characteristics of drusen and pigmentary

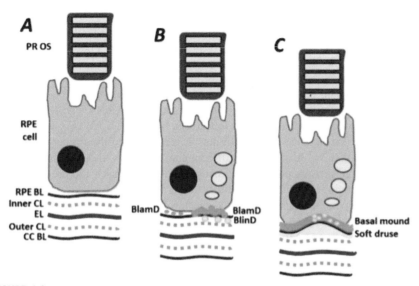

FIGURE 4.2

Development of subclinical deposits and soft drusen. In this cartoon, the healthy configuration is shown on the left. With aging (middle diagram), basal laminar deposits accumulate (internal to the RPE basement membrane) and vacuoles appear within RPE cells; early basal linear deposits (external to the RPE basement membrane) may also develop. The right-hand side shows more extensive BlinD coalescing to form soft drusen. (PR OS, photoreceptor outer segment; RPE, retinal pigment epithelium; BL, basal lamina that is, basement membrane of RPE; CL, collagenous layer; EL, elastic layer; CC, choriocapillaris; BlamD, basal laminar deposit; BlinD, basal linear deposit).

Modified from Khan KN, Mahroo OA, Khan RS, et al. Differentiating drusen: drusen and drusen-like appearances associated with ageing, age-related macular degeneration, inherited eye disease and other pathological processes. Prog Retin Eye Res. 2016;53:70–106. https://doi.org/10.1016/j.preteyeres.2016.04.008.

changes are identifiable signs correlating with the evolution of subretinal deposits and RPE function. Histologically, the drusen with trichrome present collagen-like materials, while with periodic acid Schiff stain they appear to be glycoproteins. Ultrastructurally, these small deposits between the plasma membrane and RPE basement membrane (basal lamina) are named basal laminar deposits (BlamD). Whereas, the materials as membranous collections visualized by electron microscopy between the basement membrane and the inner collagenous layer of Bruch's membrane are termed as basal linear deposits (BLinD) (Fig. 4.2B). Based on a histological study with postmortem eyes, Sarks et al. found that a continuous layer of early BlamD precedes the first appearance of BLinD.[21] They incisively pointed out that the presence of both BLinD and early BlamD represents the threshold of early AMD. At this point, the fundus is still normal. Because AMD progression depends on the degree of membranous debris accumulation, the large membranous deposit manifests as intermediate or large drusen clinically. When late BlamD appears, it heralds severe RPE damage and corresponds to clinical pigmentary changes. Whereas, if the membranous deposit process is limited to BLinD and basal mounds that are focal membranous accumulations internal to the basement membrane,[17] the fundus may remain normal or present as pigmentary change alone, because RPE integrity may be still intact. On the other hand, the progressively thickening of BLinD may lead to clinically visible soft drusen (Fig. 4.2C).[22] While, membranous debris production in some eyes could not progress beyond the formation of basal mounds (Fig. 4.2C).[21] In summary, different characteristics of drusen including intermediate/large drusen, pigmentary changes, and soft drusen represent membranous accumulation at different cellular structures of RPE and indication of disease progression. Epidemiologic studies showed that a large amount of membranous debris, in the appearance of large drusen and soft drusen are at the highest risk of developing late AMD over a 5- or 10-year period. If the clinical sign is pigmentary changes alone, the lower rate of late AMD development was observed over the same period.[23,24] The latter suggests that the membranous deposit process is limited to the formation of BLinD and basal mounds.

Drusen can be further defined by their boundaries including hard drusen with distinct demarcation, soft drusen with poor demarcation, and confluent drusen without clear boundaries (Fig. 4.3). Hard drusen are discrete and well-defined focal areas containing hyalinization of the RPE-Bruch's membrane complex. Soft drusen share the same materials with BLinD, but BLinD is diffusely distributed. Soft drusen can coalesce to form confluent drusen. Both soft and confluent drusen are associated with a high risk of late AMD development.[22]

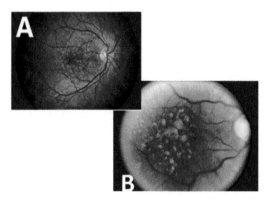

FIGURE 4.3

Fundus photograph of eyes with nonexudative AMD showing (A) numerous hard drusen and (B) soft and confluent drusen.

Modified from Abdelsalam A, Del Priore L, Zarbin MA. Drusen in age-related macular degeneration: pathogenesis, natural course, and laser photocoagulation-induced regression. Surv Ophthalmol. 1999;44(1):1–29. https://doi.org/10.1016/s0039-6257(99)00072-7.

Drusenoid pigment epithelial detachment

Clinically observed soft drusen represent the progressive process of membranous deposit, because soft drusen composition resembles both plasma lipoproteins and outer segment.[25,26] Histologically soft drusen is the same as BLinD (Fig. 4.4).

The progressive BLinD forming thickened inner portion of Bruch's membrane with overlying RPE can separate from the rest of Bruch's membrane, resulting in pigment epithelial detachment (PED). This pathological splitting between the inner layer and the rest layers of Bruch's membrane demonstrated by OCT and histologic study is named as drusenoid PED (Fig. 4.5).[27] Drusenoid PED can be seen in both nonexudative and neovascular AMD.

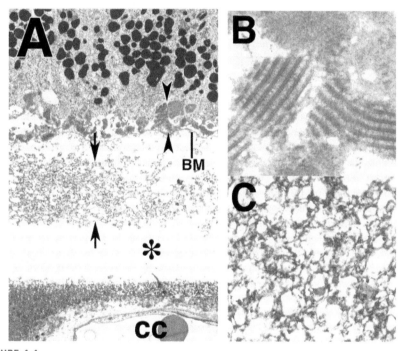

FIGURE 4.4

(A) Soft drusen from basal linear deposit (BlinD between arrows and in C with higher power view) located between the RPE basement membrane (BM) and the inner aspect of Bruch's membrane. A thin layer of basal laminar deposit (BlamD between arrowheads and in B) is present between the RPE and the RPE basement membrane. The detachment of BlinD (asterisk) is probably an artifact (cc is choriocapillaris) (original magnification, 2,8003). (B) Higher-power view of BlamD with wide-spaced collagen that has a periodicity of 100 nm (original magnification, 40,0003). (C) Higher-power view of BlinD with granular and vesicular material (original magnification, 19,0003).[22]

Modified from Abdelsalam A, Del Priore L, Zarbin MA. Drusen in age-related macular degeneration: pathogenesis, natural course, and laser photocoagulation-induced regression. Surv Ophthalmol. 1999;44(1):1–29.
https://doi.org/10.1016/s0039-6257(99)00072-7.

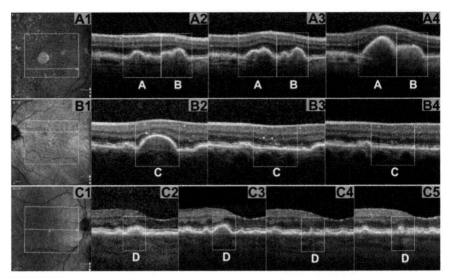

FIGURE 4.5

Change of maximum height (MaxH) of drusenoid PED lesion (DL) viewed by SD-OCT. A, Example of MaxH increase. A1, Infrared image showing B-scan location on the fundus at baseline. A2–A4, OCT B-scans where MaxH of DL (A) and DL (B) was located. A2, MaxH for DL of 96 (A) and 93 μm (B) at baseline. A3, MaxH for DL of 119 (A) and 81 μm (B) at 6 months after baseline. A4, MaxH for DL of 303 (A) and 132 μm (B) 27 months after baseline. B, Example of MaxH decrease. B1, Infrared image showing B-scan location on the fundus at baseline. B2–B4, OCT B-scans where the MaxH (C) is located. B2, MaxH for DL of 197 μm (C) at baseline. B3, MaxH for DL (C) decreased to 0 μm 10 months after baseline. B4, MaxH for DL (C) remained at 0 μm 15 months after baseline. C, Example of MaxH fluctuated. C1, Infrared image showing B-scan location on the fundus at baseline. C2–C4, OCT B-scans where MaxH of DL (D) is located. C2, MaxH for DL of 76 μm (C) baseline. C3, MaxH for DL of 115 μm (C) 10 months after baseline. C4, MaxH for DL of 68 μm (C) 18 months after baseline. B5, MaxH for DL of 87 μm (C) 44 months after baseline.

Modified from Ouyang Y, Heussen FM, Hariri A, Keane PA, Sadda SR. Optical coherence tomography–based observation of the natural history of drusenoid lesion in eyes with dry age-related macular degeneration. Ophthalmology. *2013;120(12):2656–2665. https://doi.org/10.1016/j.ophtha.2013.05.029.*

Curcio raised a very important question that whether soft drusen has position predilection for macula.[19] Sarks et al. observed that soft drusen of elderly patients are located within or just beyond the inner macula (within 3-mm diameter area).[28] In a histology study of postmortem eyes with nonexudative AMD, BLinD is more abundant than subretinal drusenoid deposits under the fovea.[29] Based on the pathology data of 760 eyes with AMD from 450 patients, both BlamD and BLinD at macula are positively associated with choroidal neovascularization.[30] Although the underlying mechanisms of soft drusen's predilection for macula is currently unknown, longitudinal observation of BLinD/soft drusen at macula is critical for disclose of AMD progression.

Clinical characteristics of drusen by multimodal imaging techniques

In recent years, multimodal imaging techniques in addition to color fundus photograms have been used in the clinic for the identification of drusen and other retinal deposits. These techniques include near-infrared reflectance (NIR), fundus autofluorescence (FAF), fluorescein angiography (FA), indocyanine green angiography (ICG), and OCT.[31] The distinct features of drusen by using each technique not only facilitate the detection of drusen but also gain an insight into the mechanisms of drusen formation. Hard drusen appear as discrete yellow-white mound-like elevation with a clear border on color fundus photography. The size of hard drusen could be ranging from small to large in diameter (Figs. 4.3A and 4.6C). In contrast, soft drusen are generally larger than hard drusen, have an ill-defined border with the tendency of confluence (Figs. 4.3B and 4.6E). Under FAF examination, drusen show hyper-autofluorescence, likely due to the accumulation of lipofuscin in the overlying

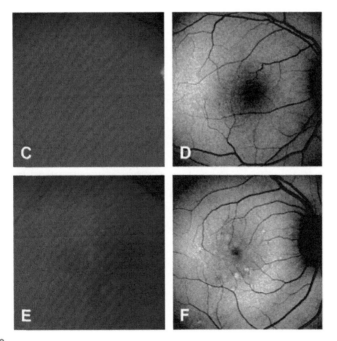

FIGURE 4.6

Hard drusen (in fundus photo, C) show minimal increase in autofluorescent intensity in FAF (D). Large and confluent drusen (in fundus photo, E) present hyper-autofluorescence in FAF (F).

Modified from Schmitz-Valckenberg S, Fleckenstein M, Scholl HPN, Holz FG. Fundus autofluorescence and progression of age-related macular degeneration. Surv Ophthalmol. *2009;54(1):96–117.*
https://doi.org/10.1016/j.survophthal.2008.10.004.

RPE layer (Fig. 4.6D and F). However, Schmitz-Valckenberg et al. pointed out that alterations of the FAF signal are not necessarily associated with corresponding fundus photo or angiographic drusen. It suggests that FAF findings represent an independent measure of disease stage and activity.[32]

Histologically, hard drusen, both at central and peripheral location, are associated with atrophy or loss of overlying RPE. Although hard drusen appearance on FA can vary, typically hard drusen show hyperfluorescence in the early phase. Afterward, there are no significant changes of fluorescent intensity through the early to late phase, likely due to a phenomenon of window defect on FA (Fig. 4.7).[31] The window defect is caused by overlying RPE atrophy or RPE loss.

The appearance of soft and confluent drusen and drusenoid PED shows slow and homogenous staining and pooling of the fluorescein dye in the sub-RPE space at the late phase (Fig. 4.8). On color fundus photograms, soft drusen are deposits under the retina with ill-defined border, often larger than 63 μm and confluent (Fig. 4.8). FA imaging reveals fluorescein staining of soft drusen. The composition of soft drusen is the same as BLinD that is rich in membrane deposits.[33]

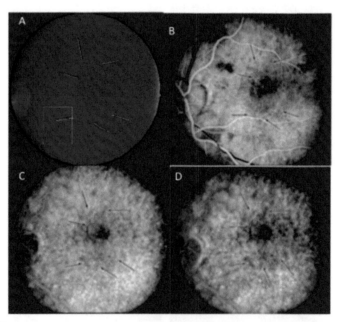

FIGURE 4.7

Representative color photograph (upper left) and fundus fluorescein angiogram images with hard drusen ranging from small to large size. No significant differences are noted in hyperfluorescent lesion size between arteriovenous (upper right), late venous (lower left), and washout phases (lower right).

Modified from Russell SR, Gupta RR, Folk JC, Mullins RF, Hageman GS. Comparison of color to fluorescein angiographic images from patients with early-adult onset grouped drusen suggests drusen substructure. Am J Ophthalmol. 2004;137(5):924–930. https://doi.org/10.1016/j.ajo.2003.12.043.

Color Fundus Photo   **Fluorescein Angiography**

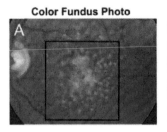 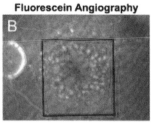

FIGURE 4.8

Large and confluent soft drusen of a 77-year-old man. A, Color fundus photograph. B, Late-phase fluorescein angiogram showing a staining of drusen.

Modified from Sikorski BL, Bukowska D, Kaluzny JJ, Szkulmowski M, Kowalczyk A, Wojtkowski M. Drusen with accompanying fluid underneath the sensory retina. Ophthalmology. 2011;118(1):82–92. https://doi.org/10.1016/j.ophtha.2010.04.017.

Currently, SD-OCT can precisely characterize the structure of drusen, which is superior to traditional imaging modalities such as color fundus photo and FA. By using SD-OCT, the shape of RPE elevation, internal reflectivity between RPE and choroid, homogeneity of reflectivity of dursen, and presence or absence of foci of hyper-reflectivity of drusen were analyzed.[34] These characterizations by OCT may be exemplified by the following Fig. 4.9B: druse 1, concave shape; drusen 2,

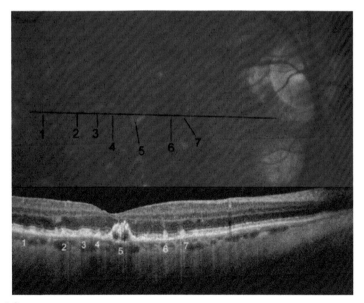

FIGURE 4.9

(Top) Seven drusen through a line on color photo to correlate with tomographic appearance. (Bottom) Drusen numbered in the color photo corresponding the numbers in a superimposed SD-OCT B-scan through fovea.

Modified from Khanifar AA, Koreishi AF, Izatt JA, Toth CA. Drusen ultrastructure imaging with spectral domain optical coherence tomography in age-related macular degeneration. Ophthalmology. 2008;115(11): 1883–1890. https://doi.org/10.1016/j.ophtha.2008.04.041.

3, 4, convex shape; drusen 6 and 7, saw-toothed shape; drusen 1, 2, 3, 4, 6 and 7, medium reflectivity; druse 5, high reflectivity; drusen 1 to 7 except for 5, homogenous internal reflectivity; druse 5, nonhomogenous internal reflectivity; focus of hyperreflectivity of druse 5, suggesting a calcific druse.[34,35]

Cuticular drusen

In addition to hard and soft drusen, there is another type of drusen named cuticular drusen (CD). CD were represented as numerous, small (25–75 μm), dot-like drusen that occur both in macula and periphery.[17] CD were characterized by a distinct "starry sky" appearance on FA (Fig. 4.10B). Previously CD were named as basal laminar drusen, which was believed to be a misnomer, because histologically CD were cellular aggregations located between the basal lamina of the RPE, and the inner collagenous layer of Bruch's membrane (Fig. 4.2).[36] Therefore, Russell et al. named this kind of deposits as "early adult onset, grouped drusen."[36] On color fundus photos, the small individual CD can be mistaken for hard drusen, but they could be distinguished from hard drusen with numerous cluster appearance (Fig. 4.10A). CD can also be mistaken for soft drusen when they coalesce. As a result color fundus photography is not sufficiently sensitive for CD detection. Small CD appear discrete hypoautofluorescent dots, while larger CD show

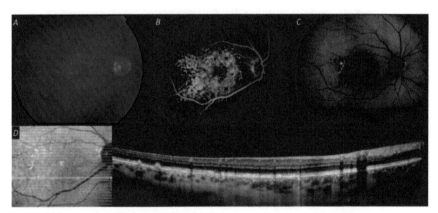

FIGURE 4.10

Images from the right eye of a 47-year-old man with cuticular drusen. A, Color fundus photograph showing drusen and pigmentary change. B, Fluorescein angiogram (at 27 s after dye injection) showing the characteristic "starry sky" appearance. C, Short-wavelength AF showing a mixture of hypo and hyper-autofluorescence. D, Horizontal enhanced depth OCT scan with corresponding infrared reflectance image.

Modified from Khan KN, Mahroo OA, Khan RS, et al. Differentiating drusen: drusen and drusen-like appearances associated with ageing, age-related macular degeneration, inherited eye disease and other pathological processes. Prog Retin Eye Res. 2016;53:70–106. https://doi.org/10.1016/j.preteyeres.2016.04.008.

hyperautofluorescence, depending on the status of RPE disturbance (Fig. 4.10C).[37] When CD are large, NIR and red-free photos may be useful for detection because these techniques increase the contrast with RPE (Fig. 4.10D). CD have a prolate shape and moderate hyperrefractivity on OCT. Larger CD seem to erode into RPE layer, resulting in a thin covering of RPE at the apex of a curricular druse (Fig. 4.10D).

In a recent study, a consecutive series of patients with CD were followed for the development of geographic atrophy (GA) and choroidal neovascularization (CNV) longitudinally. GA developed in 19.0% of eyes and CNV in 4.8% of eyes. The cumulative estimated 5-year incidence developing GA and CNV was 28.4% and 8.7%, respectively.[38] The risk of late AMD in patients with CD suggests CD are part of the overall clinical spectrum of AMD.

Reticular pseudodrusen/subretinal drusenoid deposits

In Chapter 2, reticular pseudodrusen (RPD), that is, subretinal drusenoid deposits (SDDs) were introduced. SDD/RPD have drawn great attention because they are an independent risk factor for AMD. SDD/RPD have different histologic location and composition from conventional drusen. SDD/RPDs present the subretinal location and the penetration of deposits through the outer limiting membrane into the outer nuclear layer. The penetration of SDD/RPD materials is the morphologic evidence of visual disturbance of involved individuals. SDD/RPDs are rich in photoreceptor outer segment proteins and immune cells. In contrast to conventional drusen, SDD/RPDs are due to a lack of lipid composition.[39] Clinical detection of SDD/RPD is dependent on multimodal imaging. Based on NIR, FAF, and color fundus examinations, there are three subtypes of SDD/RPD including dot and ribbon subtypes. By NIR examination, dot SDD/RPDs, the most common subtype, appear hyporeflective, or hyperreflective center surrounded by a hyporeflective annulus, thus called a target appearance (see Fig. 2.4 of Chapter 2). OCT demonstrates subretinal deposits forming sharp peaks pointing the photoreceptor bands (see Fig. 2.5 of Chapter 2). Ribbon SDD/RPD, that is, the original descriptions of reticular pseudodrusen, appear broad interlacing ribbons in the color fundus. OCT shows subretinal materials forming broad rounded elevation (Fig. 4.11).[40]

Drusen and SDD/RPD characterization by multimodal imaging techniques are summarized in Table 4.1.

Nonexudative AMD

AMD is divided into two main types as dry (nonexudative) and wet (neovascular) AMD. Dry AMD is the most common form, comprising around 90% of diagnosed disease cases. GA is the advanced stage of dry AMD. The clinical classification and

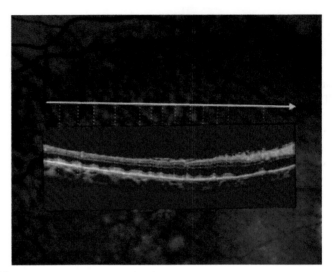

FIGURE 4.11

Ribbon pseudodrusen detected by color fundus photo and OCT. The color photograph shows the superior macula of an 83-year-old patient with ribbon pseudodrusen. Inset: An OCT scan taken at the position of the green arrow shows subretinal drusenoid deposits corresponding to ribbon pseudodrusen. Subretinal accumulation of material forms broad, rounded elevations.

Modified from Spaide RF, Ooto S, Curcio CA. Subretinal drusenoid deposits AKA pseudodrusen. Surv Oph-thalmol. 2018;63(6):782–815. https://doi.org/10.1016/j.survophthal.2018.05.005.

severity scale were described in Table 2.1 of Chapter 2 and Table 3.1 of Chapter 3; in short, drusen, pigmentary changes and GA are critical signs of nonexudative AMD. Dry AMD is a chronic disorder. The clinical signs approximately follow chronological sequence. First, intermediate to large soft drusen may become confluent (Fig. 4.12A).[41] Hyper-pigmentary or hypo-pigmentary foci appear at the posterior pole. Then, a sharply circumscribed area of RPE atrophy along with variable loss of choriocapillaris follows. Gradually enlarged RPE atrophic areas and more exposed larger choroidal vessels become evident. At this point, geographic atrophy may be diagnosed (Fig. 4.12B).[41] GA is gradually encroaching to fovea. The vision impairment of GA patients depends on whether the fovea is involved. The evolution of preexisting drusen consists of regression of preexisting drusen and development of drusenoid PED (Fig. 4.13).[42] The possible mechanism for spontaneous drusen regression involves RPE atrophy.[19] In the OCT era the signs of atrophy of outer retina in dry AMD can be more accurately defined, which will be further discussed in AMD diagnosis sections in Chapter 5.

The symptoms of dry AMD patients could range from asymptomatic to severe vision impairment. The gradually impaired vision undergoes over months and years. Vision impairment is usually bilateral, but often asymmetrical. Vision may fluctuate with better vision in bright light.

Table 4.1 Drusen and pseudodrusen characterization with multimodal imaging techniques.

	Color fundus photo	NIR	FAF	FA	ICG	SD-OCT	Histologic location
Hard drusen	Yellow-white mound-like elevations, clear border, small to large size	NS	HyperAF	Window defect	NS	Dome-shaped elevation	BlamD
Soft drusen	Ill-defined border, larger than 63 μm or confluent	NS	HyperAF	Staining, pooling	Staining	Dome-shaped PED	BlinD
Cuticular drusen	Numerous small dot-like	Visible due to increased contrast	Small hypoAF large hyperAF	Starry sky	Early hyperfluo	Prolate, thin RPE cover	BlamD and inner BM
SDD/ RPDs	Bluish-white deposits, delineated dots, or confluent dots	Hyporeflective dots, target configuration	Common hypoAF few hyperAF	Early defects in CC filling	Hypofluo mid/late	Subretinal	SDD
	Interlocking ribbon/reticular	Faint hyporeflective ribbon	Ill-defined hypoAF	Early defects in CC filling	Hypofluo mid/late		SDD

Abbreviations: BlamD, *basal laminar deposits;* BLinD, *basal linear deposits;* BM, *Bruch's membrane;* CC, *choriocapillaris;* FA, *fluorescein angiography;* FAF, *fundus autofluorescence;* hyperAF, *hyperautofluorescence;* hypoAF, *hypoautofluorescence;* hyperfluo, *hyperfluorescence;* hypofluo, *hypofluorescence;* NIR, *near-infrared reflectance;* NS, *not specific;* RPD, *reticular pseudodrusen;* SDD, *subretinal drusenoid deposits;* SD-OCT, *spectral-domain optic coherence tomography.*

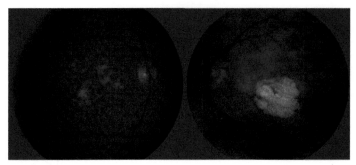

FIGURE 4.12

Evolving nonexudative AMD followed chronologic order. (Left) intermediate to large soft drusen became confluent. (Right) Geographic atrophy encroached fovea of left eye.

Modified from Mehta S. Age-related macular degeneration. Prim Care. *2015;42(3):377–391.*

https://doi.org/10.1016/j.pop.2015.05.009.

Neovascular AMD

Wet (neovascular) AMD is less common than dry AMD, but is associated with rapid vision loss. The main manifestations are CNV and CNV-associated PED, intra and subretinal fluid. Based on recent literature, retinal angiomatous proliferation (RAP) and polypoidal choroidal vasculopathy are considered as subtypes of wet AMD.[43] CNV is caused by various etiologies. Herein, the discussion is only limited to CVN arising de novo as the primary lesion of wet AMD.

The signs of CNV, based on color fundus examination, may be identifiable as a grey-green or pinkish-yellow lesion. In some cases, the lesion is slightly elevated in contrast to the lesion of dry AMD. In the CNV eye or fellow eye, coexisting medium to large size drusen are typical sign of wet AMD. If no druse is found in either eye, the etiology of CVN needs to be questioned (see the differential diagnosis of CNV in Chapter 6). Localized intraretinal and subretinal fluid at macula are common signs of active CNV, which may be associated with cystoid macular edema. In some cases, because of a large amount of intra- and subretinal lipid, extensive exudate is obvious. Various types of hemorrhage are common, including subretinal, intraretinal, sub-RPE, preretinal/retrohyaloid, vitreous hemorrhage. It seems that the size and location in the proximity of macula of subretinal hemorrhage (SRH) are determinative factors for visual outcome. A small amount of SRH can be cleaned with minimal damage. Large SRH may cause damage to the retina because of iron toxicity on the photoreceptors and RPE, inflammation induced by mononuclear/macrophage migration, macular atrophy (Fig. 4.14 BL19.6 & M65) and fibrovascular scar formation, etc.[44] Therefore, the absorption process of hemorrhage due to CNV needs to be monitored closely.

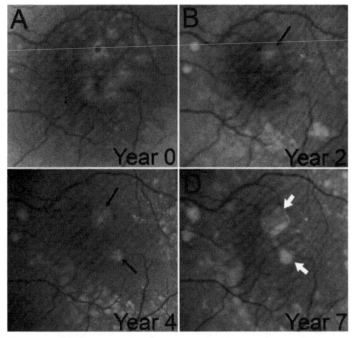

FIGURE 4.13

Fundus changes occurring in the left eye of a 73-year-old man with a drusenoid PED (DPED) that progressed to GA during the course of the study. A, Fundus at year 0: Centrally located DPED is present with hyperpigmentary changes. B, at year 2, most of the DPED has disappeared and a new area of hypopigmentation has emerged (black arrow). C, at year 4, an additional area of hypopigmentation has arisen (black arrows). In the meantime, several preexisting drusen disappeared and the hyperpigmentary changes seen earlier have decreased. D, at year 7, areas of GA have emerged from earlier patches of hypopigmentation that have enlarged and coalesced. GA, geographic atrophy; DPED, drusenoid pigment epithelial detachment.

Modified from Cukras C, Agrón E, Klein ML, et al. Natural history of drusenoid pigment epithelial detachment in age-related macular degeneration: age-related eye disease study report no. 28. Ophthalmology. 2010;117(3): 489–499. https://doi.org/10.1016/j.ophtha.2009.12.002.

PED is a frequent finding associated with AMD. The subtypes of PED consisting of drusenoid, serous, hemorrhagic, and fibrovascular are found in the context with or without CNV of AMD patients. Retinal and subretinal "disciform" scar can be seen as a sequelae of involuted wet AMD (Fig. 4.14 BL8.1 & M7).

The symptoms of wet AMD consist of acute or subacute painless vision loss. Intraocular hemorrhage may cause positive central scotoma. The patients of wet AMD also often complain metamorphopsia, a type of distorted vision.[44,45]

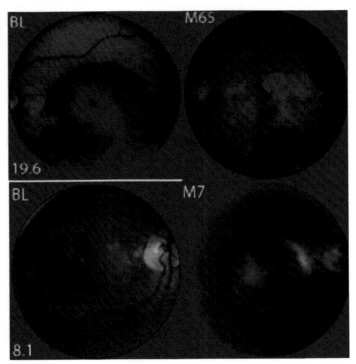

FIGURE 4.14

CNV in neovascular AMD. Patient A (Top) presenting large preretinal and subretinal hemorrhage at posterior pole (photo BL 19.6); After absorption of blood, in addition to residual blood and pigmentary changes, a larger macular atrophy is present (M65); Patient B (Bottom) showing the evolution of CNV after subretinal hemorrhage (BL 8.1), resulting fibrotic scar (M7).

Modified from Kherani S, Scott AW, Wenick AS, et al. Shortest distance from fovea to subfoveal hemorrhage border is important in patients with neovascular age-related macular degeneration. Am J Ophthalmol. 2018; 189:86–95. https://doi.org/10.1016/j.ajo.2018.02.015.

Retinal pigment epithelial detachment associated with and without CNV

PED, a separation between RPE with the inner collagenous layer of Bruch's membrane and the rest of Bruch's membrane, is caused by disruption of the physiological forces maintaining this adhesion.[46] The etiologies of this disruption are various including (1) degenerative process in Bruch's membrane during appearance of drusenoid formation, (2) serous fluid accumulation, (3) hemorrhage due to CNV beneath RPE, and (4) fibrovascular membrane growth.

Drusenoid PED described above (Fig. 4.13) can be a Bruch's membrane splitting between the inner layer and the rest of the layers. The clinical sign is dynamic changes of confluent soft drusen and drusenoid formation without evidence of CNV.

Serous PED is typically seen in central serous chorioretinopathy (CSC) (Fig. 4.15). CSC belongs to a spectrum of pachychoroidal disorders associated with

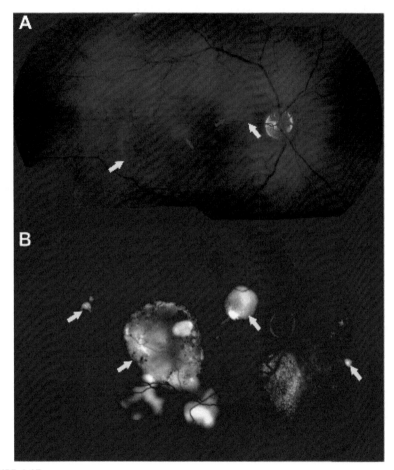

FIGURE 4.15

Multiple serous PED associated with central serous chorioretinopathy, a PED with non-CNV etiology. A, multiple serous PEDs with a pale border of subretinal fluid (*yellow arrows*) and dome-shaped elevation with turbid subretinal fluid (*red arrows*). B, Fluorescein angiography images revealed focal areas of hyper-fluorescence (blowouts) within PEDs (*red arrows*). The size of PEDs ranged from 0.2 to 3 disc diameters, and there was leakage evident from a large PED adjacent to the inferior vascular arcade.

Modified from Balaratnasingam C, Freund KB, Tan AM, et al. Bullous variant of central serous chorioretinopathy: expansion of phenotypic features using multimethod imaging. Ophthalmology. 2016;123(7):1541–1552. https://doi.org/10.1016/j.ophtha.2016.03.017.

or without CNV.[47] By the similar mechanisms of CSC,[48] a purely exudative accumulation of fluid between Bruch membrane and RPE, that is, serous PED is a clinical sign of wet AMD. Hemorrhagic PED is caused by bleeding beneath the RPE in wet AMD. A retrospective cohort study showed the visual outcome of hemorrhagic PED is poorer among different subtypes of PED.[49] Fibrovascular membrane complex, occult CNV that occupies the space beneath the RPE, and the development of this complex causing hemorrhage and serous fluid together contribute to PED formation.

In Fig. 4.16 serous PED appears as an orange dome-shaped elevation, often with a pale border of subretinal fluid. Association of pigmentary changes indicate chronicity. The coexistence of blood, lipid exudate, chorioretinal folds, fibrosis and irregular subretinal fluid indicate underlying CNV (Fig. 4.16). The symptoms include blurred vision and metamorphopsia.[50]

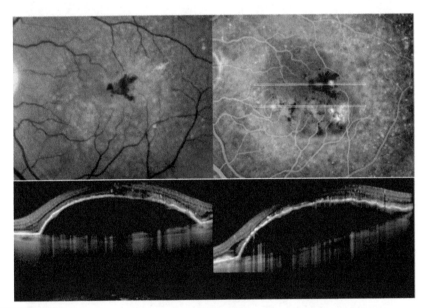

FIGURE 4.16

Hemorrhagic PED associated with intra- and subretinal hemorrhage (Top left). During early fluorescein angiography (FA), the PED showed generalized decreased fluorescence with two areas, indicating fluorescence blockage. Later in the FA, there was a generalized increase in fluorescence within the PED, indicating pooling (Top right). The two lines correspond to sections examined with the EDI OCT (Bottom left and right). At the margin of PED, small amount of intra- and subretinal hemorrhage were shown (Bottom left and right).

Modified from Spaide RF. Enhanced depth imaging optical coherence tomography of retinal pigment epithelial detachment in age-related macular degeneration. Am J Ophthalmol. 2009;147(4):644–652. https://doi.org/ 10.1016/j.ajo.2008.10.005.

Retinal pigment epithelial tear

An RPE tear generally occurs at the junction of the attached and detached PPE layer. RPE tear is a complication of PED and a clinical sign associated with wet AMD. The most common cause is a vascularized PED in patients with neovascular AMD. Although RPE tears can develop spontaneously in vascularized PEDs, most recent cases have been associated with anti-VEGF injections.[51] The cumulated fluid within the PED creates hydrostatic pressure to the RPE and stretches it. When the hydrostatic pressure increases the PED increases as well. Contraction of the CNV beneath RPE applies tractional forces to RPE in the context of enlarged PED. After anti-VEGF therapy owing to increasing contraction of the choroidal neovascular membrane, the tractional force to RPE is further aggravated. Thus, it tears already strained RPE layer under PED.

RPE tear is best seen by multimodal imaging such as color fundus photo, FA and OCT (Fig. 4.17, upper three showing pretear and bottom three showing posttear). The sign of RPE tear consists of a crescent-shaped pale area of RPE dehiscence, which is next to a darker area corresponding to the retracted and folded RPE flap (Fig. 4.17 lower middle two). Posttear OCT is shown in Fig. 4.17 bottom OCT.[51] When fovea is involved, the primary symptom of RPE tear is a sudden loss of vision followed by a long-term visual impairment.

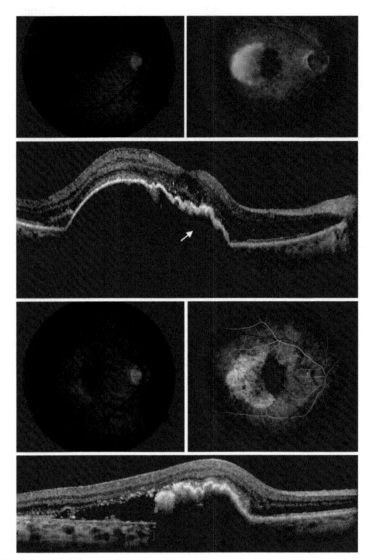

FIGURE 4.17

Color fundus photography, fluorescein angiography, and optical coherence tomography (OCT) illustrating retinal pigment epithelium (RPE) tear formation after intravitreal bevacizumab injection for neovascular age-related macular degeneration. (Top) Baseline color fundus photograph (top left) and late fluorescein angiogram (top right) of the right eye showing a vascularized pigment epithelial detachment (PED). (Image at the second row) Pretear OCT shows hyperreflective material consistent with choroidal neovascularization (CNV) adherent to the undersurface of the PED and associated with severe contractile folds in the RPE (*arrow*). Subretinal fluid can be seen over the opposite edge of the PED, adjacent to a segment of bare RPE. (Images at the third row) Color fundus photograph (left image) and fluorescein angiogram (right image) after 1 bevacizumab injection illustrate an RPE tear. (Bottom) Posttear OCT demonstrates persistent adherence of the CNV to the retracted and folded RPE.

Modified from Nagiel A, Freund KB, Spaide RF, Munch IC, Larsen M, Sarraf D. Mechanism of retinal pigment epithelium tear formation following intravitreal anti-vascular endothelial growth factor therapy revealed by spectral-domain optical coherence tomography. Am J Ophthalmol. 2013;156(5):981–988.e2. https://doi.org/10.1016/j.ajo.2013.06.024.

References

1. Ko TH, Fujimoto JG, Schuman JS, Paunescu LA, Kowalevicz AM, Hartl I, Drexler W, Wollstein G, Ishikawa H, Duker JS. Comparison of ultrahigh- and standard-resolution optical coherence tomography for imaging macular pathology. *Ophthalmology.* 2005; 112(11):1922.e1−15. https://doi.org/10.1016/j.ophtha.2005.05.027

2. Gao H, Hollyfield JG. Aging of the human retina. Differential loss of neurons and retinal pigment epithelial cells. *Invest Ophthalmol Vis Sci.* 1992;33(1):1−17.

3. Curcio CA, Millican CL, Allen KA, Kalina RE. Aging of the human photoreceptor mosaic: evidence for selective vulnerability of rods in central retina. *Invest Ophthalmol Vis Sci.* 1993;34(12):3278−3296.

4. Nivison-Smith L, Wang H, Assaad N, Kalloniatis M. Retinal thickness changes throughout the natural history of drusen in age-related macular degeneration. *Optom Vis Sci.* 2018;95(8):648−655. https://doi.org/10.1097/OPX.0000000000001256.

5. Curcio CA, Messinger JD, Sloan KR, Mitra A, McGwin G, Spaide RF. Human chorioretinal layer thicknesses measured in macula-wide, high-resolution histologic sections. *Invest Ophthalmol Vis Sci.* 2011;52(7):3943−3954. https://doi.org/10.1167/iovs.10-6377.

6. Loduca AL, Zhang C, Zelkha R, Shahidi M. Thickness mapping of retinal layers by spectral-domain optical coherence tomography. *Am J Ophthalmol.* 2010;150(6): 849−855. https://doi.org/10.1016/j.ajo.2010.06.034.

7. Trinh M, Tong J, Yoshioka N, Zangerl B, Kalloniatis M, Nivison-Smith L. Macula ganglion cell thickness changes display location-specific variation patterns in intermediate age-related macular degeneration. *Invest Ophthalmol Vis Sci.* 2020;61(3):2. https://doi.org/10.1167/iovs.61.3.2.

8. Doustar J, Torbati T, Black KL, Koronyo Y, Koronyo-Hamaoui M. Optical coherence tomography in Alzheimer's disease and other neurodegenerative diseases. *Front Neurol.* 2017;8:701. https://doi.org/10.3389/fneur.2017.00701.

9. Koronyo Y, Biggs D, Barron E, et al. Retinal amyloid pathology and proof-of-concept imaging trial in Alzheimer's disease. *JCI Insight.* 2017;2(16). https://doi.org/10.1172/jci.insight.93621.

10. Garcia-Martin E, Bambo MP, Marques ML, et al. Ganglion cell layer measurements correlate with disease severity in patients with Alzheimer's disease. *Acta Ophthalmol.* 2016;94(6):e454−459. https://doi.org/10.1111/aos.12977.

11. Ehrlich R, Harris A, Kheradiya NS, Winston DM, Ciulla TA, Wirostko B. Age-related macular degeneration and the aging eye. *Clin Interv Aging.* 2008;3(3):473−482. https://doi.org/10.2147/cia.s2777.

12. Lipecz A, Miller L, Kovacs I, et al. Microvascular contributions to age-related macular degeneration (AMD): from mechanisms of choriocapillaris aging to novel interventions. *Geroscience.* 2019;41(6):813−845. https://doi.org/10.1007/s11357-019-00138-3.

13. Spaide RF, Fujimoto JG, Waheed NK, Sadda SR, Staurenghi G. Optical coherence tomography angiography. *Progress in Retinal and Eye Research.* 2018;64:1−55. https://doi.org/10.1016/j.preteyeres.2017.11.003.

14. Wakatsuki Y, Shinojima A, Kawamura A, Yuzawa M. Correlation of aging and segmental choroidal thickness measurement using swept source optical coherence tomography in healthy eyes. *PLoS One.* 2015;10(12):e0144156. https://doi.org/10.1371/journal.pone.0144156.

15. Chirco KR, Sohn EH, Stone EM, Tucker BA, Mullins RF. Structural and molecular changes in the aging choroid: implications for age-related macular degeneration. *Eye*. 2017;31(1):10−25. https://doi.org/10.1038/eye.2016.216.

16. Pettenkofer M, Scherm P, Feucht N, Wehrmann K, Lohmann CP, Maier M. Choriocapillaris flow density negatively correlates with advancing age on spectral-domain optical coherence tomography angiography. *Ophthalmic Surg Lasers Imag Retina*. 2019; 50(5):302−308. https://doi.org/10.3928/23258160-20190503-07.

17. Khan KN, Mahroo OA, Khan RS, et al. Differentiating drusen: drusen and drusen-like appearances associated with ageing, age-related macular degeneration, inherited eye disease and other pathological processes. *Prog Retin Eye Res*. 2016;53:70−106. https://doi.org/10.1016/j.preteyeres.2016.04.008.

18. Ferris FL, Wilkinson CP, Bird A, et al. Clinical classification of age-related macular degeneration. *Ophthalmology*. 2013;120(4):844−851. https://doi.org/10.1016/j.ophtha.2012.10.036.

19. Curcio CA. Antecedents of soft drusen, the specific deposits of age-related macular degeneration, in the biology of human macula. *Invest Ophthalmol Vis Sci*. 2018;59(4): AMD182−AMD194. https://doi.org/10.1167/iovs.18-24883.

20. Schlanitz F, Baumann B, Sacu S, et al. Impact of drusen and drusenoid retinal pigment epithelium elevation size and structure on the integrity of the retinal pigment epithelium layer. *Br J Ophthalmol*. 2019;103(2):227−232. https://doi.org/10.1136/bjophthalmol-2017-311782.

21. Sarks S, Cherepanoff S, Killingsworth M, Sarks J. Relationship of basal laminar deposit and membranous debris to the clinical presentation of early age-related macular degeneration. *Invest Ophthalmol Vis Sci*. 2007;48(3):968. https://doi.org/10.1167/iovs.06-0443.

22. Abdelsalam A, Del Priore L, Zarbin MA. Drusen in age-related macular degeneration: pathogenesis, natural course, and laser photocoagulation-induced regression. *Surv Ophthalmol*. 1999;44(1):1−29. https://doi.org/10.1016/s0039-6257(99)00072-7.

23. Wang JJ, Foran S, Smith W, Mitchell P. Risk of age-related macular degeneration in eyes with macular drusen or hyperpigmentation: the blue mountains eye study cohort. *Arch Ophthalmol*. 2003;121(5):658−663. https://doi.org/10.1001/archopht.121.5.658.

24. Ferris FL, Davis MD, Clemons TE, et al. A simplified severity scale for age-related macular degeneration: AREDS report no. 18. *Arch Ophthalmol*. 2005;123(11):1570−1574. https://doi.org/10.1001/archopht.123.11.1570.

25. Sarks JP, Sarks SH, Killingsworth MC. Evolution of geographic atrophy of the retinal pigment epithelium. *Eye*. 1988;2(Pt 5):552−577. https://doi.org/10.1038/eye.1988.106.

26. Sarks JP, Sarks SH, Killingsworth MC. Evolution of soft drusen in age-related macular degeneration. *Eye*. 1994;8(Pt 3):269−283. https://doi.org/10.1038/eye.1994.57.

27. Ouyang Y, Heussen FM, Hariri A, Keane PA, Sadda SR. Optical coherence tomography−based observation of the natural history of drusenoid lesion in eyes with dry age-related macular degeneration. *Ophthalmology*. 2013;120(12):2656−2665. https://doi.org/10.1016/j.ophtha.2013.05.029.

28. Sarks SH, Arnold JJ, Sarks JP, Gilles MC, Walter CJ. Prophylactic perifoveal laser treatment of soft drusen. *Aust N Z J Ophthalmol*. 1996;24(1):15−26. https://doi.org/10.1111/j.1442-9071.1996.tb01546.x.

29. Curcio CA, Messinger JD, Sloan KR, McGwin G, Medeiros NE, Spaide RF. Subretinal drusenoid deposits in non-neovascular age-related macular degeneration: morphology,

prevalence, topography, and biogenesis model. *Retina (Philadelphia, Pa)*. 2013;33(2): 265−276. https://doi.org/10.1097/IAE.0b013e31827e25e0.

30. Green WR, Enger C. Age-related macular degeneration histopathologic studies. The 1992 Lorenz E. Zimmerman lecture. *Ophthalmology*. 1993;100(10):1519−1535. https://doi.org/10.1016/s0161-6420(93)31466-1.

31. Russell SR, Gupta RR, Folk JC, Mullins RF, Hageman GS. Comparison of color to fluo-rescein angiographic images from patients with early-adult onset grouped drusen suggests drusen substructure. *Am J Ophthalmol*. 2004;137(5):924−930. https://doi.org/10.1016/j.ajo.2003.12.043.

32. Schmitz-Valckenberg S, Fleckenstein M, Scholl HPN, Holz FG. Fundus autofluores-cence and progression of age-related macular degeneration. *Surv Ophthalmol*. 2009; 54(1):96−117. https://doi.org/10.1016/j.survophthal.2008.10.004.

33. Sikorski BL, Bukowska D, Kaluzny JJ, Szkulmowski M, Kowalczyk A, Wojtkowski M. Drusen with accompanying fluid underneath the sensory retina. *Ophthalmology*. 2011; 118(1):82−92. https://doi.org/10.1016/j.ophtha.2010.04.017.

34. Khanifar AA, Koreishi AF, Izatt JA, Toth CA. Drusen ultrastructure imaging with spec-tral domain optical coherence tomography in age-related macular degeneration. *Ophthalmology*. 2008;115(11):1883−1890. https://doi.org/10.1016/j.ophtha.2008.04.041.

35. Leuschen JN, Schuman SG, Winter KP, et al. Spectral-domain optical coherence tomog-raphy characteristics of intermediate age-related macular degeneration. *Ophthalmology*. 2013;120(1):140−150. https://doi.org/10.1016/j.ophtha.2012.07.004.

36. Russell SR, Mullins RF, Schneider BL, Hageman GS. Location, substructure, and composition of basal laminar drusen compared with drusen associated with aging and age-related macular degeneration. *Am J Ophthalmol*. 2000;129(2):205−214. https://doi.org/10.1016/s0002-9394(99)00345-1.

37. Meyerle CB, Smith RT, Barbazetto IA, Yannuzzi LA. Autofluorescence of basal laminar drusen. *Retina (Philadelphia, Pa)*. 2007;27(8):1101−1106. https://doi.org/10.1097/IAE.0b013e3181451617.

38. Sakurada Y, Parikh R, Gal-Or O, et al. Cuticular drusen: risk of geographic atrophy and macular neovascularization. *Retina*. 2020;40(2):257−265. https://doi.org/10.1097/IAE.0000000000002399.

39. Greferath U, Guymer RH, Vessey KA, Brassington K, Fletcher EL. Correlation of histo-logic features with in vivo imaging of reticular pseudodrusen. *Ophthalmology*. 2016; 123(6):1320−1331. https://doi.org/10.1016/j.ophtha.2016.02.009.

40. Spaide RF, Ooto S, Curcio CA. Subretinal drusenoid deposits AKA pseudodrusen. *Surv Ophthalmol*. 2018;63(6):782−815. https://doi.org/10.1016/j.survophthal.2018.05.005.

41. Mehta S. Age-related macular degeneration. *Prim Care*. 2015;42(3):377−391. https://doi.org/10.1016/j.pop.2015.05.009.

42. Cukras C, Agrón E, Klein ML, et al. Natural history of drusenoid pigment epithelial detachment in age-related macular degeneration: age-related eye disease study report no. 28. *Ophthalmology*. 2010;117(3):489−499. https://doi.org/10.1016/j.ophtha.2009.12.002.

43. Cheung CMG, Lai TYY, Ruamviboonsuk P, et al. Polypoidal choroidal vasculopathy: definition, pathogenesis, diagnosis, and management. *Ophthalmology*. 2018;125(5): 708−724. https://doi.org/10.1016/j.ophtha.2017.11.019.

44. Kherani S, Scott AW, Wenick AS, et al. Shortest distance from fovea to subfoveal hem-orrhage border is important in patients with neovascular age-related macular

degeneration. *Am J Ophthalmol.* 2018;189:86—95. https://doi.org/10.1016/j.ajo.2018.02.015.

45. Kulkarni A, Kuppermann B. Wet age-related macular degeneration. *Adv Drug Deliv Rev.* 2005;57(14):1994—2009. https://doi.org/10.1016/j.addr.2005.09.003.

46. Balaratnasingam C, Freund KB, Tan AM, et al. Bullous variant of central serous chorioretinopathy: expansion of phenotypic features using multimethod imaging. *Ophthalmology.* 2016;123(7):1541—1552. https://doi.org/10.1016/j.ophtha.2016.03.017.

47. Marchese A, Arrigo A, Sacconi R, et al. Spectrum of choroidal neovascularisation associated with dome-shaped macula. *Br J Ophthalmol.* 2019;103(8):1146—1151. https://doi.org/10.1136/bjophthalmol-2018-312780.

48. Wasmuth S. Pathogenetische Konzepte zur Pigmentepithelabhebung bei exsudativer AMD. *Ophthalmologe.* 2010;107(12):1109—1114. https://doi.org/10.1007/s00347-010-2142-7.

49. Hartnett ME, Weiter JJ, Garsd A, Jalkh AE. Classification of retinal pigment epithelial detachments associated with drusen. *Graefes Arch Clin Exp Ophthalmol.* 1992;230(1):11—19. https://doi.org/10.1007/bf00166756.

50. Spaide RF. Enhanced depth imaging optical coherence tomography of retinal pigment epithelial detachment in age-related macular degeneration. *Am J Ophthalmol.* 2009;147(4):644—652. https://doi.org/10.1016/j.ajo.2008.10.005.

51. Nagiel A, Freund KB, Spaide RF, Munch IC, Larsen M, Sarraf D. Mechanism of retinal pigment epithelium tear formation following intravitreal anti-vascular endothelial growth factor therapy revealed by spectral-domain optical coherence tomography. *Am J Ophthalmol.* 2013;156(5):981—988.e2. https://doi.org/10.1016/j.ajo.2013.06.024.

Diagnosis of age-related macular degeneration

5

History and risk factors of AMD

Age-related macular degeneration (AMD) is a clinical diagnosis based on characteristic macular findings in individuals over 50 years old.[1] Age is one of the most important diagnostic criteria for AMD. The Beaver Dam Eye Study compared the 5-year incidence and progression of AMD in people aged 75 years or older to the group of people in 43–54 years. The incidence of developing large drusen (125–249 μm) was 8.3 times higher in the former group. The same trend was observed in other pathological changes in these two age groups as the following: larger drusen (>250 μm), 32 times; soft indistinct drusen, 9 times; pigmentary changes, 14.3 times higher, respectively.[2] Because of the much more increased incidences of macular degenerative lesions with age, the AMD-like signs in younger persons may prompt us for the workup of a differential diagnosis of AMD.

In addition to age, the history of other risk factors including ethnic specificity, smoking, hypertension, dietary factors, and aspirin is sensible to be considered in the diagnostic workup for AMD.[3,4] A recent meta-analyses and literature review on the global prevalence of AMD revealed that, among the population age ranging 45–85 years, the global prevalence of any type of AMD was approximately 8.7%. If AMD is categorized into early and late stages, the prevalence of early AMD was 8.0% and that of late AMD was 0.4%.[3] To analyze the impact of ethnic differences on the prevalence of AMD, it was noticed that early AMD was more common in individuals of European ancestry (8.8%) than in Asians (6.8%). Whereas the prevalence of the late stage of AMD did not differ significantly between Europeans (0.59%) and Asians (0.56%). Among individuals of African ancestry, the prevalence of any AMD was the lowest.[5] A recent study on AMD-associated visual impairment among Europeans, an encouraged report showed that the prevalence of blindness and visual impairment among European patients with AMD is on the decrease. It is likely to be contributed by improved diagnostic procedures, that is, earlier diagnosis of late AMD and the earlier introduction of anti-VEGF therapy.[4]

In some previous studies, it was believed that women are at increased risk of developing AMD, particularly those women who have a longer life span.[6] However, after age effects were excluded, the analysis of recent studies showed that sex was not markedly associated with the prevalence of AMD.[6] Numerous epidemiology

Age-Related Macular Degeneration. https://doi.org/10.1016/B978-0-12-822061-0.00012-8

studies addressed the relationship between cigarette smoking and AMD. There is reasonably consistent evidence that smoking cigarettes results in an increased risk of the disease. Based on the summary of these studies, the odds ratio was ~2.0, meaning that smoking roughly doubles the risk of AMD.[6] High dietary fat intake theoretically may increase the risk of developing AMD. The elevated levels of cholesterol due to high dietary fat may have an adverse impact on choroidal circulation. The exceeded fat deposition in Bruch's membrane may affect transport functions of retinal pigment epithelium (RPE).[7] However, the dietary factors as biochemical markers for AMD have not been consistently proven.[6] Based on meta-analyses and systematic reviews, an association between other risk factors and AMD was calculated. Some case-controlled studies did identify a significant association between hypertension and late AMD.[8] Aspirin may increase the risk of neovascular AMD, though the evidence is limited.[9] Other factors such as cataract surgery, blue iris, and exposure to sunlight are suspected, but their influence remains uncertain.[6,8]

In terms of the risk factors for age-related macular degeneration, age and genetic make-up are the most important risk factors identified to date. Over the next decade, more novel genes that are involved in the development of AMD might be identified and validated. The question that whether antioxidant vitamin and mineral supplementation prevents or delays the development of the disease will be answered as the results of large ongoing trials become available. Other risk factors such as alcohol consumption, estrogen replacement, and lifetime light exposure require further study. Studies with large numbers of late-stage disease are needed to provide the power to investigate moderate risks.[6,8] In summary, obtaining the history and risk factors of each individual is essential for clinicians to start the diagnostic process and establish communication with patients.

Drusen examined by multimodal imaging technique

Drusen are the hallmark of AMD. However, few small drusen alone without pigmentary changes, based on the classification of AMD, are considered as normalcy.[10] Meanwhile, in the study of geographic atrophy evolution, even when typical drusen is absent, diffuse mottling of small pigment clumps or microreticular pattern of small lines in aged eyes are still evidence of early AMD.[11] Therefore, both drusen (>medium drusen) and pigmentary changes are required as diagnostic criteria of early AMD.[10] Drusen are rare before the age of 40, but are common by the sixth decade. Drusen are extracellular deposits located between the RPE and Bruch's membrane.[12] The distribution is highly variable. Drusen may be confined to the macula, and may encircle it around the macular periphery. They may also be seen in the midperipheral or peripheral area. The size of drusen, the composition of drusen,[12] and the pigmentary abnormalities are also highly variable. Therefore, the examination of drusen and drusen-associated progression of macular changes require multimodal imaging studies. In this section, the clinical features of various drusen examined by multimodal imaging techniques are referred to Chapter 4, Table 4.1.

Dry AMD diagnosed by multimodal imaging techniques
Color fundus photography

Using color fundus photography (CFP) obtains equivalent information as that of bio-microscopic examination. CFP illustrates different subtypes of macular drusen (e.g., medium and large, hard and soft, and scattered and confluent) and drusen location, number, and area of involvement. CFP is a sensitive imaging technique showing pigmentary abnormalities, for example, various patterns of hyper- and hypo-pigmentation, indicating loss of RPE. As areas indicated by black dashed boxes in Fig. 5.1A and B middle, the sharply delineated area of hypopigmentation with

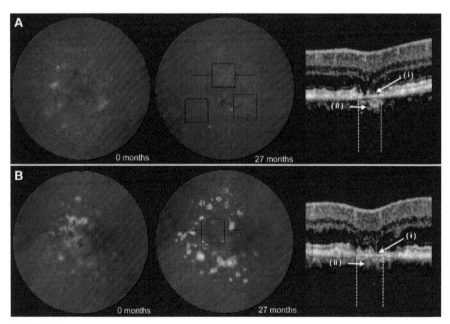

FIGURE 5.1

Color fundus photographs of the two participants (A and B) at the initial examination and at 27 months, illustrating the regression of drusen with resultant development of atrophy detected on spectral-domain optical coherence tomography (SD-OCT) scans, taken through the region indicated by a black dashed line at 27 months and shown on the right side. These areas of atrophy were visible as clinically defined geographic atrophy (GA) on color fundus photography (CFP) for the first participant at 27 months (A middle, three areas indicated by black dashed boxes), but not for the second participant (B), because there was no sharply delineated area of hypopigmentation with choroidal vessels visible at its base. On SD-OCT, they displayed features including the loss of the inner-segment ellipsoid (EZ) and retinal pigment epithelium (RPE) bands (i), increased signal transmission below Bruch's membrane (BrM) (ii), and loss of the outer nuclear layer (ONL) and external limiting membrane (ELM).

Modified from Wu Z, Luu CD, Ayton LN, et al. Optical coherence tomography-defined changes preceding the development of drusen-associated atrophy in age-related macular degeneration. Ophthalmology. *2014;121(12): 2415–2422. doi: 10.1016/j.ophtha.2014.06.034.*

choroidal vessels are typical geographic atrophy (GA). The GA lesions typically gradually expand and encroach upon the fovea. At this point, central visual functions deteriorate significantly.[14]

However, there are limitations of CFP, including variability of pigmentation and drusen appearance, lack of depth resolution of fundus, and lack of detailed quantitative information.[15,16] In spite of these limitations and the emergence of newer imaging modalities, CFP remains applicable in routine clinic and large clinical trials. It must be realized that the application of CFP in future studies is necessary because it allows for comparisons with earlier studies regarding AMD classification criteria Chapter 3, Table 3.1) and for validation of the newer techniques.

Fundus autofluorescence

Fundus autofluorescence (FAF) is a specific modality for the evaluation of GA because it provides high-contrast retinal images detecting RPE atrophy. Atrophic areas represent decreased autofluorescence (hypoautofluorescence) due to the loss of the RPE cells. Because of the demarcation between areas of RPE loss and neighboring areas of relatively intact photoreceptors and RPE, semiautomated quantification of atrophic areas by FAF is applicable. As a result, FAF has been used as a morphologic marker for the progression of GA in clinical studies.[17] FAF imaging technique that employs a confocal scanning laser ophthalmoscope with a blue light excitation wavelength filter (488 nm) and an emission filter of 500–521 nm is currently the most commonly used method for FAF. However, FAF imaging is susceptible to media opacities, thus it is difficult to observe the fovea with macular pigment that absorbs blue light. Meanwhile, the blue light causes patient discomfort.[18] The following FAF photographs of six patients are excellent examples that quantitatively monitoring the progression of GA. In a literature review, the median of GA progression monitored by FAF is ~ 1.78 mm^2/year (Fig. 5.2).[19]

Optical coherence tomography

Nascent onset of outer retina atrophy

Spectral-domain optical coherence tomography (SD)-OCT provides high-resolution, optical cross-sectional, and *en face* analysis of the retina, RPE, and choroid with depth-resolved segmentation. It has been used most frequently in retinal clinics. It has been validated to assess and quantify atrophy and has been used as a critical adjunct in large AMD clinical studies.[16] With anatomic tracking functions, overlay of baseline and follow-up images enable an analysis of the evolution of dry AMD. Therefore, longitudinal SD-OCT examination is a sensitive technique that can detect structural alteration of drusen-associated atrophy before GA appearance identified by either CFP or FAF. Using OCT, Wu et al. found that "immature GA" represents as subsidence of the outer plexiform layer and inner nuclear layer, and a funnel-shaped band within the outer plexiform layer shown in

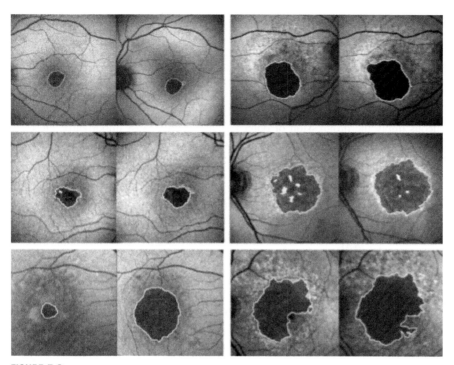

FIGURE 5.2

Examples of atrophy enlargement over time in six patients with GA attributable to AMD for the fundus autofluorescence (FAF) patterns (showing in left two columns and right two columns). Each pattern is shown in pairs with baseline FAF image (left) and follow-up FAF image (right). Atrophic areas are outlined in white in each image. Time between image pairs and atrophy progression rates are described in the following: (Upper left) Left eye of a 78-year-old patient with no FAF abnormalities (none). Minimal atrophy enlargement is observed (0.02 mm^2/year, follow-up 12 months). (Middle left) Right eye of a 77-year-old patient with only small areas of focally increased autofluorescence at the margin of the atrophic patch (focal). Slow atrophy progression over time can be detected (0.36 mm^2/year, follow-up 15 months). (Lower left) Right eye of a 66-year-old patient for the patchy pattern (atrophy progression 1.84 mm^2/year) (patchy). Note that follow-up (25.2 months) between the images is much longer compared to the other examples. (Upper right) Right eye of a 55-year-old patient with diffuse fine granular FAF pattern surrounding atrophy (diffuse). Moderate growth of atrophy is noticed over time (1.71 mm^2/year, follow-up 12 months). (Middle right) Left eye of a 76-year-old patient with a band of increased autofluorescence surrounding the geographic atrophy (banded). High atrophy progression is observed (2.52 mm^2/year, follow-up 18 months). (Lower right) Left eye of a 64-year-old patient with a diffuse trickling FAF pattern (diffuse, tricking) with very high atrophy enlargement over time (3.78 mm^2/year, follow-up 18 months).

Modified from Holz FG, Bindewald-Wittich A, Fleckenstein M, Dreyhaupt J, Scholl HPN, Schmitz-Valckenberg S. Progression of geographic atrophy and impact of fundus autofluorescence patterns in age-related macular degeneration. Am J Ophthalmol. *2007;143(3):463–472.e2. doi: 10.1016/j.ajo.2006.11.041.*

Fig. 5.1A (upper right). In this OCT image, an outer-retina atrophy that is a hyper-reflectivity of drusen-associated area is only mildly evident.[14]

Outer retinal atrophy at the location of drusenoid lesions

The evolution of drusenoid lesion can be monitored by using OCT with a grading system. Internal reflectivity of drusenoid lesion is graded as homogeneous verse heterogeneous. The existing data show that changes from homogeneous to heterogeneous imply the progression of outer retinal atrophy. Most importantly, OCT can detect any increased hyperreflective foci of outer retina at the location of drusenoid, an indicator of developing atrophy (Fig. 5.3).[20]

Outer retinal tubulation

OCT can detect outer retinal tubulation (ORT). ORT is thought to be consisted of degenerative photoreceptors aggregated into the tubular structure (Fig. 5.4). ORT represents roundish hyporeflective spaces, often around the margin of GA or neovascular complex.[21,22]

Outer retinal corrugations

Outer retinal corrugations (ORCs) is an OCT description of an undulating hyper-reflective layer of the outer retina.[23] OCT reveals ORCs as wide-based mound-like structures with flattened apices characterized by a hyporeflective and heterogeneous interior and an overlying hyperreflective exterior (Fig. 5.5).[24] The OCT features of ORCs demonstrate the evolution of drusenoid pigment epithelial detachment (PED) of dry AMD (Fig. 4.5 in Chapter 4). In the study by Tan et al., these OCT structures were redescribed as "plateaus" due to collapse of drusenoid PED, previously ascribed to persistent large amount of BLamD materials.[23,25] Therefore, ORCs are

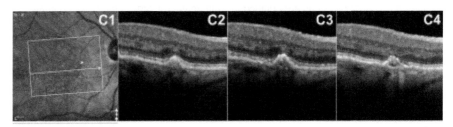

FIGURE 5.3

Case C represents a new atrophy onset-related changes of internal reflectivity of drusenoid lesion (IRDL). C1, Infrared image showing B-scan location on the fundus at baseline. C2, OCT B-scan showing IRDL graded as homogeneous. C3, OCT B-scan showing IRDL changed to heterogeneous without the presence of atrophy 9 months after baseline. C4, OCT B-scan showing the presence of hyper-reflective foci of outer retina 21 months after baseline.

Modified from Ouyang Y, Heussen FM, Hariri A, Keane PA, Sadda SR. Optical coherence tomography—based observation of the natural history of drusenoid lesion in eyes with dry age-related macular degeneration. Ophthalmology. 2013;120(12):2656—2665. doi: 10.1016/j.ophtha.2013.05.029.

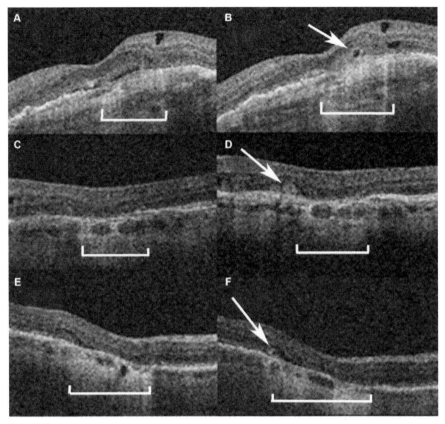

FIGURE 5.4

Longitudinal observation of outer retinal tubulations (ORTs) by SD-OCT images. At week 56 (A, C, E) and week 104 (B, D, F) in three eyes without ORTs at week 56 but with ORTs (arrows) at week 104. The ORTs are seen adjacent to areas of geographic atrophy, seen as photoreceptor layer thinning above an area of increased light penetration into the choroid (brackets).

Modified from Lee JY, Folgar FA, Maguire MG, et al. Outer retinal tubulation in the comparison of age-related macular degeneration treatments trials (CATT). Ophthalmology. 2014;121(12):2423-2431. doi:10.1016/ j.ophtha.2014.06.013.

irregular elevations of the RPE/Bruch membrane complex, a sequelae of drusenoid lesion evolution.

Splitting of the RPE/Bruch's membrane complex

Splitting of the RPE/Bruch's membrane complex (SRBC), ORT, and ORC are the three common OCT microstructural findings mainly in atrophic AMD. Based on the study by Moussa et al., splitting of the RPE/Bruch's membrane complex band without fluid may indicate a higher risk for progression to GA,[26] correlating with

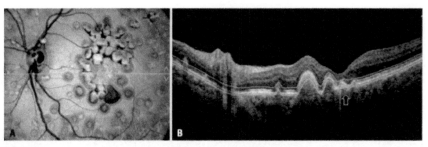

FIGURE 5.5

en face OCT images obtained from a patient with large drusen, representing outer retinal corrugations. (A) Structural en face OCT with upper segmentation line located at the avascular outer retina and lower segmentation line placed at the subretinal pigment epithelium (RPE) space showing a hyper-reflective center surrounded by a hypo-reflective halo, bordered by hyper-reflective and hypo-reflective rings, similar to the donut effect. (B) Corresponding OCT B-scan of (A) showing the corrugations with medium and homogeneous internal reflectivity under the RPE, as well as marked thinning of the outer nuclear and ellipsoid layers. A small area of RPE atrophy as seen under the horizontal foveal scan, identified as reverse shadowing (black arrow). No fluid accumulation is observed.

Modified from Roberti NC, Dias de JRO, Novais EA, Regatieri CS, Belfort Jr R. Large colloid drusen analyzed with structural en face optical coherence tomography. Arq Bras Oftalmol. 2017;80(2). doi: 10.5935/0004-2749.20170029.

faster atrophy enlargement, larger size increment, and multifocal patches of atrophy. In real practice, OCT features of SRBC and tricking pattern on FAF, showing RPE abnormalities and a thinner choroid,[27] not only can help diagnose GA but also predict GA growth (Fig. 5.6).[28] Notably, SRBC might be an analog of the "double-layer" sign detected by OCT.[29] This sign has been reported to be associated with subclinical type 1 MNV. Therefore, the double-layer sign is a predictive factor for nonexudative neovascular AMD in the patients with atrophic AMD.[30]

Staging GA progression by OCT

The above descriptions have focused on OCT features of drusen, inner and outer layers of retina, and the junction between atrophy and its neighbor tissues. The progression of GA needs a standard OCT diagnostic system, because future studies will require consistent definitions for comparison. Sadda et al. in 2018 summarized expert opinions on the consensus nomenclature and definition of different stages of GA based on OCT data (Fig. 5.7).[13] The staging of atrophic AMD and nomenclature are presented in Table 5.1.[13,14]

By using these OCT guidelines, the cases in Fig. 5.8 met the criteria for diagnosis of complete RPE and outer retinal atrophy (cRORA).[13]

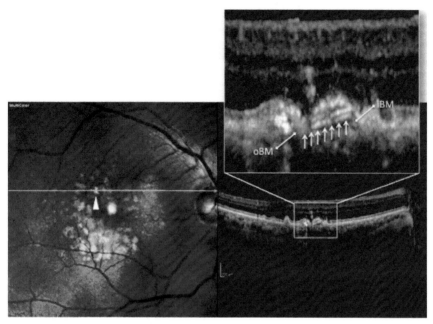

FIGURE 5.6

Color fundus photography and SD-OCT scan of a patient with nonexudative age-related macular degeneration. CFP (left) shows a regressing calcific drusen (ar), and tracked SD-OCT image (right) shows an intense multilaminar hyperreflective signal (arrows) beneath the RPE layer, splitting the RPE/Bruch's membrane complex. *Abbreviation*: oBM, *outer Bruch's membrane.*

Modified from Querques G, Georges A, Ben Moussa N, Sterkers M, Souied EH. Appearance of regressing drusen on optical coherence tomography in age-related macular degeneration. Ophthalmology. 2014;121(1): 173–179. doi: 10.1016/j.ophtha.2013.06.024.

Fellow eye with geographic atrophy

AMD is a bilateral disease with variable asymmetry. Single eye involvement of GA is a strong predictor of GA in the fellow eye. Based on AREDS, the median period for developing GA in the fellow eye was estimated at 7 years.[31] Once the presence of GA in both eyes, the intereye progression rates are compatible.[31,32] This explains why the compatible or similar intereye progression rates may be used for intrapersonal control when a single eye is recruited for a GA clinical trial.

OCT is a unique tool for diagnosing, staging, and predicting GA. OCT has provided information for predicting the progression of the disease (e.g., enlargement rates of GA over time) and may be used for monitoring potential therapeutic interventions. However, drawbacks of OCT need to be pointed out as follows: a limited scan field, dependence on image quality for interpretation, imperfect automated image segmentation. Therefore, fewer large studies have used SD-OCT in comparison with CFP and FAF to study the features of nonexudative AMD. To validate the

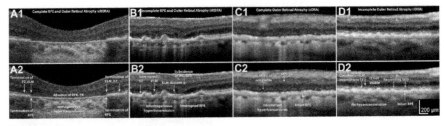

FIGURE 5.7

Representative OCT demonstrating the four terms (A–D) for atrophy defined by the Classification of Atrophy Meetings. Rows 1 and 2 show each OCT without (upper row) and with (lower row) annotations of an identical OCT, respectively. (A) Images obtained from an 83-year-old white woman, A1, A2, Complete RPE and outer retinal atrophy (cRORA) is defined by a zone of homogeneous choroidal hypertransmission and absence of the RPE band measuring 250 µm or more with overlying OR thinning and loss of photoreceptors (PRs). No signs of an RPE tear are evident. B1, B2, For incomplete RPE and OR atrophy (iRORA), some hypertransmission is evident but is discontinuous; the RPE band is present but irregular or interrupted. Interrupted ELM and EZ evidences PR degeneration. The inner nuclear layer and outer plexiform layer exhibit subsidence. Criteria for cRORA are not met. C1, C2, Complete OR atrophy (cORA) is defined by continuous nonvisibility of the EZ and IZ and severe thinning of the outer retina, in the setting of an intact RPE band. Hypertransmission associated with RPE degeneration is intermittent. D1, D2. Incomplete OR atrophy (iORA) demonstrating continuous ELM and detectable EZ disruption in the setting of regressing subretinal drusenoid deposits (SDDs), with detectable thinning of the outer retina, an intact RPE band, and no hypertransmission.

Modified from Sadda SR, Guymer R, Holz FG, et al. Consensus definition for atrophy associated with age-related macular degeneration on OCT: classification of atrophy report 3. Ophthalmology. *2018;125(4):537–548. doi: 10.1016/j.ophtha.2017.09.028.*

Table 5.1 Criteria for diagnosis of RPE and outer retinal atrophy on OCT.[13]

	SD-OCT B-scan characteristics
Complete RPE and outer retinal atrophy (cRORA)	Zone of choroidal hypertransmission and loss of RPE band >250 µm with OR thinning and loss of PR, excluding scrolled RPE of RPE tear
Incomplete RPE and outer retinal atrophy (iRORA)	Zone of discontinuous hypertransmission, disruption of RPE band and OR atrophy, interrupted ELM, EZ, and PR degeneration. Criteria for cRORA are not met. The ONL, HFL, OPL, and INL subside in parallel to the ELM, creating a funnel
Complete outer retinal atrophy (cORA)	Continuous loss of ELM, and EZ or IZ and severe thinning of the OR, with an intact RPE band. Hypertransmission associated with RPE degeneration is intermittent
Incomplete outer retinal atrophy (iORA)	Continuous ELM and detectable EZ disruption with subretinal drusenoid deposits (SDDs), with detectable thinning of the OR, an intact RPE band, and no hypertransmission

Abbreviation: ELM, external limiting membrane; EZ, ellipsoid zone; HFL, Henle fiber layer; INL, inner nuclear layer; IZ, inner digitation zone; ONL, outer nuclear layer; OPL, outer plexiform layer; OR, outer retina; PR, photoreceptor; RPE, retinal pigment epithelium; SDD, subretinal drusenoid deposits.
Modified from Sadda SR, Guymer R, Holz FG, et al. Consensus definition for atrophy associated with age-related macular degeneration on OCT: classification of atrophy report 3. Ophthalmology. *2018; 125(4):537–548. doi: 10.1016/j.ophtha.2017.09.028.*

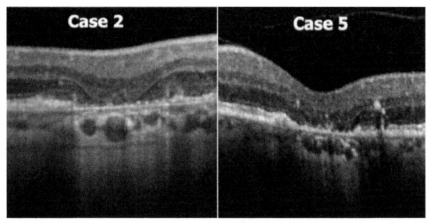

FIGURE 5.8

OCT images for the two patients were evaluated by the criteria described in Table 5.1. Cases 2 and 5 met these criteria and were diagnosed as complete retinal pigment epithelium (RPE) and outer retinal atrophy (cRORA), with choroidal hypertransmission and attenuation of the RPE band with thinning of the overlying retina in a region exceeding 250 μm in diameter.

Modified from Sadda SR, Guymer R, Holz FG, et al. Consensus definition for atrophy associated with age-related macular degeneration on OCT: classification of atrophy report 3. Ophthalmology. 2018;125(4):537–548. doi: 10.1016/j.ophtha.2017.09.028.

imaging findings of dry AMD, other than CFP, FAF, and OCT, near-infrared reflectance (NIR) and near-infrared autofluorescence have been used to detect RPE atrophy as valuable adjuncts to the diagnosis of dry AMD.

Fluorescein angiography

Fluorescein angiography (FA) has been the gold standard method to detect and assess the wet AMD, but this modality may also readily identify drusen and GA, particularly for differential diagnosis of wet and dry AMD. The FA features of drusen have been summarized in Table 4.1 of Chapter 4 including drusen staining. GA can typically represent a "window defect" by FA (Fig. 5.9), because of atrophic RPE unmasking of background fluorescence of choriocapillaris.[33]

Diagnosis of neovascular AMD from FA era to OCT era

Neovascularization, a signature of wet AMD, together with geographic atrophy (GA) represent the late stages of AMD. In Chapter 4, clinical signs of choroidal neovascularization (CNV) and associated components such as drusen, PED, exudate, hemorrhage, fibrosis, and RPE tear were studied mainly based on FA, known as in FA era. This section is focusing on the diagnosis of neovascular AMD based

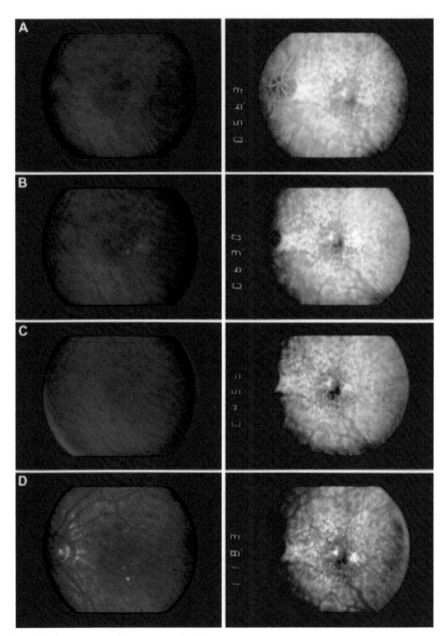

FIGURE 5.9

Color fundus photographs (CFPs, left column) and corresponding fluorescein angiograms (right column) over time from a subject with GA. The subject's visual acuity remained 20/32 or better at all visits. A, On CFP (year 0), there were soft confluent drusen. Corresponding FA demonstrated a staining pattern. B, One year later, the appearance of on the recent consensus nomenclature system with multimodal imaging techniques, known as in OCT era. In the context of neovascular AMD, the coexisting components of atrophic AMD are also emphasized because both macular atrophy and neovascularization can contribute to the severe vision impairment.[34]

Diagnosis of wet AMD with fluorescein angiography and OCT

FA has been the gold standard method to diagnose CNV for decades. First, diagnosis of CNV should be urgently made by FA if clinical suspicion exists. Second, CNV subtypes are classified by fluorescein angiographic features and validated by OCT angiography (OCTA) and indocyanine green angiography (ICGA).

Occult CNV, that is, newly defined type 1 macular neovascularization (type 1 MNV), is the most common type of CNV ($\sim$80%). On FA, the occult CNV has ill-defined regions representing stippled hyperfluorescence, that is, "late leakage of an undetermined source" (Fig. 5.10). On OCT, type 1 MNV represents areas of neovascular complexes arising from the choroid, showing an elevation of the RPE by material with heterogeneous reflectivity (Fig. 5.10).[35] OCT shows vascular elements below the level of the RPE layer. ICGA demonstrates hyperfluorescent plaque choroidal new vessels (Fig. 5.10).

Classic CNV, that is, newly defined type 2 MNV, is the second common type of CNV ($\sim$20%) in wet AMD. Classic CNV originates from the choroid, traverses Bruch's membrane and the RPE layer, and then proliferates in the subretinal space. Because of its anatomic location above the RPE layer, in the early phase of FA, it fills with dye in a well-defined "lacy" hyper-fluorescence pattern. In 1–2 min, both the intensity and size of hyperfluorescent lesion are increased, indicating the dye leaks into the subretinal space (Fig. 5.11). Most CNV due to wet AMD is subfoveal. Extrafoveal CNV is defined as >200 μm from the center of the foveal avascular zone on FA.[34,36]

Predominantly or minimally classic CNV, that is, newly defined mixed type 1 and type 2 MNV, is present when the classic component is greater or less than 50% of the lesion, respectively. OCT shows mixed type 1 and type 2 MNV together.

Figure 5.9 Continued

the drusen on CFP has become more confluent and an area of depigmentation or incipient atrophy has developed just temporal to the fovea. The FA shows a corresponding area of hyperfluorescence in a staining pattern consistent with drusen. C, Incident GA was detected at year 2. The CFP again shows a focal area of depigmentation with well-defined borders just temporal to the fovea in the same location that was occupied by confluent drusen the previous year. In this case, the sharp borders of the window defect on FA confirm the presence of GA area. D, One year after detection of GA (year 3), the area of GA becomes larger and more apparent on CFP alone, The FA again confirms the presence of GA.

Modified from Brader HS, Ying G-S, Martin ER, Maguire MG, Complications of Age-Related Macular Degeneration Prevention Trial (CAPT) Research Group. Characteristics of incident geographic atrophy in the complications of age-related macular degeneration prevention trial. Ophthalmology. 2013;120(9):1871–1879. doi: 10.1016/j.ophtha.2013.01.049.

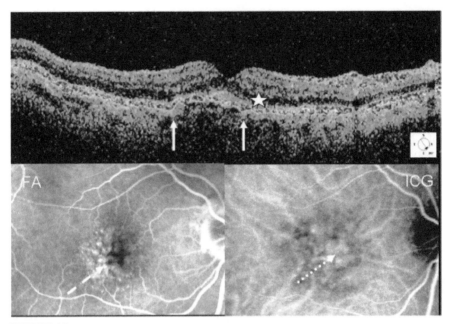

FIGURE 5.10

OCT identification of apparently isolated occult choroidal new vessels. (Top) OCT results showing slightly prominent elevation (*arrow*) of the pigment epithelium along with changes in the RPE band, which is thickened and irregular. Note the minimal intraretinal fluid accumulation (star). (Bottom left) Fluorescein angiogram showing occult choroidal new vessels with predominantly temporal hyperfluorescence (*arrow*). (Bottom right) Scanning laser ophthalmoscopy (SLO) indocyanine green angiography (ICGA) image showing hyperfluorescent subfoveal plaque choroidal new vessels (arrow).

Modified from Coscas F, Coscas G, Souied E, Tick S, Soubrane G. Optical coherence tomography identification of occult choroidal neovascularization in age-related macular degeneration. Am J Ophthalmol. 2007;144(4): 592–599.e2. doi: 10.1016/j.ajo.2007.06.014.

OCTA demonstrates neovascularization in the sub-RPE and subretinal compartments. For instance, in Fig. 5.12,[34] the classic component larger than 50% of the lesion is present, so that it is called predominantly classic CNV. Clinically, it may be difficult to differentiate the mixed type 1 and 2 MNV from type3 MNV (Fig. 5.12D).

Retinal angiomatous proliferation (RAP), that is, newly defined type 3 MNV, is a variant of wet AMD. The neovascularization initially originates from the retinal circulation, typically the deep capillary plexus, and grows toward the outer retina. Eventually, an aberrant connection between the retinal and the choroidal circulation has been established, that is, a retinal-choroidal anastomosis. Fig. 5.13A of this chapter and Fig. 3.11 in Chapter 3 show a diagram of retinal proliferative vessels posteriorly with the formation of retinal-choroidal anastomosis lesion. This pathologic process is proved by ICGA (Fig. 5.13B).[34]

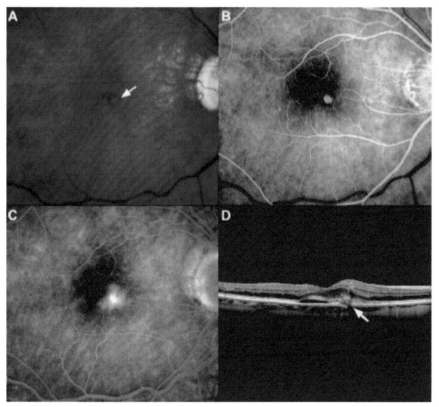

FIGURE 5.11

Images showing type 2 macular neovascularization. (A) Fundus photograph from a 74-year-old showing a hyperpigmented ring in the fovea (*arrow*). (B and C), Early-phase fluorescein angiogram showing (B) a well-defined lesion with late leakage and (C) obscuration of the borders of the neovascular lesion. (D and B) scan OCT showing the outer retinal lesion with extension of subretinal fluid under the fovea. The ingrowth site through the retinal pigment epithelium is evident (*arrow*).

Modified from Spaide RF, Jaffe GJ, Sarraf D, et al. Consensus nomenclature for reporting neovascular age-related macular degeneration data: consensus on neovascular age-related macular degeneration nomenclature study group. Ophthalmology. 2019. doi: 10.1016/j.ophtha.2019.11.004.

Based on examinations using FA and ICGA, RAP is defined as three stages. Stage 1, intraretinal neovascularization, showing telangiectatic retinal vessels and small angiomatous lesions, typically associated with intra-, sub-, and preretinal hemorrhage, edema, and exudate (Fig. 5.14A, E, and F). Subretinal neovascularization, in Stage 2, extends into the subretinal space associated with increased edema and exudate. A serous PED may be present (Fig. 5.14C and D). CNV in Stage 3 originates from choroid with retinal-choroidal anastomosis (Fig. 5.14G and H). OCT

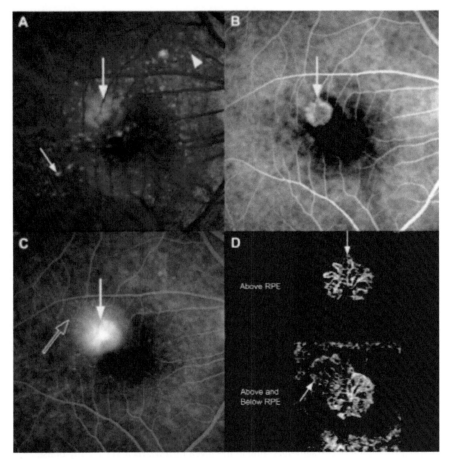

FIGURE 5.12

Images showing mixed type 1 and type 2 macular neovascularization. (A) Fundus photograph from 62-year-old showing a region of yellowish exudation (larger arrow). Note the drusen (smaller arrow) and pseudodrusen (ar). (B) Early-phase fluorescein angiogram showing a well-defined area of neovascularization (vertical arrow). (C) Later-phase fluorescein angiogram showing pronounced leakage from the well-defined neovascularization and some punctate leakage from and adjacent area (open arrow). (D) *en face* OCTA showing two perspectives: (Top) above the level of RPE, the well-defined lesion seen in the fluorescein angiogram is evident (vertical arrow); (Bottom) the slab section was deepened to include visualization of neovascularization below the RPE. The neovascularization above the RPE, seen as the well-defined lesion, is type 2, and the deeper proliferation, below the RPE, is type 1 macular neovascularization.

Modified from Spaide RF, Jaffe GJ, Sarraf D, et al. Consensus nomenclature for reporting neovascular age-related macular degeneration data: consensus on neovascular age-related macular degeneration nomenclature study group. Ophthalmology. 2019. doi: 10.1016/j.ophtha.2019.11.004.

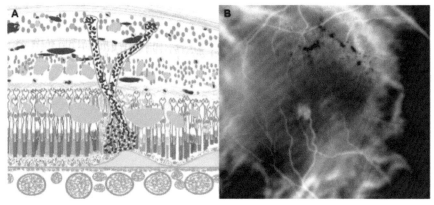

FIGURE 5.13

Type 3 macular neovascularization. (A) Diagram showing proliferation of vessels posteriorly with formation of what has been called an angiomatous lesion. The vessels supplying the blood flow to the angiomatous proliferation remodel into larger feeding and draining vessels. The edema and hemorrhage in the retina are from both the neovascularization and to increased local tissue levels of vascular endothelial growth factor. Some evidence is present that the retinal pigment epithelium monolayer may not be intact, even before penetration of new vessels into the basal laminar or basal linear material. (B) Comparative indocyanine green angiographic image of a patient with an established retinal choroidal anastomosis lesion.

Modified from Spaide RF, Jaffe GJ, Sarraf D, et al. Consensus nomenclature for reporting neovascular age-related macular degeneration data: consensus on neovascular age-related macular degeneration nomenclature study group. Ophthalmology. *2019. doi: 10.1016/j.ophtha.2019.11.004.*

shows hyper-reflectivity from the middle retina toward to level of the RPE associated with intraretinal edema (Fig. 5.14B−D). OCTA shows the down growth of new vessels toward the level of the RPE (Fig. 5.14H).[34]

Just using FA and ICGA is difficult to differentiate the mixed type 1 and 2 MNV from type 3 MNV. Therefore, in a recent comparative study by using FA, ICGA, and OCTA, the characteristics of RAP were analyzed. This study showed that OCTA is superior to FA and ICGA in acquiring more detailed information about the location and the precise layer of lesions (Fig. 5.14H).[37]

Polypoidal choroidal vasculopathy (PCV) is another variant of wet AMD, that is, a newly defined variant of type 1 MNV. PCV is less likely to manifest soft drusen, cuticular drusen, and reticular pseudodrusen. PCV is commonly seen in Asian populations and more in women than men (5:1).[38] This disease is often bilateral but tends to be asymmetrical. The presence of prominent hemorrhage should lead to consideration of PCV, particularly if there is an absence of drusen and the patient is relatively young. Based on ICGA findings, PCV is characterized by a branching vascular network of inner choroidal vessels with multiple terminal aneurysmal protrusions (Fig. 5.15).[39] Recent EDI-OCT reveals thick choroids in PCV contrary to

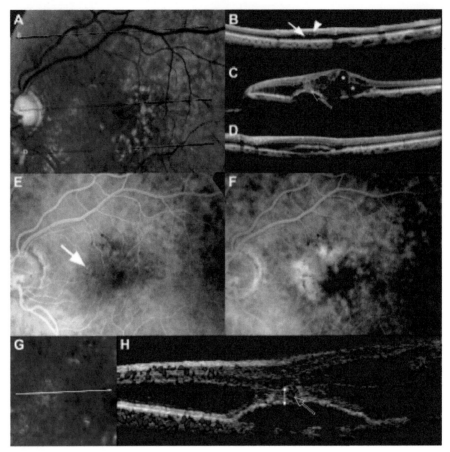

FIGURE 5.14

Images showing type3 macular neovascularization with prominent edema and hemorrhage. (A) Fundus photograph from an 87-year-old showing dozens of small fleck hemorrhages in the superior and nasal macula. The *blue arrows* show the location of the structural OCT scans. (B) OCT scan of the section through the superior arcade showing the expansion of the inner nuclear layer (ar) and Henle's fiber layer from edema fluid (*arrow*). (C) OCT scan of the section through the superior parafovea revealing edema of inner nuclear layer and Henle's fiber layer with cystoid spaces (yellow and green asterisks, respectively). Hyperreflectivity within the retina overlying the apex of RPE (*arrow*) is evident. Note the edema nasal and temporal to the area of neovascularization is greater than that immediately surrounding the new vessels. (D) OCT scan of the inferior macula showing edematous thickening of the retina and subretinal fluid. (E) Fluorescein angiogram showing a small area of hyperfiuorescence corresponding to the hyperrefiective area in (C). (F) Later fiuorescein angiogram showing pooling of dye in cystoid spaces as well as diffuse staining well away from the area highlighted by the *arrow* in (E). (G) Fundus photograph of magnification of the central portion of the involved macula showing the numerous isolated hemorrhages, many of which were in the inner retina. The *green arrow* shows the section captured by the OCT angiogram in (H). (H) OCTA showing the small focus neovascularization found within the outer retina (*open arrow*). The vertical double arrow is 150 μm. Note that the hemorrhages do not colocalize with the neovascularization.

Modified from Spaide RF, Jaffe GJ, Sarraf D, et al. Consensus nomenclature for reporting neovascular age-related macular degeneration data: consensus on neovascular age-related macular degeneration nomenclature study group. Ophthalmology. *2019. doi: 10.1016/j.ophtha.2019.11.004.*

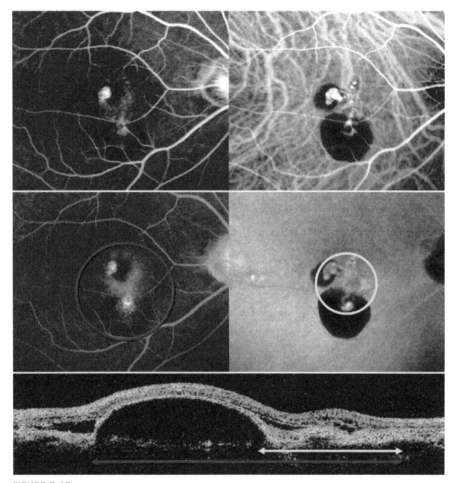

FIGURE 5.15

Angiographic and OCT findings of polypoidal choroidal vasculopathy (PCV). (Top left) The early phase of FA. (Top right) The ICGA results. Polypoidal vascular lesions and branched vascular networks in a "string-pearls" configuration clearly are detectable on ICGA, but not on FA. (Second row left) The red circle in the late-phase FA image indicates the FA-guided greatest linear dimension (GLD). (Second row right) In the late-phase ICGA image, the lesion of network vasculature is more prominent. The yellow circle indicates ICGA-guided GLD. (Third row) Vertical scan of OCT shows details of the lesions including intra- and subretinal fluid, and a large serous PED. The *yellow arrow* indicates the PCV vascular lesion (ICGA GLD) that does not include the large serous PED. The FA GLD is indicated by a *red arrow*.

Modified from Otani A, Sasahara M, Yodoi Y, et al. Indocyanine green angiography: guided photodynamic therapy for polypoidal choroidal vasculopathy. Am J Ophthalmol. 2007;144(1):7–14.e1. doi: 10.1016/ j.ajo.2007.03.014.

choroidal thinning in eyes with typical neovascular AMD.[40] The presence of choroidal thickening and hyperpermeability of choroidal veins in patients with PCV indicates a link between this entity and the pachychoroid disease spectrum, in particular pachychoroid neovasculopathy (PNV).

Vitreous hemorrhage occurs more often in association with PCV than in non-PCV wet AMD (Fig. 5.16).[41] Therefore, PCV was initially called a posterior uveal bleeding syndrome.

Wet AMD is associated with other neovascularization-related presentations including intraretinal fluid (IRF), subretinal fluid (SRF), lipid (hard exudate), subretinal hyperreflective materials (SHRMs), hemorrhage, and fibrosis. All of the above are biomarkers for validation of the diagnosis and monitoring follow-ups in the management of neovascularization.

IRF and SRF are difficult to be detected by CFP and FA. It is true in some cases, fluorescein "pooling" may be seen in cystoid spaces in the retina by FA. However, in the OCT era, IRF and SRF can be detected rapidly by new modalities. IRF representing cystoid spaces in the retina is typically accompanied by increased retinal thickening. SRF shows the separation of the neurosensory retina from the RPE by hypo-reflective fluid. Representative OCT findings of IRF and SRF are shown in Fig. 5.14B—D).

Hard exudates are yellow-white globular materials in or under the retina, resulting from lipoprotein particles due to chronic vascular leakage. OCT cross-section shows that hyperreflective foci are located at intraretinal, subretinal, or sub-RPE spaces, which are present in Fig. 5.17E (temporal to the fovea) or nasal to the fovea, respectively.[42]

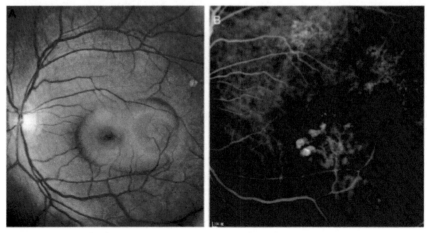

FIGURE 5.16

Fundus color photograph, indocyanine green angiography (ICGA) images of a naïve PCV. (A) Presentation of submacular hemorrhage. (B) ICGA at baseline demonstrates several PCV lesions.

Modified from Lin T-C, Hwang D-K, Lee F-L, Chen S-J. Visual prognosis of massive submacular hemorrhage in polypoidal choroidal vasculopathy with or without combination treatment. J Chin Med Assoc. 2016;79(3): 159–165. doi: 10.1016/j.jcma.2015.11.004.

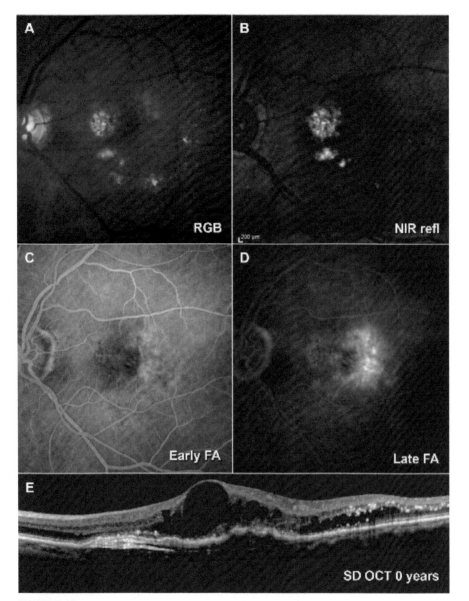

FIGURE 5.17

Multimodal imaging of hard exudates in neovascular AMD. (A) Color fundus photograph (CFP) showing yellow-gray exudation just nasal to the fovea and circinate yellow exudates at the temporal to the fovea. (B) Near-infrared reflectance (NIR) scanning laser ophthalmoscope image showing hyperreflectivity of the yellow-gray exudates nasal to the fovea. (C) Early fluorescein angiogram showing hyperfluorescence temporal to the fovea consistent with neovascularization. (D) Late FA showing late leakage, also consistent with neovascularization. (E) SD-OCT scan through the fovea showing the onion sign nasal to the fovea, consisting of multiple layered hyperreflective lines below RPE. There are multiple intraretinal and subretinal hyperreflective foci temporal to the fovea.

Modified from Pang CE, Messinger JD, Zanzottera EC, Freund KB, Curcio CA. The onion sign in neovascular age-related macular degeneration represents cholesterol crystals. Ophthalmology. 2015;122(11):2316–2326. doi: 10.1016/j.ophtha.2015.07.008.

SHRMs, likely comprising serum, fibrin, and inflammatory cells, are detected in subretinal space by OCT. SHRMs are hyperreflective in comparison with fluid. They were not revealed before the OCT era. Therefore, in the FA era, it is difficult to differentiate SHRM from the scar tissue on CFP. The clinical significance of SHRM detection is that the worse visual outcome of wet AMD is associated with the larger size of SHRM (Fig. 5.18), because large SHRMs herald the severe damage of the RPE layer.[43]

In the FA era, retinal hemorrhage in patients with wet AMD may be inferred as subretinal and sub-RPE spaces. Whereas OCT scan demonstrates the exact location of blood. Fibrosis appears to be hyperreflective and usually in the subretinal or sub-RPE spaces on OCT.

Taken together, AMD is a common, chronic, progressive degenerative disease in older individuals. AMD affects the photoreceptor/RPE/Bruch's membrane/choriocapillaris complex of macula. The diagnostic purpose is to find the patients at an early stage and to classify the patients with advanced stages for appropriate treatment. Acquiring history and risk factors is a prerequisite for making a diagnosis

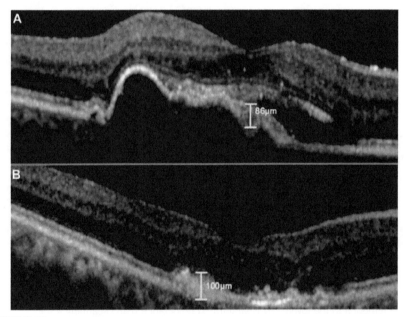

FIGURE 5.18

(A) OCT scan showing SHRM thickness (86 μm) that is distinguishable from the underlying RPE layer. (B) OCT scan showing subretinal hyperreflective material (100 μm) that is indistinguishable from underlying RPE layer.

Modified from Willoughby AS, Ying G, Toth CA, et al. Subretinal hyperreflective material in the comparison of age-related macular degeneration treatments trials. Ophthalmology. *2015;122(9):1846–1853.e5. doi: 10.1016/j.ophtha.2015.05.042.*

of AMD. Clinical examination is usually sufficient to establish a diagnosis or at least a clinical suspicion of AMD, although subtle macular abnormalities are best detected with the help of ancillary tests. From the era of FA including color fundus photography, that equivalent to biomicroscopic examination, along with FA to the era of OCT including multimodal imaging techniques, the more sensitive and specific detection of abnormal macula neurovascular complex can be achieved.

References

1. Mehta S. Age-related macular degeneration. *Prim Care*. 2015;42(3):377−391. https://doi.org/10.1016/j.pop.2015.05.009.
2. Klein R, Klein BE, Jensen SC, Meuer SM. The five-year incidence and progression of age-related maculopathy: the Beaver Dam eye study. *Ophthalmology*. 1997;104(1): 7−21. https://doi.org/10.1016/s0161-6420(97)30368-6.
3. Jonas JB, Cheung CMG, Panda-Jonas S. Updates on the epidemiology of age-related macular degeneration. *Asia Pac J Ophthalmol*. 2017;6(6):493−497. https://doi.org/10.22608/APO.2017251.
4. Colijn JM, Buitendijk GHS, Prokofyeva E, et al. Prevalence of age-related macular degeneration in Europe: the past and the future. *Ophthalmology*. 2017;124(12): 1753−1763. https://doi.org/10.1016/j.ophtha.2017.05.035.
5. Klein R, Klein BEK, Knudtson MD, et al. Prevalence of age-related macular degeneration in 4 racial/ethnic groups in the multi-ethnic study of atherosclerosis. *Ophthalmology*. 2006;113(3):373−380. https://doi.org/10.1016/j.ophtha.2005.12.013.
6. Evans JR. Risk factors for age-related macular degeneration. *Prog Retin Eye Res*. 2001; 20(2):227−253. https://doi.org/10.1016/s1350-9462(00)00023-9.
7. Rojas B, Ramírez AI, Salazar JJ, et al. Low-dosage statins reduce choroidal damage in hypercholesterolemic rabbits. *Acta Ophthalmol*. 2011;89(7):660−669. https://doi.org/10.1111/j.1755-3768.2009.01829.x.
8. Chakravarthy U, Wong TY, Fletcher A, et al. Clinical risk factors for age-related macular degeneration: a systematic review and meta-analysis. *BMC Ophthalmol*. 2010;10:31. https://doi.org/10.1186/1471-2415-10-31.
9. Small KW, Garabetian CA, Shaya FS. Macular degeneration and aspirin use. *Retina*. 2017;37(9):1630−1635. https://doi.org/10.1097/IAE.0000000000001475.
10. Ferris FL, Davis MD, Clemons TE, et al. A simplified severity scale for age-related macular degeneration: AREDS report no. 18. *Arch Ophthalmol*. 2005;123(11):1570−1574. https://doi.org/10.1001/archopht.123.11.1570.
11. Sarks JP, Sarks SH, Killingsworth MC. Evolution of geographic atrophy of the retinal pigment epithelium. *Eye*. 1988;2(Pt 5):552−577. https://doi.org/10.1038/eye.1988.106.
12. Bergen AA, Arya S, Koster C, et al. On the origin of proteins in human drusen: the meet, greet and stick hypothesis. *Prog Retin Eye Res*. 2019;70:55−84. https://doi.org/10.1016/j.preteyeres.2018.12.003.
13. Sadda SR, Guymer R, Holz FG, et al. Consensus definition for atrophy associated with age-related macular degeneration on OCT: classification of atrophy report 3. *Ophthalmology*. 2018;125(4):537−548. https://doi.org/10.1016/j.ophtha.2017.09.028.
14. Wu Z, Luu CD, Ayton LN, et al. Optical coherence tomography-defined changes preceding the development of drusen-associated atrophy in age-related macular degeneration. *Ophthalmology*. 2014;121(12):2415−2422. https://doi.org/10.1016/j.ophtha.2014.06.034.

15. Garrity ST, Sarraf D, Freund KB, Sadda SR. Multimodal imaging of nonneovascular age-related macular degeneration. *Invest Ophthalmol Vis Sci.* 2018;59(4):AMD48−AMD64. https://doi.org/10.1167/iovs.18-24158.

16. Holz FG, Sadda SR, Staurenghi G, et al. Imaging protocols in clinical studies in advanced age-related macular degeneration: recommendations from classification of atrophy consensus meetings. *Ophthalmology.* 2017;124(4):464−478. https://doi.org/10.1016/j.ophtha.2016.12.002.

17. Yung M, Klufas MA, Sarraf D. Clinical applications of fundus autofluorescence in retinal disease. *Int J Retina Vitreous.* 2016;2:12. https://doi.org/10.1186/s40942-016-0035-x.

18. Fleckenstein M, Mitchell P, Freund KB, et al. The progression of geographic atrophy secondary to age-related macular degeneration. *Ophthalmology.* 2018;125(3):369−390. https://doi.org/10.1016/j.ophtha.2017.08.038.

19. Holz FG, Bindewald-Wittich A, Fleckenstein M, Dreyhaupt J, Scholl HPN, Schmitz-Valckenberg S. Progression of geographic atrophy and impact of fundus autofluorescence patterns in age-related macular degeneration. *Am J Ophthalmol.* 2007;143(3):463−472.e2. https://doi.org/10.1016/j.ajo.2006.11.041.

20. Ouyang Y, Heussen FM, Hariri A, Keane PA, Sadda SR. Optical coherence tomography−based observation of the natural history of drusenoid lesion in eyes with dry age-related macular degeneration. *Ophthalmology.* 2013;120(12):2656−2665. https://doi.org/10.1016/j.ophtha.2013.05.029.

21. Lee JY, Folgar FA, Maguire MG, et al. Outer retinal tubulation in the comparison of age-related macular degeneration treatments trials (CATT). *Ophthalmology.* 2014;121(12):2423−2431. https://doi.org/10.1016/j.ophtha.2014.06.013.

22. Zweifel SA, Engelbert M, Laud K, Margolis R, Spaide RF, Freund KB. Outer retinal tubulation: a novel optical coherence tomography finding. *Arch Ophthalmol.* 2009;127(12):1596−1602. https://doi.org/10.1001/archophthalmol.2009.326.

23. Tan ACS, Astroz P, Dansingani KK, et al. The evolution of the plateau, an optical coherence tomography signature seen in geographic atrophy. *Invest Ophthalmol Vis Sci.* 2017;58(4):2349−2358. https://doi.org/10.1167/iovs.16-21237.

24. Roberti NC, Dias de JRO, Novais EA, Regatieri CS, Belfort Jr R. Large colloid drusen analyzed with structural en face optical coherence tomography. *Arq Bras Oftalmol.* 2017;80(2). https://doi.org/10.5935/0004-2749.20170029.

25. Ooto S, Vongkulsiri S, Sato T, Suzuki M, Curcio CA, Spaide RF. Outer retinal corrugations in age-related macular degeneration. *JAMA Ophthalmol.* 2014;132(7):806−813. https://doi.org/10.1001/jamaophthalmol.2014.1871.

26. Moussa K, Lee JY, Stinnett SS, Jaffe GJ. Spectral domain optical coherence tomography-determined morphologic predictors of age-related macular degeneration-associated geographic atrophy progression. *Retina.* 2013;33(8):1590−1599. https://doi.org/10.1097/IAE.0b013e31828d6052.

27. Lindner M, Bezatis A, Czauderna J, et al. Choroidal thickness in geographic atrophy secondary to age-related macular degeneration. *Invest Ophthalmol Vis Sci.* 2015;56(2):875−882. https://doi.org/10.1167/iovs.14-14933.

28. Querques G, Georges A, Ben Moussa N, Sterkers M, Souied EH. Appearance of regressing drusen on optical coherence tomography in age-related macular degeneration. *Ophthalmology.* 2014;121(1):173−179. https://doi.org/10.1016/j.ophtha.2013.06.024.

29. Sato T, Kishi S, Watanabe G, Matsumoto H, Mukai R. Tomographic features of branching vascular networks in polypoidal choroidal vasculopathy. *Retina.* 2007;27(5):589−594. https://doi.org/10.1097/01.iae.0000249386.63482.05.

30. Shi Y, Motulsky EH, Goldhardt R, et al. Predictive value of the OCT double-layer sign for identifying subclinical neovascularization in age-related macular degeneration. *Ophthalmology*. 2019;3(3):211−219. https://doi.org/10.1016/j.oret.2018.10.012.

31. Lindblad AS, Lloyd PC, Clemons TE, et al. Change in area of geographic atrophy in the age-related eye disease study: AREDS report number 26. *Arch Ophthalmol*. 2009; 127(9):1168−1174. https://doi.org/10.1001/archophthalmol.2009.198.

32. Fleckenstein M, Schmitz-Valckenberg S, Adrion C, et al. Progression of age-related geographic atrophy: role of the fellow eye. *Invest Ophthalmol Vis Sci*. 2011;52(9): 6552−6557. https://doi.org/10.1167/iovs.11-7298.

33. Brader HS, Ying G-S, Martin ER, Maguire MG, Complications of Age-Related Macular Degeneration Prevention Trial (CAPT) Research Group. Characteristics of incident geographic atrophy in the complications of age-related macular degeneration prevention trial. *Ophthalmology*. 2013;120(9):1871−1879. https://doi.org/10.1016/j.ophtha.2013. 01.049.

34. Spaide RF, Jaffe GJ, Sarraf D, et al. Consensus nomenclature for reporting neovascular age-related macular degeneration data: consensus on neovascular age-related macular degeneration nomenclature study group. *Ophthalmology*. 2019. https://doi.org/ 10.1016/j.ophtha.2019.11.004.

35. Coscas F, Coscas G, Souied E, Tick S, Soubrane G. Optical coherence tomography identification of occult choroidal neovascularization in age-related macular degeneration. *Am J Ophthalmol*. 2007;144(4):592−599.e2. https://doi.org/10.1016/j.ajo.2007.06.014.

36. Wachtlin J, Stroux A, Wehner A, Heimann H, Foerster MH. Photodynamic therapy with verteporfin for choroidal neovascularisations in clinical routine outside the TAP study. One- and two-year results including juxtafoveal and extrafoveal CNV. *Graefes Arch Clin Exp Ophthalmol*. 2005;243(5):438−445. https://doi.org/10.1007/s00417-004-1071-z.

37. Mao J, Cheng D, Lin J, Chen Y, Lv Z, Shen L. Evaluating retinal angiomatous proliferation with optical coherence tomography angiography. *Ophthalmic Surg Lasers Imag Retina*. 2020;51(3):136−144. https://doi.org/10.3928/23258160-20200228-02.

38. Yanagi Y, Foo VHX, Yoshida A. Asian age-related macular degeneration: from basic science research perspective. *Eye*. 2019;33(1):34−49. https://doi.org/10.1038/s41433-018-0225-x.

39. Otani A, Sasahara M, Yodoi Y, et al. Indocyanine green angiography: guided photodynamic therapy for polypoidal choroidal vasculopathy. *Am J Ophthalmol*. 2007;144(1): 7−14.e1. https://doi.org/10.1016/j.ajo.2007.03.014.

40. Chung SE, Kang SW, Lee JH, Kim YT. Choroidal thickness in polypoidal choroidal vasculopathy and exudative age-related macular degeneration. *Ophthalmology*. 2011; 118(5):840−845. https://doi.org/10.1016/j.ophtha.2010.09.012.

41. Lin T-C, Hwang D-K, Lee F-L, Chen S-J. Visual prognosis of massive submacular hemorrhage in polypoidal choroidal vasculopathy with or without combination treatment. *J Chin Med Assoc*. 2016;79(3):159−165. https://doi.org/10.1016/j.jcma.2015.11.004.

42. Pang CE, Messinger JD, Zanzottera EC, Freund KB, Curcio CA. The onion sign in neovascular age-related macular degeneration represents cholesterol crystals. *Ophthalmology*. 2015;122(11):2316−2326. https://doi.org/10.1016/j.ophtha.2015.07.008.

43. Willoughby AS, Ying G, Toth CA, et al. Subretinal hyperreflective material in the comparison of age-related macular degeneration treatments trials. *Ophthalmology*. 2015; 122(9):1846−1853.e5. https://doi.org/10.1016/j.ophtha.2015.05.042.

Differential diagnosis of age-related macular degeneration

6

Drusen, pigmentary changes, retinochoroidal atrophy, and macular neovascularization are the most characteristic age-related macular degeneration (AMD)-like manifestations. Meanwhile, numerous fundus diseases may share these features. Therefore, in a real clinic, it is imperative to differentiate these fundus diseases in which there is considerable overlap with AMD manifestations. In the differential diagnosis of AMD, acquiring patients' age, family history, history of risk factors, and present medical history is always the prerequisite. Then, the imaging study and ancillary testing follow. In the multimodal imaging era, selective ancillary tests are needed in general, because the differentiated points among these diseases have been understood.

Differential diagnosis of dry AMD

Many conditions may mimic nonneovascular AMD, exemplified by pathologic myopia, pachychoroid spectrum diseases, macular dystrophies, hydroxychloroquine toxicity, and cancer-associated retinopathy.[1]

Pathologic myopia comprises multiple ocular tissue pathologies due to the elongation of the axial length of the eyeball (AXL). The fundus lesions of pathologic myopia may show several similarities to those of AMD. A myopic conus is an early change in the posterior fundus of highly myopic eyes. The mechanical expansion in the peri-papillary sclera results in a concentric depigmentation at para-papillary region, the so-called myopic conus (Fig. 6.1C). β-parapapillary atrophy (β-PPA) is a parapapillary region of visible large choroidal vessels and sclera caused by lacking of retinal pigment epithelium (RPE). β-PPA without Bruch's membrane (BrM), a subtype of β-PPA, is called PPA$_{-BM}$, that is, parapapillary γ zone. PPA$_{-BM}$ has been considered as a result of mechanical stretching in the peripapillary sclera and border tissues during axial elongation. Therefore, the existence of PPA$_{-BM}$, that is, γ zone may be a marker of the presence of high myopia.[3] A posterior staphyloma is an outward protrusion of all layers of the posterior eye globe. The age and the AXL have been found to be highly correlated with the development and progression of staphylomas.[4] The incidence of staphyloma is high in older people with pathologic myopia (96.7% in those > 50 years old). The simplified meta-analysis of pathologic myopia (META-PA) classification represents an evolution process from "dry"

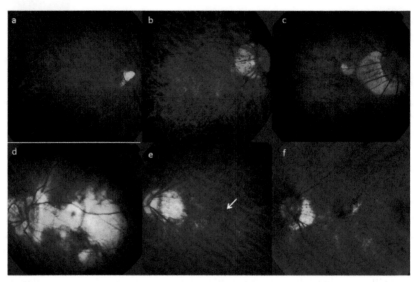

FIGURE 6.1

Myopic maculopathy classification according to META-PM study based on color fundus photographs. Category 1 maculopathy is characterized by a tessellated fundus, in which the outline of choroidal vessels is easily visible throughout the posterior pole (A) Category 2 maculopathy is characterized by diffuse chorioretinal atrophy, in which the posterior pole appears yellowish-white in appearance (B) Category 3 maculopathy is characterized by patchy chorioretinal atrophy (black arrowheads), which appears as well-defined, grayish-white lesions. In this photograph, inferior myopic conus exists (C) Category 4 is characterized by macular atrophy, which appears as a well-defined, round grayish-white chorioretinal atrophic lesion around a regressed fibrovascular membrane (D) Lacquer crake (*white arrow*) is one of the plus lesions and appears as a yellowish thick linear pattern (E) Fuchs spot (*black arrow*) is a pigmented spot representing the scarring phase of myopic choroidal neovascularization (F).

Modified from Ohno-Matsui K, Lai TYY, Lai C-C, Cheung CMG. Updates of pathologic myopia. Prog Retin Eye Res. *2016;52:156–187. doi: 10.1016/j.preteyeres.2015.12.001.*

pathologic myopia to "wet" pathologic myopia. The "dry" stages include tessellated fundus, diffuse chorioretinal atrophy, patchy chorioretinal atrophy, and macular atrophy (Fig. 6.1A–D).[2] The "wet stages" consist of lacquer cracks and myopic choroidal neovascularization (CNV) (Fig. 6.1E–F).[2] Based on the Singapore Indian Eye Study (2013), a population-based, cross-sectional study of Indians aged 40–84 years living in Singapore, there is the differential association between the prevalence of myopia and AMD.[5] Although high myopia shares overlapping fundus features with AMD, myopic eyes are less likely to have AMD. Therefore, these two diseases should be differentially diagnosed to be managed based on the underlying causes of each.

Pachychoroid disease is a spectrum of disorders that represent attenuation of the choriocapillaris, thickened choroid with dilated choroidal veins and functionally disturbed RPE homeostasis.[6,7] The following four disease groups are resided in this spectrum. First, pachychoroid pigment epitheliopathy (PPE) is a condition characterized by fundus autofluorescence (FAF) and OCT-detected RPE changes that occurred in the regions of choroidal thickening.[8] In the clinic, these changes had been observed in fellow eyes of patients with unilateral acute central serous chorioretinopathy (CSC). Therefore, the patients with PPE were frequently misdiagnosed as having inactive classic CSC, early AMD, pattern dystrophies, or inflammatory chorioretinopathies or retinal pigment epitheliitis.[9] PPE is usually asymptomatic. The pigmentary changes of PPE represent mottling pigmentation, isolated "drusenoid" RPE elevation viewed by OCT, and an absence of soft drusen. FAF shows mottled hypo- and hyper-autofluorescent areas correlated with foci of RPE thickening.[10] These multimodal imaging features are useful for differential diagnosis of PPE from AMD. Second, CSC is a common disease featured as serous retinal detachment with or without serous pigment epithelial detachment (PED) and in the presence or absence of thickened choroid (Fig. 6.2).[11] CSC may be misinterpreted as nonneovascular AMD, because it could produce RPE changes similar to those in AMD. CSC occurs mainly in young to middle-aged men. Typical manifestations include solitary and localized neurosensory retinal detachment and serous PEDs, which should be differentiated from AMD. FA demonstrates one or multiple focal leaks at the level of the RPE in "ink-blot" or "smoke-stack" patterns (Fig. 6.2C).[11,12] As spectral-domain optical coherence tomography (SD-OCT) becomes the primary modality for diagnosis and differential diagnosis of CSC, the OCT-measurable features of CSC have been summarized as follows: thinning of the choriocapillaris layer accompanied by thickened subfoveal choroid and dilated large choroidal vessels; serous PED with RPE hypertrophy and hypotrophy; elevated PED indicating leakage site; shaggy photoreceptors representing elongated photoreceptor outer segments; intraretinal hyperreflective deposits in OPL, ONL, external limiting membrane (ELM), and inner segment/outer segment (IS/OS) band. The chronic CSC may be associated with cystoid macular degeneration (Fig. 6.2).[11,12] The rest of the diseases in the pachychoroid spectrum, that is, pachychoroid neovasculopathy and polypoidal choroidal vasculopathy, will be discussed in the section of differential diagnosis of wet AMD vide infra.

Macular dystrophies are a group of genetic macular diseases that impair central vision. Some forms of macular dystrophy appear in childhood, and other forms appear in adulthood. Genetically, they are monogenic with specific inheritance patterns. Macular dystrophies have heterogeneous clinical presentations. In the differential diagnosis of AMD, only macular dystrophies with AMD-like features appearing in adulthood will be discussed. Pattern dystrophies of RPE present as various forms of reticular or butterfly-shaped pigmentary changes of macula. One of the forms is called butterfly-shaped pigment dystrophy of the fovea. The best imaging study for this pattern dystrophy is FAF that shows lesions with pigmented center surrounded by a depigmented zone at macula (Fig. 6.3).[13] It is caused by mutations in the *peripherin/RDS* gene, mostly with heterogeneous genotype.[13]

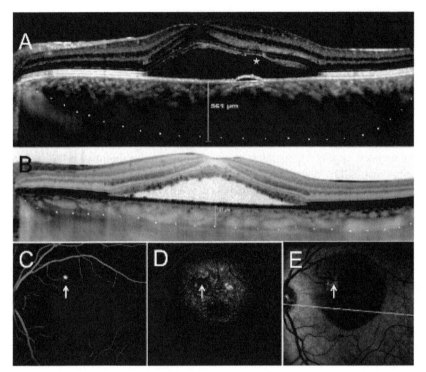

FIGURE 6.2

Acute CSC in two cases, with increased and normal choroidal thickness. (A) SD-OCT in a 32-year-old male patient with acute CSC showing increased choroidal thickness (measured subfoveally at 560 μm in green letters) and eroded photoreceptor outer segments over the leakage site (star), visible as a small pigment epithelial detachment. (B—E) SD-OCT of a 36-year old male patient with normal refractive status showing acute CSC and a subfoveal choroidal thickness within normal range (181 μm in green letters). The elongated photoreceptor outer segments showing the sign of "shaggy photoreceptors. At the leakage site evidenced by fluorescein angiography (*arrow*) (C), a diminished fundus autofluorescence (D) and a moderate increased infrared reflectance (E) indicated local RPE modifications. Autofluorescence was globally increased over the detached area due to the accumulation of autofluorescent material in outer segments.

Modified from Daruich A, Matet A, Dirani A, et al. Central serous chorioretinopathy: recent findings and new physiopathology hypothesis. Prog Retin Eye Res. 2015;48:82—118. doi: 10.1016/j.preteyeres.2015.05.003.

Adult-onset foveomacular vitelliform dystrophy (AFVD) is characterized by bilateral yellowish one or multiple macular lesions that are round and typically one-third disc diameter in size. When subfoveal lesions are large, they could be misdiagnosed as Best vitelliform macular dystrophy (BVMD) or AMD (Fig. 6.4A).[14] Using FA to examine AFVD shows a hypofluorescent center surrounded by a small hyperfluorescent ring. Some larger, less pigmented lesions

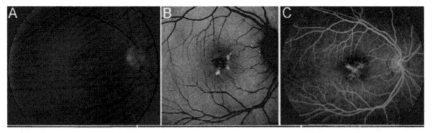

FIGURE 6.3

Pattern dystrophies caused by mutations in the peripherin/RDS gene. (A−C) Butterfly-shaped pigment dystrophy of the fovea. (A) Color fundus photograph of a 62-year-old patient carrying an Arg220fsX34 mutation in peripherin/RDS. A butterfly-shaped lesion is observed in the fovea, containing areas of increased and decreased pigmentation. On a fundus autofluorescence (FAF) image (B), some parts of the lesion display increased AF, whereas AF is decreased in other parts. (C) Fluorescein angiogram of the same patient. Hyperfluorescent areas correspond with the depigmentated areas at ophthalmoscopy, while hypofluorescent parts largely coincide with the pigmented parts of the lesion. The visual acuity in this patient was 20/20.

Modified from Boon CJF, den Hollander AI, Hoyng CB, Cremers FPM, Klevering BJ, Keunen JEE. The spectrum of retinal dystrophies caused by mutations in the peripherin/RDS gene. Prog Retin Eye Res. 2008;27(2): 213−235. doi: 10.1016/j.preteyeres.2008.01.002.

may show a central, patchy hyperfluorescence with late staining (Fig. 6.4B and C).[14] FAF shows lesions in AFVD are hyper-autofluorescent. On SD-OCT, lesions are located between the neuroretina and RPE, with a variable amount of hyperreflective material accumulated in the subretinal space (Fig. 6.4D and E). This material corresponds to the yellowish material seen on color fundus photographs (CFP). Unlike BVMD, AFVD presents as normal or near-normal EOG.[15] AFVD is associated with autosomal dominant inheritance with the most common mutations in the *PRPH2* gene.

Stargardt disease, a hereditary retinal dystrophy, is characterized with irregular yellowish flecks at macula. If the flecks are widely scattered throughout the fundus with central sparing, the condition is referred to as *fundus flavimaculatus*. Both Stargardt disease and *fundus flavimaculatus* are resulted from the mutation of the same genes. The most common one mutated is *ABCA4* gene. Based on longitudinal studies, the clinical presentation of Stargardt disease varies (Fig. 6.5).[16] In Fig. 6.5 (from left to right) paramacular yellowish flecks and "beaten-bronze" central macular atrophy are transformed into multiple patches of macular atrophy. In the process of diagnosis and differential diagnosis, the funduscopic findings require validation by FA showing "dark choroid" and FAF demonstrating elevated background autofluorescence, etc.[17]

There are numerous fundus disorders that may mimic dry AMD because of the presence of drusen, pigmentary changes, and macular atrophic lesions. In addition to the common conditions such as pathologic myopia, pachychoroid diseases, and

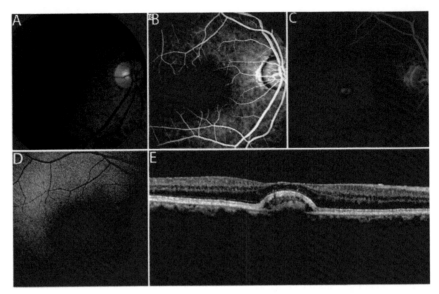

FIGURE 6.4

Multimodal imaging of adult-onset foveomacular vitelliform dystrophy. (A) Color fundus photograph showing a typical yellowish vitelliform foveal lesion; the size of the lesion is approximately one-fourth of the disc diameter. (B) Fluorescein angiogram showing blocked fluorescence in the foveal center surrounded by a transmission defect in the early phase of the angiogram. Several small drusen are also visible in the color (A) and early-phase fluorescein angiogram (B). (C) In the late phase of the angiogram, the lesion exhibits staining. (D and E) Fundus autofluorescence imaging reveals hyper-autofluorescence at the site of the vitelliform lesion (D), whereas OCT reveals a corresponding dome-shaped hyperreflective subretinal lesion (E).

Modified from Chowers I, Tiosano L, Audo I, Grunin M, Boon CJF. Adult-onset foveomacular vitelliform dystrophy: a fresh perspective. Prog Retin Eye Res. *2015;47:64–85. doi: 10.1016/j.preteyeres.2015.02.001.*

macular dystrophies, several other disorders are listed in Table 6.1 for the purpose of differential diagnosis.

Macular telangiectasia type 2, also called MacTel 2, belongs to a spectrum of idiopathic juxtafoveal telangiectatic disorders. MacTel 2, symptomatically similar to dry AMD progression, shows bilateral gradual loss of central vision, metamorphosia, positive scotoma, and reading difficulties (Fig. 6.6D and F). Multimodal imaging studies show the presence of pigmentary changes and abnormal telangiectatic vessels often at the temporal to macula (Fig. 6.6A and B). The features that help to differentiate MacTel 2 from AMD are as follows: onset at an earlier age; absence of drusen, abnormal foci limited to the parafovea and predominantly temporal to the fovea; depletion of macular pigment detected by FAF; and retinal thinning (usual no thickening) with loss of ELM and ellipsoid zone (EZ) by SD-OCT imaging (Fig. 6.6).[18]

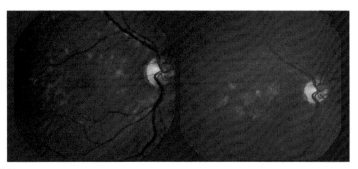

FIGURE 6.5

Longitudinal follow-up from 1997 to 2011 by fundus photographs of a representative case of Stargardt disease. Color fundus photographs show foveal mottling surrounded by confluent flecks at baseline (left) and multiple areas of macular atrophy at follow-up (right). The patient presented with clinically significant electrophysiologic deterioration.

Modified from Fujinami K, Lois N, Davidson AE, et al. A longitudinal study of stargardt disease: clinical and electrophysiologic assessment, progression, and genotype correlations. Am J Ophthalmol. *2013;155(6): 1075–1088.e13. doi: 10.1016/j.ajo.2013.01.018.*

Table 6.1 Differential diagnosis of non-neovascular AMD.

	Distinguished manifestations and data from ancillary tests
Pathologic myopia	Tessellated fundus, myopic conus, prominent β-PPA without BM (β-PPA$_{-BM}$), posterior staphyloma, chorioretinal atrophy, lacquer cracks in patients with high AXL
Pachychoroid spectrum diseases: Pachychoroid pigment epitheliopathy	In posterior pole, mottling pigmentation, isolated "drusenoid" RPE accumulation viewed by OCT, but absence of soft drusen, the pigmented foci frequently seen in fellow eyes of patients with unilateral acute CSC
Central serous chorioretinopathy	CSC occurring mainly in young to middle-aged men, CFP, FAF, and OCT showing solitary and localized neurosensory retinal detachment, serous PED, and shaggy photoreceptors
Macular dystrophies: Pattern dystrophy	Symmetrical, specific pattern- pigmentary changes of macula, best seen by FAF, confirmed by variants in *peripherin/RDS* gene
Vitelliform macular dystrophy	Central vitelliform lesion without surrounding drusen; autofluorescence changes within lesions; hyperreflective accumulation in subretinal space on SD-OCT, presenting in adulthood, confirmed by mutations in *PRPH2* gene

Continued

Table 6.1 Differential diagnosis of non-neovascular AMD.—*cont'd*

	Distinguished manifestations and data from ancillary tests
Stargardt disease	Paracentral yellowish flecks, central "beaten bronze" atrophy; "dark choroid" by FA; confirmed by mutations in *ABCA4* gene
Miscellaneous: MacTel 2	Bilateral juxtafoveal telangiectatic disorder, an earlier age at onset, no drusen, foci limited to the parafovea and temporal to the fovea; depletion of macular pigment, and retinal thinning with loss of outer retinal layers
Hydroxychloroquine toxicity	HCQ toxicity causing pigmentary abnormalities, presenting as bull's-eye retinopathy, OCT and FAF morphological tests and Humphry VF10-2 and multifocal ERG functional tests are complementary
Cancer-associated retinopathy	Visual disturbance, pigmentary changes, positive antiretina antibody, and ERG abnormalities in patients who may have a history of cancer
Myotonic dystrophy	DM1, an adult-onset hereditary, systemic disease, affecting retina with presentation of pattern pigmentary changes

Abbreviations: β-PPA, *β-parapapillary atrophy;* AXL, *axial length;* BM, *Bruch's membrane;* CFP, *color fundus photography;* CSC, *Central Serous Chorioretinopathy;* DM1, *myotonic dystrophy type 1;* ERG, *electroretinogram;* FAF, *fundus autofluorecence;* HCQ, *hydroxychloroquine;* MacTel 2, *Macular Telangiectasia type 2;* PED, *pigment epithelial detachment;* PPE, *Pachychoroid pigment epitheliopathy.*

Hydroxychloroquine (HCQ) possesses a low risk of retinal toxicity that increases dramatically only with a cumulative dose of >1000 g. HCQ toxicity targets ganglion cells and photoreceptors that probably secondary to the negative effect of HCQ on RPE cells.[19] HCQ toxicity causes pigmentary abnormalities or lipofuscin accumulation. The bull's-eye retinopathy and OCT characteristics expressed in HCQ toxicity may have similar imaging features as that identified with dry AMD (Fig. 6.7).[20]

Cancer-associated retinopathy (CAR) is another group of patients with pigmentary changes of the retina. CAR is the most common intraocular paraneoplastic syndrome. The average age of symptom onset in patients with CAR is ∼65 years. The Fundus examination in CAR varies from unremarkable to findings of optic nerve pallor, attenuated retinal arterioles, and RPE thinning and mottling in the disease course. In addition to RPE abnormalities, both CAR and AMD patients reside in the same age bracket. The accurate, timely diagnosis for CAR and differential diagnosis such as AMD may give a therapeutic opportunity to patients.[21] In the clinic, anti-retinal antibody testing and electroretinogram (ERG), are extremely helpful in establishing the diagnosis of CAR.

Myotonic dystrophy type 1 (DM1) is the most frequent adult-onset muscular dystrophy. DM1 is a multisystem disorder, which affects, besides the skeletal muscle,

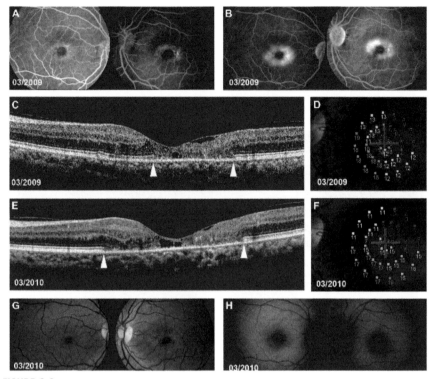

FIGURE 6.6

Clinically characteristic MacTel type 2 features. In fluorescein angiography (A and B), perifoveal blood vessels appear telangiectatic during early-stage (A) and leaky during late-stage (B) imaging. The optical coherence tomography (OCT) and microperimetry of the left eye in 2009 (C and D) and 2010 (E and F) show a loss of external limiting membrane (ELM) and break in the IS/OS (arrowheads) and loss of function predominantly in the temporal macula. Color fundus images (G) and autofluorescence (H) also were recorded.

Modified from Powner MB, Gillies MC, Zhu M, Vevis K, Hunyor AP, Fruttiger M. Loss of Müller's cells and photoreceptors in macular telangiectasia type 2. Ophthalmology. 2013;120(11):2344–2352. doi: 10.1016/ j.ophtha.2013.04.013.

other organs and tissues including the eye. The macular alterations in DM1 comprise reticular and butterfly-shaped pigmentary changes,[22] which share some similarities of retinal findings of nonneovascular AMD (Fig. 6.8).[23]

In summary, various degenerative and dystrophic diseases of the retina, with pigmentary abnormalities, lipofuscin accumulation, and chorioretinal atrophy, may have similar clinical features as dry AMD. Therefore, those conditions that may mimic dry AMD are listed in Table 6.1.

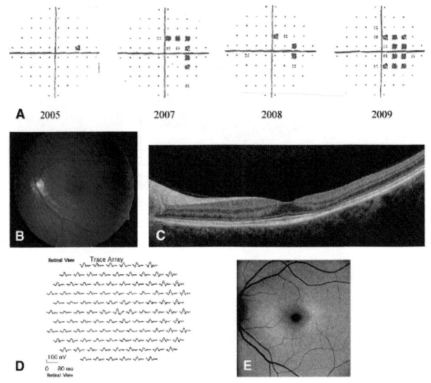

FIGURE 6.7

Case of HCQ toxicity illustrating the relative sensitivity of different screening tests. SD-OCT, mfERG, and FAF showed damage both nasally and temporally, although field loss was only nasal. The patient is a 48-year-old woman who took 400 mg HCQ/day (8 mg/kg) for most of 25 years. No visual symptoms. All images are from the left eye in 2009, except for visual fields. (A) Automated 10-2 visual fields from 2005 to 2009. From 2005 to 2008, the abnormalities were judged of no clinical significance. In 2009, nasal parafoveal scotomas were obvious, and she was referred to a specialist. (B) Fundus photograph (and retinal examination) shows no bull's-eye retinopathy. (C) Spectral domain-OCT shows parafoveal thinning of photoreceptor layers and loss of the inner-/outer-segment line. (D) Multifocal ERG trace array shows decreased parafoveal waveform amplitudes (confirmed by ring ratio analysis of amplitudes in the parafovea relative to other regions). (E) Fundus autofluorescence is increased in a bull's-eye pattern by FAF.

Modified from Marmor MF, Kellner U, Lai TYY, Lyons JS, Mieler WF. Revised recommendations on screening for chloroquine and hydroxychloroquine retinopathy. Ophthalmology. *2011;118(2):415–422. doi: 10.1016/ j.ophtha.2010.11.017.*

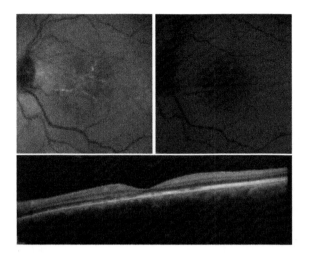

FIGURE 6.8

Myotonic dystrophy type 1 (DM1) with butterfly pattern dystrophy. Infrared imaging (IR), fundus autofluorescence (FAF) and SD-OCT of a patient with butterfly pattern dystrophy. The lesion was hyperreflective at IR (upper left) and hyperautofluorescent at FAF (upper right). (Bottom) SD-OCT shows a hyperreflective layer between the photoreceptor inner/ outer segments (IS/OS) junction and the retinal pigment epithelium, disruption of the IS/ OS junction and of the external limiting membrane (ELM), thinning of the outer nuclear layer (ONL) nasally to the fovea and accentuation of the foveal depression.

Modified from Abed E, D'Amico G, Rossi S, Perna A, Bianchi MLE, Silvestri G. Spectral domain optical coherence tomography findings in myotonic dystrophy. Neuromusc Disord. *2020;30(2):144–150. doi: 10.1016/j.nmd.2019.11.012.*

Differential diagnosis of neovascular AMD

Many conditions associated with disruption of the RPE/Bruch's membrane/chorio-capillaris complex may cause secondary CNV, which mimic those of neovascular AMD.

On the severe end of pachychoroid disease spectrum, clinical features could consist of leakage, exudation, and CNV. In CSC, subretinal fluid is frequently seen and easily confused with a sign of wet AMD. Contently, EDI-OCT (enhanced depth imaging OCT) reveals a thickened choroid in CSC and typically thin choroidal layer in AMD as described earlier.

Pachychoroid neovasculopathy (PNV) that resides in the spectrum of pachychoroid diseases is defined as the occurrence of type 1 (sub-RPE) choroidal neovascularization in eyes with PPE or CSC.[10] The differential diagnosis of AMD from PNV is a challenge. However, multimodal imaging techniques could facilitate this process. FAF displays pigmentary changes and the absence of drusen. ICGA shows dilated choroidal vessels and occult sub-RPE neovascular membrane. The proof-of-concept

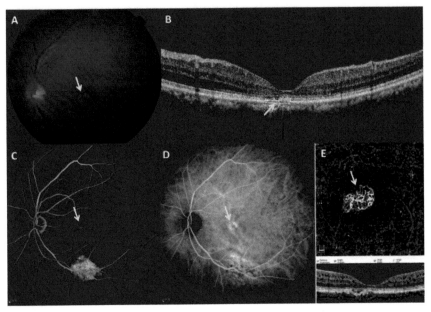

FIGURE 6.9

Multimodal images of the left eye of a 53-year-old man with pachychoroid neovasculopathy. Fundus photography (A) shows subretinal orange and yellow mass within the macula (arrowed). OCT (B) reveals a shallow irregular pigment epithelial detachment with moderate internal reflectivity (arrowed) and thickened choroid. FA (C) shows macular hyperfluorescence and mottled hyperfluorescence (*arrows*) and inferior hyperfluorescent area owing to RPE damage in central serous chorioretinopathy. Indocyanine green angiography (D) shows choroidal neovascularization at the macular region (arrowed) and inferior hyperfluorescent area. OCTA (E) shows the presence of new vessels with a shape of sparse tangled hyperreflective filamentous structures in the choriocapillaris region (arrowed).

Modified from Shen C, Zhang J, Tian J, Liu Y, Zhao H. Optical coherence tomography angiography for visualization of retinal capillary plexuses in pachychoroid neovasculopathy. Can J Ophthalmol. *2020. doi: 10.1016/j.jcjo.2020.09.016.*

features demonstrated by EDI-OCT and/or OCTA show shallow PED at the region of thicken choroid, which is differential evidences of PNV (Fig. 6.9).[24,25]

Polypoidal choroidal vasculopathy (PCV), an entity of pachychoroid disease spectrum as well as a variant of neovascular AMD, has distinct clinical features such as type 1 MNV in combination with thickened choroid and the absence of drusen. The diagnosis of PCV by multimodal imaging technique has been described in Chapter 5. In this section, the differential evidences of PCV from typical neovascular AMD are briefly summarized in Table 6.2 vide infra.

The frequency of lacquer cracks in pathologic myopic eyes is about 4.3%−15.5%. Lacquer crack is an important risk factor for myopic CNV development,[26] because

Table 6.2 Differential diagnosis of neovascular AMD.

	Distinguished manifestations and data from ancillary tests
Pachychoroid spectrum diseases	
Pachychoroid neovasculopathy	Type 1 MNV in eyes with PPE or CSC eyes, no or minimal drusen, OCT showing small SRF and shallow PED located at overlying thickened choroid
Polypoidal choroidal vasculopathy	Type 1 MNV common in Asian people, with thickened subfoveal choroid and without drusen, OCT signs including irregular PED, thick choroid and subretinal fluid, ICGA showing polyps.
Pathologic myopia	Lacquer cracks, myopic CNV, i.e., type 2 MNV, myopic macular retinoschisis
Angioid streaks	Gray or dark linear lesions radiating outwards for the peri-papillary area, with multiple systemic associations, complicated by CNV
Ocular histoplasmosis	Multiple macular "histo spots," peripapillary atrophy and absence of vitritis, complicated with different types of MNV
Toxoplasmic retinochoroiditis	A single focus of fluffy white retinitis, recurrent foci adjacent to old scar, severe vitritis, vasculitis, optic disc edema, occasionally complicated by CNV
Serpiginous-like choroiditis	Bilateral posterior uveitis starting around optic disc, recurrence is usually contiguous with or adjacent to existing lesions, resulting in extensive chorioretinal atrophy, complicated by CNV and subretinal fibrosis
Macular dystrophy Sorsby fundus dystrophy	Bilateral hereditary fundus dystrophy, in the early course (in 30s) at midperipheral numerous small to medium-sized drusen with symptoms of nyctalopia, in late course (in 50s) exudative maculopathy secondary to CNV at approximately 40 years of age
Acquired vitelliform lesions	AVLs caused by various etiologies such as vitelliform macular dystrophy and AMD, CNV is a common complication of AVLs, CNV develops when vitelliform lesions collapse, the subtype of CNV is type 1 MNV
Peripheral exudative hemorrhagic chorioretinopathy	Temporal peripheral exudative hemorrhagic elevated lesions, unlike PCV, PEHCR representing abnormal choroidal vascular network and polyp-like telangiectasia in periphery, best validated by wide-field ICGA
Traumatic CNV	Traumatic history of eye globe, particularly choroidal rupture, or excessive retinal laser therapy
Intraocular tumor-related CNV	Consideration about choroidal melanoma, choroidal nevus, choroidal hemangioma and metastatic tumors
Idiopathic CNV	Young patients with clinical features of CNV without primary ocular or systemic diseases, responding well to anti-VEGF

Abbreviations: anti-VEGF, *anti-vascular endothelium growth factor;* CSC, *Central Serous Chorioretinopathy;* hist, *histoplasmosis;* MNV, *macular neovascularization;* PCV, *Polypoidal choroidal vasculopathy;* PED, *pigment epithelial detachment;* PEHCR, *Peripheral exudative hemorrhagic chorioretinopathy;* PPE, *Pachychoroid pigment epitheliopathy;* SRF, *subretinal fluid.*

lacquer cracks represent ruptures in Bruch's membrane. Stretching of the tissue due to axial elongation appears to play an important role in the pathogenesis of lacquer cracks (Fig. 6.1E). In a longitudinal study, 13.3% of eyes with lacquer cracks develop myopic CNV, and 42.7% develop patchy chorioretinal atrophy.[27] Myopic CNV usually represents minimal subretinal fluid or exudative changes. The diagnosis of myopic CNV can be confirmed by FA and SD-OCT (Fig. 6.10).[28] FA findings in myopic CNV usually demonstrate well-defined hyperfluorescence in the early phase with leakage in the late phase in a classic CNV pattern of leakage (Fig. 6.10C and D).[28]

Angioid streaks represent discrete irregular breaks in Bruch's membrane (BrM) of eye, associated with calcified BrM and atrophic overlying RPE. 50% of patients with angioid streaks have a systemic disorder. There is a mnemonic **PEPSI**, which represents the major systemic associations of angioid streaks. First, pseudoxanthoma elasticum (**PXE**) is a hereditary connective tissue disease. The degenerative elastic fibers are seen in the skin, cardiovascular system, and most commonly, the angioid streaks in the eye (Fig. 6.11).[29] The blinding complication of PXE is the development of CNV.[29] Second, **E**hler-Danlos syndrome (EDS) is a rare, autosomal dominant collagen disorder. Only the subtype of ocular scoliotic EDS is associated with angioid streaks.[30] Angioid streaks occur in about 2% among patients with EDS. Third, **P**aget disease is a chronic, progressive bone disease, in which excessive metabolism of resorption and formation of bone is characteristic. Fourth, **s**ickle cell disease and other hemoglobinopathies occasionally associated with angioid streaks, followed by **i**diopathic and miscellaneous associations.

Ocular histoplasmosis is considered as a fungal uveitis that follows inhalation of *Histoplasma capsulatum* (*H. capsulatum*). Pulmonary involvement is the most common feature of this infection. Based on epidemiology studies, *H. capsulatum* has been implicated as the infectious etiology by positive skin antigen testing, but has not been established as a direct pathogen with certainty. Therefore, ocular histoplasmosis is also called presumed ocular histoplasmosis syndrome (POHS). POHS is usually asymptomatic unless macular CNV is developed. The classic triad of fundus features includes multiple white atrophic chorioretinal "histo spots" of 200 µm in size (Fig. 6.12. Top left); peripapillary atrophy and usually absence of vitritis. CNV occurs in less than 5% of affected eyes. CNV is frequently seen in association with previous macular histo spots. Subretinal fluid, hemorrhage, and fibrovascular membrane complicated with macular neovascularization, which could be type 1, 2, or 3 MNV, cause decreased vision of the affected eyes (Fig. 6.12 top, middle, and bottom OCT rows).[31]

Toxoplasmic retinochoroiditis (TRC) is the most common cause of posterior segment uveitis.[32] The pathogen, Toxoplasma gondii, is an obligate, intracellular parasitic protozoan. The clinical signs of active TRC comprise focal necrotizing retinochoroiditis with moderate to severe vitritis (Fig. 6.13A and B). Recurrent disease is indicated by an adjacent retinochroidal scar. SD-OCT shows thickened inner layers of retina (Fig. 6.13C). CNV could be a late complication of toxoplasmic retinochoroiditis based on a handful cohort studies (Fig. 6.14).[33]

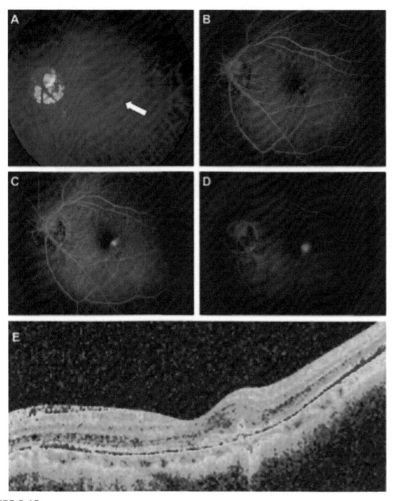

FIGURE 6.10

Clinical features of a typical choroidal neovascularization secondary to pathological myopia. (A) Color fundus photograph of the left eye showing greyish lesion (arrow) with negligible exudation; (B) Early phase of fluorescein angiogram showing a tiny well-defined hyperfluorescence with minimal leakage in late phases (C and D) typical of myopic CNV; (E) Optical coherence tomography showing hyper-reflective lesion corresponding to myopic CNV located above the retinal pigment epithelial cell layer (Type 2 CNV).

Modified from Neelam K, Cheung CMG, Ohno-Matsui K, Lai TYY, Wong TY. Choroidal neovascularization in pathological myopia. Prog Retin Eye Res. 2012;31(5):495–525. doi: 10.1016/j.preteyeres.2012.04.001.

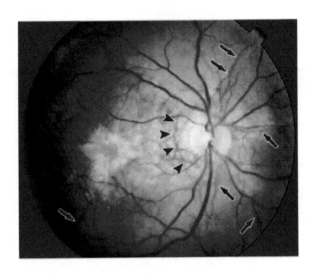

FIGURE 6.11

Angioid streaks in the right fundus of a 47-year-old man with pseudoxanthoma elasticum. Arrows point to broad streaks, resembling larger vessels. On the left side of the disk arrowheads indicate more circumferential smaller streaks. There is a scar in the fovea leading to enhanced visibility of the luteal pigmentation. On its left are hemorrhages from a choroidal neovascularization.

Modified from Hu X, Plomp AS, van Soest S, Wijnholds J, de Jong PTVM, Bergen AAB. Pseudoxanthoma elasticum: a clinical, histopathological, and molecular update. Surv Ophthalmol. *2003;48(4):424–438. doi: 10.1016/S0039-6257(03)00053-5.*

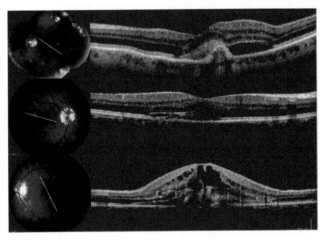

FIGURE 6.12

SD-OCT features of choroidal neovascularization in POHS. 1. Sub-RPE choroidal neovascularization: The hyperreflective band corresponding to the RPE appears elevated (type 1 MNV in upper panel). 2. Subretinal choroidal neovascularization: There is an accumulation of fluid between the ellipsoid zone and RPE hyperreflective bands (type 2 MNV in middle panel). 3. Retinal angiomatous choroidal neovascularization: The RPE hyperreflective band is elevated and intraretinal fluid is present, as well as fluid occupying the subretinal space (type 3 MNV in bottom panel).

Modified from Diaz RI, Sigler EJ, Rafieetary MR, Calzada JI. Ocular histoplasmosis syndrome. Surv Ophthalmol. *2015;60(4):279–295. doi: 10.1016/j.survophthal.2015.02.005.*

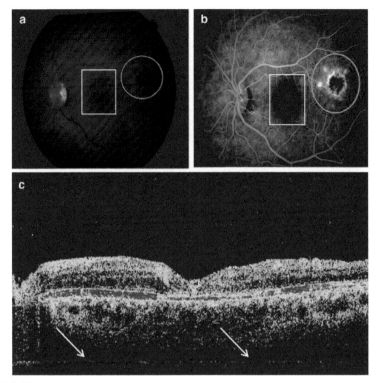

FIGURE 6.13

Images of a Brazilian patient with toxoplasmic retinochoroiditis. (a) Fundus photography showing a satellite lesion (*yellow square*) of activity suggestive of retinochoroiditis toxoplasmosis in the macula region and a healed retinochoroiditis lesion (*blue circle*); (b) FA showing a satellite lesion suggestive of activity of toxoplasmosis (*yellow rectangle*) in the macula region and a healed retinochoroiditis lesion (*blue circle*); (c) increases in the thickness of the inner retinal layers in perimacular regions (*arrows*) seen by optical coherence tomography.

Modified from Previato M, Frederico FB, Murata FHA, et al. A Brazilian report using serological and molecular diagnosis to monitoring acute ocular toxoplasmosis. BMC Res Notes. *2015;8:746. doi: 10.1186/s13104-015-1650-6.*

Serpiginous choroiditis (SC) is a recurrent posterior uveitis involving outer retina (RPE) and inner choroid (choriocapillaris) with unknown etiology. With numerous recurrences, serpiginous chorioretinal lesions heal and extend centrifugally around the center of optic nerve head to macula (Fig. 6.15 top left and right). In Fig. 6.15 (top right), the scaring lesion after recurrences is seen on the temporal to the disc, while an active grey-white, fluffy lesion with subretinal hemorrhage at inferior margin is observed at the nasal to the disc. FA shows type 2 MNV in Fig. 6.15 (middle right, bottom left, and right). In the angiographic transit from the middle to late

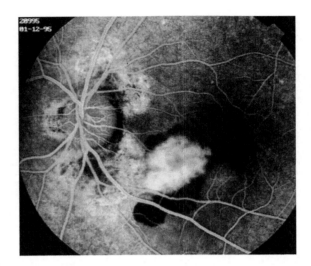

FIGURE 6.14

FA showing hyperfluorescence in choroidal neovascularization secondary to toxoplasmic retinochoroiditis.

Modified from Atmaca LS, Simsek T, Batioglu F. Clinical features and prognosis in ocular toxoplasmosis. Jpn J Ophthalmol. 2004;48(4):386–391. doi: 10.1007/s10384-003-0069-0.

phase, the hyperfluorecent area and intensity are gradually increasing at the nasal to the disc, documenting CNV.[34]

Sorsby fundus dystrophy (SFD) is a subtype of macular dystrophy that mimics neovascular AMD because of its exudative nature. SFD has autosomal dominant inheritance with allelic variation in the gene *TIMP3*. Early presentation is in the third decade with yellow small to medium-sized drusen-like deposits along the vascular arcades and midperiphery (Fig. 6.16 left and middle). In the fifth decade, an exudative maculopathy secondary to CNV may be developed (Fig. 6.16 right), leading to severe loss of vision.[35]

Acquired vitelliform lesion (AVL) is an umbrella term describing yellowish subretinal material accumulation caused by multiple etiologies such as adult-onset foveomacular vitelliform dystrophy (AFVD), basal laminar or cuticular drusen, pattern dystrophy, chronic CSC, macular vitreous traction, and AMD.[36] The major reason for vision impairment in patients with AVLs is either CNV or foveal atrophy, in which the foveal atrophy is a stronger determiner. Based on the study of the growth and resorption cycle of AVLs, AVLs associated with AMD have a higher chance of CNV development than that with AFVD. Whereas CNV develops most commonly when vitelliform lesions collapse or resorb. Therefore, the collapse of vitelliform lesions is a predictor for CNV development. The common subtype of CNV associated with AVLs is type 1 MNV (Fig. 6.17).[37]

Peripheral exudative hemorrhagic chorioretinopathy (PEHCR) is a bilateral, temporal peripheral fundus disease with unknown etiology. The CFP and ICGA

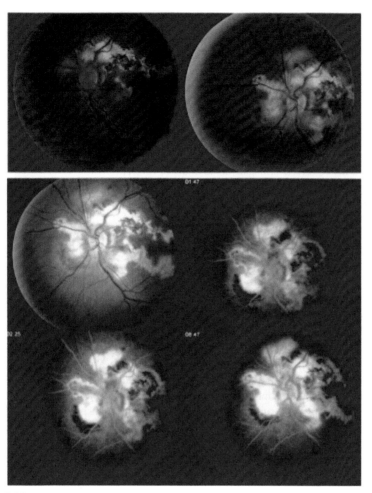

FIGURE 6.15

Top: Fundus photography showing development of choroidal neovascular lesion (arrow). Bottom (2 rows): Fundus fed-free photography and fluorescein angiography of choroidal neovascularization secondary to serpiginous choroiditis.

Modified from Lim W-K, Buggage RR, Nussenblatt RB. Serpiginous Choroiditis. Survey of Ophthalmology. *2005; 50(3):231-244. doi:10.1016/j.survophthal.2005.02.010.*

findings of PEHCR show abnormal choroidal vascular network and polyp-like telangiectatic lesions, but no evident CNV in the periphery (Fig. 6.18).[38,39,40] In contrast to PEHCR, PCV demonstrates abnormal choroidal vascular network and polyp-like CNV in the posterior fundus. Thus, there is a comment that PEHCR could be a peripheral variant of exudative AMD.[41] Nevertheless, the extensive exudate and hemorrhage of PEHCR require a differential diagnosis from exudative AMD, particularly PCV and choroidal melanoma.[38,39]

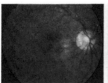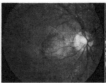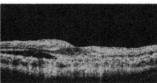

FIGURE 6.16

Color Fundus photographs showing CNV in Sorsby fundus dystrophy. (Left) Extrafoveal CNV. (Right) Subfoveal extension of the membrane. SD-OCT showing subretinal fluid in another patient with CNV secondary to Sorsby fundus dystrophy. The subretinal fluid was visualized before clinical or angiographic evidence of CNV.

Modified from Sivaprasad S, Webster AR, Egan CA, Bird AC, Tufail A. Clinical course and treatment outcomes of sorsby fundus dystrophy. Am J Ophthalmol. 2008;146(2):228–234.e2. doi: 10.1016/j.ajo.2008.03.024.

Traumatic choroidal neovascularization

Traumatic CNV occurs in patients (5%—10%) with choroidal rupture following severe blunt ocular injuries (Fig. 6.19).[42] In a large 5-year cohort study, patients with traumatic CNV secondary to choroidal rupture were treated with intravitreal anti-VEGF therapy. The treatment is safe and effective for CNV regression. Compared to neovascular AMD fewer injections are needed to control this disease.[43]

Intraocular tumor-related CNV

As described earlier, various lesions located in the macular region can mimic neovascular AMD, making challenges in establishing a proper diagnosis. In the retinal clinic, the most significant challenge is a differential diagnosis of AMD with posterior pole tumors including choroidal melanoma, choroidal nevus, choroidal hemangioma, and metastatic tumors. The diagnosis and differential diagnosis of intraocular tumors may be referred to the extensive reviews by Shields et al.[39,44,45]

Idiopathic choroidal neovascularization

Idiopathic choroidal neovascularization (ICNV) was characterized by a solitary focus of subretinal neovascularization at or near the fovea in.[46] Although this kind of lesion simulates the neovascular membrane seen in the presumed ocular histoplasmosis syndrome, no apparent primary ocular or systemic diseases can be detected. It had been reported that the disease was self-limited over a variable period of time, but may result in extensive scarring with loss of central vision before anti-VEGF therapy emerged. Nowadays, intravitreal anti-VEGF treatment can improve the visual outcome of patients with ICNV.[46,47]

The conditions associated with CNV may be categorized for differential diagnosis of neovascular AMD based on etiology (Table 6.2). CNV may masquerade as degenerative diseases such as pathologic myopia, angioid streaks, and peripheral exudative hemorrhagic chorioretinopathy; heredo-degenerative diseases, for example, macular dystrophy and vitelliform maculopathy; inflammatory diseases such as ocular histoplasmosis syndrome, toxoplasmic retinochoroiditis, and serpiginous choroiditis; traumatic CNV; Intraocular tumor-related CNV and idiopathic CNV.

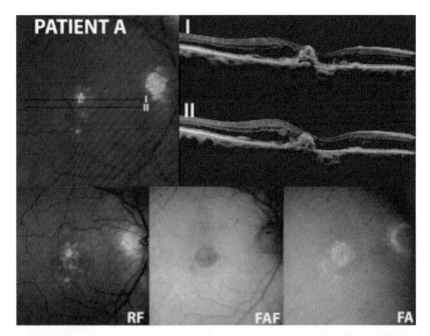

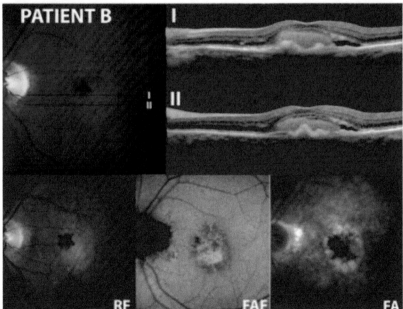

FIGURE 6.17

CNV in acquired vitelliform lesions (AVLs) in two patients. Ophthalmoscopic, OCT, red-free, fundus autofluorescence (FAF), and fluorescein angiogram findings of neovascularization that developed after resorption of an AVL (Patient A) and during the presence of an AVL (Patient B).

Modified from Balaratnasingam C, Hoang QV, Inoue M, et al. Clinical characteristics, choroidal neo-vascularization, and predictors of visual outcomes in acquired vitelliform lesions. Am J Ophthalmol. 2016;172: 28–38. doi: 10.1016/j.ajo.2016.09.008.

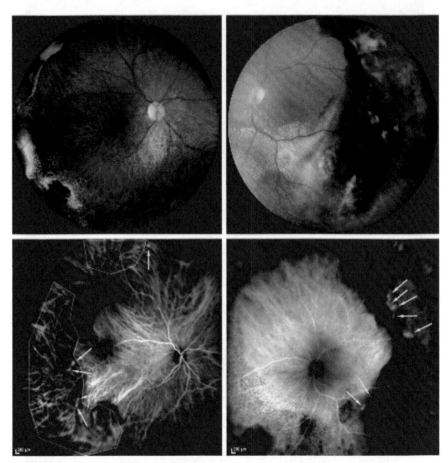

FIGURE 6.18

Extensive abnormal choroidal vascular network and numerous peripheral polyp-like choroidal telangiectasis in a patient with bilateral PEHCR. (Top left) Right eye with peripheral fibrosis in the temporal superior quadrant and hemorrhagic and lipid exudation in the temporal inferior quadrant. (Top right) Left eye with extensive serosanguineous exudation and hemorrhage in the temporal and inferior quadrants. (Bottom left) Wide-field ICGA of the right eye at 3 min revealed 2 areas of abnormal choroidal vascular networks (line), associated with 5 polyp-like telangiectatic lesions (*arrows*) at the border. (Bottom right) ICGA revealed 7 polyp-like lesions (*arrows*) in the left eye, seen only on the late frames (image shown: 14 min) because of partial masking by the subretinal hemorrhage. In both eyes, no evident CNV was found.

Modified from Mantel I, Schalenbourg A, Zografos L. Peripheral exudative hemorrhagic chorioretinopathy: pol-ypoidal choroidal vasculopathy and hemodynamic modifications. Am J Ophthalmol. *2012;153(5):910–922.e2.*

doi: 10.1016/j.ajo.2011.10.017.

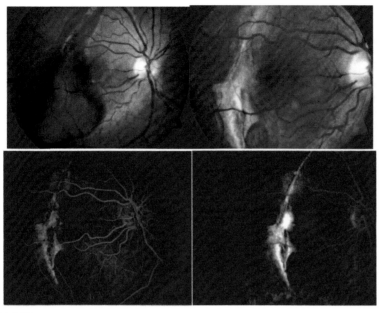

FIGURE 6.19

Color fundus photography of right eye a 28-year-old male who had severe blunt eye trauma, the initial presentation showing choroidal rupture temporal to the fovea and subretinal hemorrhage with macular involvement (top left); After 3 months, juxtafoveal lesion in the choroidal rupture area with subretinal fluid and fibrosis, corresponding to CNV (top right); Fluorescein angiography showing leakage at early phase (bottom left) and sustained exudation of the lesion in late phase (bottom right), demonstrating CNV.

Modified from Valldeperas X, Bonilla R, Romano MR, de la Cámara J. Use of intravitreal bevacizumab for the treatment of choroidal neovascularization secondary to choroidal rupture. Arch Soc Esp Oftalmol. *2011;86(11): 380—383. doi: 10.1016/j.oftal.2011.05.019.*

References

1. Garrity ST, Sarraf D, Freund KB, Sadda SR. Multimodal imaging of nonneovascular age-related macular degeneration. *Invest Ophthalmol Vis Sci.* 2018;59(4):AMD48. https://doi.org/10.1167/iovs.18-24158.
2. Ohno-Matsui K, Lai TYY, Lai C-C, Cheung CMG. Updates of pathologic myopia. *Prog Retin Eye Res.* 2016;52:156—187. https://doi.org/10.1016/j.preteyeres.2015.12.001.
3. Sung MS, Heo H, Piao H, Guo Y, Park SW. Parapapillary atrophy and changes in the optic nerve head and posterior pole in high myopia. *Sci Rep.* 2020;10(1):4607. https://doi.org/10.1038/s41598-020-61485-2.
4. Gözüm N, Cakir M, Gücukoglu A, Sezen F. Relationship between retinal lesions and axial length, age and sex in high myopia. *Eur J Ophthalmol.* 1997;7(3):277—282.

5. Pan C-W, Cheung CY, Aung T, et al. Differential associations of myopia with major age-related eye diseases. *Ophthalmology*. 2013;120(2):284—291. https://doi.org/10.1016/j.ophtha.2012.07.065.
6. Cheung CMG, Lee WK, Koizumi H, Dansingani K, Lai TYY, Freund KB. Pachychoroid disease. *Eye*. 2019;33(1):14—33. https://doi.org/10.1038/s41433-018-0158-4.
7. Akkaya S. Spectrum of pachychoroid diseases. *Int Ophthalmol*. 2018;38(5):2239—2246. https://doi.org/10.1007/s10792-017-0666-4.
8. Warrow DJ, Hoang QV, Freund KB. Pachychoroid pigment epitheliopathy. *Retina*. 2013; 33(8):1659—1672. https://doi.org/10.1097/IAE.0b013e3182953df4.
9. Pang CE, Freund KB. Pachychoroid pigment epitheliopathy may masquerade as acute retinal pigment epitheliitis. *Invest Ophthalmol Vis Sci*. 2014;55(8):5252. https://doi.org/10.1167/iovs.14-14959.
10. Dansingani KK, Balaratnasingam C, Naysan J, Freund KB. En face imaging of pachychoroid spectrum disorders with swept-source optical coherence tomography. *Retina*. 2016;36(3):499—516. https://doi.org/10.1097/IAE.0000000000000742.
11. Daruich A, Matet A, Dirani A, et al. Central serous chorioretinopathy: recent findings and new physiopathology hypothesis. *Prog Retin Eye Res*. 2015;48:82—118. https://doi.org/10.1016/j.preteyeres.2015.05.003.
12. Matsumoto H, Kishi S, Otani T, Sato T. Elongation of photoreceptor outer segment in central serous chorioretinopathy. *Am J Ophthalmol*. 2008;145(1):162—168. https://doi.org/10.1016/j.ajo.2007.08.024.
13. Boon CJF, den Hollander AI, Hoyng CB, Cremers FPM, Klevering BJ, Keunen JEE. The spectrum of retinal dystrophies caused by mutations in the peripherin/RDS gene. *Prog Retin Eye Res*. 2008;27(2):213—235. https://doi.org/10.1016/j.preteyeres.2008.01.002.
14. Chowers I, Tiosano L, Audo I, Grunin M, Boon CJF. Adult-onset foveomacular vitelliform dystrophy: a fresh perspective. *Prog Retin Eye Res*. 2015;47:64—85. https://doi.org/10.1016/j.preteyeres.2015.02.001.
15. Spaide RF, Noble K, Morgan A, Freund KB. Vitelliform macular dystrophy. *Ophthalmology*. 2006;113(8):1392—1400. https://doi.org/10.1016/j.ophtha.2006.03.023.
16. Fujinami K, Lois N, Davidson AE, et al. A longitudinal study of stargardt disease: clinical and electrophysiologic assessment, progression, and genotype correlations. *Am J Ophthalmol*. 2013;155(6):1075—1088.e13. https://doi.org/10.1016/j.ajo.2013.01.018.
17. Saksens NTM, Fleckenstein M, Schmitz-Valckenberg S, et al. Macular dystrophies mimicking age-related macular degeneration. *Prog Retin Eye Res*. 2014;39:23—57. https://doi.org/10.1016/j.preteyeres.2013.11.001.
18. Powner MB, Gillies MC, Zhu M, Vevis K, Hunyor AP, Fruttiger M. Loss of Müller's cells and photoreceptors in macular telangiectasia type 2. *Ophthalmology*. 2013;120(11): 2344—2352. https://doi.org/10.1016/j.ophtha.2013.04.013.
19. Rodriguez-Padilla JA, Hedges TR, Monson B, et al. High-speed ultra-high-resolution optical coherence tomography findings in hydroxychloroquine retinopathy. *Arch Ophthalmol*. 2007;125(6):775—780. https://doi.org/10.1001/archopht.125.6.775.
20. Marmor MF, Kellner U, Lai TYY, Lyons JS, Mieler WF. Revised recommendations on screening for chloroquine and hydroxychloroquine retinopathy. *Ophthalmology*. 2011; 118(2):415—422. https://doi.org/10.1016/j.ophtha.2010.11.017.
21. Rahimy E, Sarraf D. Paraneoplastic and non-paraneoplastic retinopathy and optic neuropathy: evaluation and management. *Surv Ophthalmol*. 2013;58(5):430—458. https://doi.org/10.1016/j.survophthal.2012.09.001.
22. Kimizuka Y, Kiyosawa M, Tamai M, Takase S. Retinal changes in myotonic dystrophy. *Clinical and follow-up evaluation*. Retina (Philadelphia, Pa). 1993;13(2):129—135.

23. Abed E, D'Amico G, Rossi S, Perna A, Bianchi MLE, Silvestri G. Spectral domain optical coherence tomography findings in myotonic dystrophy. *Neuromusc Disord.* 2020; 30(2):144–150. https://doi.org/10.1016/j.nmd.2019.11.012.

24. Shen C, Zhang J, Tian J, Liu Y, Zhao H. Optical coherence tomography angiography for visualization of retinal capillary plexuses in pachychoroid neovasculopathy. *Can J Ophthalmol.* 2020. https://doi.org/10.1016/j.jcjo.2020.09.016.

25. Amaro MH, Matos Junior RB. Pachychoroid neovasculopathy in a male patient: a case report. *Arq Bras Oftalmol.* 2015;78(6):385–387. https://doi.org/10.5935/0004-2749.2015 0102.

26. Kang HM, Koh HJ. Ocular risk factors for recurrence of myopic choroidal neovascularization: long-term follow-up study. *Retina.* 2013;33(8):1613–1622. https://doi.org/ 10.1097/IAE.0b013e318285cc24.

27. Hayashi K, Ohno-Matsui K, Shimada N, et al. Long-term pattern of progression of myopic maculopathy: a natural history study. *Ophthalmology.* 2010;117(8). https:// doi.org/10.1016/j.ophtha.2009.11.003, 1595–1611, 1611.e1-4.

28. Neelam K, Cheung CMG, Ohno-Matsui K, Lai TYY, Wong TY. Choroidal neovascularization in pathological myopia. *Prog Retin Eye Res.* 2012;31(5):495–525. https:// doi.org/10.1016/j.preteyeres.2012.04.001.

29. Hu X, Plomp AS, van Soest S, Wijnholds J, de Jong PTVM, Bergen AAB. Pseudoxanthoma elasticum: a clinical, histopathological, and molecular update. *Surv Ophthalmol.* 2003;48(4):424–438. https://doi.org/10.1016/S0039-6257(03)00053-5.

30. Malfait F, Francomano C, Byers P, et al. The 2017 international classification of the Ehlers-Danlos syndromes. *Am J Med Genet C Semin Med Genet.* 2017;175(1):8–26. https://doi.org/10.1002/ajmg.c.31552.

31. Diaz RI, Sigler EJ, Rafieetary MR, Calzada JI. Ocular histoplasmosis syndrome. *Surv Ophthalmol.* 2015;60(4):279–295. https://doi.org/10.1016/j.survophthal.2015.02.005.

32. Previato M, Frederico FB, Murata FHA, et al. A Brazilian report using serological and molecular diagnosis to monitoring acute ocular toxoplasmosis. *BMC Res Notes.* 2015;8: 746. https://doi.org/10.1186/s13104-015-1650-6.

33. Atmaca LS, Simsek T, Batioglu F. Clinical features and prognosis in ocular toxoplasmosis. *Jpn J Ophthalmol.* 2004;48(4):386–391. https://doi.org/10.1007/ s10384-003-0069-0.

34. Lim W-K, Buggage RR, Nussenblatt RB. Serpiginous choroiditis. *Surv Ophthalmol.* 2005;50(3):231–244. https://doi.org/10.1016/j.survophthal.2005.02.010.

35. Sivaprasad S, Webster AR, Egan CA, Bird AC, Tufail A. Clinical course and treatment outcomes of sorsby fundus dystrophy. *Am J Ophthalmol.* 2008;146(2):228–234.e2. https://doi.org/10.1016/j.ajo.2008.03.024.

36. Saito M, Iida T, Freund KB, Kano M, Yannuzzi LA. Clinical findings of acquired vitelliform lesions associated with retinal pigment epithelial detachments. *Am J Ophthalmol.* 2014;157(2):355–365.e2. https://doi.org/10.1016/j.ajo.2013.10.009.

37. Balaratnasingam C, Hoang QV, Inoue M, et al. Clinical characteristics, choroidal neovascularization, and predictors of visual outcomes in acquired vitelliform lesions. *Am J Ophthalmol.* 2016;172:28–38. https://doi.org/10.1016/j.ajo.2016.09.008.

38. Mantel I, Schalenbourg A, Zografos L. Peripheral exudative hemorrhagic chorioretinopathy: polypoidal choroidal vasculopathy and hemodynamic modifications. *Am J Ophthalmol.* 2012;153(5):910–922.e2. https://doi.org/10.1016/j.ajo.2011.10.017.

39. Shields CL, Salazar PF, Mashayekhi A, Shields JA. Peripheral exudative hemorrhagic chorioretinopathy simulating choroidal melanoma in 173 eyes. *Ophthalmology.* 2009; 116(3):529–535. https://doi.org/10.1016/j.ophtha.2008.10.015.

40. Mantel I, Uffer S, Zografos L. Peripheral exudative hemorrhagic chorioretinopathy: a clinical, angiographic, and histologic study. *Am J Ophthalmol.* 2009;148(6): 932–938.e1. https://doi.org/10.1016/j.ajo.2009.06.032.

41. Mashayekhi A, Shields CL, Shields JA. Peripheral exudative hemorrhagic chorioretinopathy: a variant of polypoidal choroidal vasculopathy? *J Ophthalmic Vis Res.* 2013;8(3): 264–267.

42. Valldeperas X, Bonilla R, Romano MR, de la Cámara J. Use of intravitreal bevacizumab for the treatment of choroidal neovascularization secondary to choroidal rupture. *Arch Soc Esp Oftalmol.* 2011;86(11):380–383. https://doi.org/10.1016/j.oftal.2011.05.019.

43. Barth T, Zeman F, Helbig H, Gamulescu M-A. Intravitreal anti-VEGF treatment for choroidal neovascularization secondary to traumatic choroidal rupture. *BMC Ophthalmol.* 2019;19(1):239. https://doi.org/10.1186/s12886-019-1242-7.

44. Shields CL, Furuta M, Berman EL, et al. Choroidal nevus transformation into melanoma: analysis of 2514 consecutive cases. *Arch Ophthalmol.* 2009;127(8):981–987. https://doi.org/10.1001/archophthalmol.2009.151.

45. Shields CL, Kaliki S, Rojanaporn D, Ferenczy SR, Shields JA. Enhanced depth imaging optical coherence tomography of small choroidal melanoma: comparison with choroidal nevus. *Arch Ophthalmol.* 2012;130(7):850–856. https://doi.org/10.1001/archophthalmol.2012.1135.

46. Cleasby GW. Idiopathic focal subretinal neovascularization. *Am J Ophthalmol.* 1976; 81(5):590–599. https://doi.org/10.1016/0002-9394(76)90121-5.

47. Carneiro AM, Silva RM, Veludo MJ, et al. Ranibizumab treatment for choroidal neovascularization from causes other than age-related macular degeneration and pathological myopia. *Ophthalmologica.* 2011;225(2):81–88. https://doi.org/10.1159/000317908.

Pathogenesis of age-related macular degeneration

Pathophysiology of macular neurovascular complex in AMD

The pathophysiologic process of age-related macular degeneration (AMD) primarily plays out in photoreceptor/RPE/Bruch's membrane/choriocapillaris (PR/RPE/BrM/CC) complex in the macular region. In this complex, retinal pigment epithelium (RPE), the central component, is a neuro-epithelial monolayer that acts as a metabolic interface between the choroid and the neurosensory retina.[1] The RPE cells are connected by tight intercellular junctions, forming the outer blood−retina barrier. On the apical side, the photoreceptor cells line the RPE with interdigitated microvilli. RPE cell density consistently decreases with eccentricity from the fovea. The mean ratio of the cone-to-RPE cell decreases from 16.6 at the foveal center to less than 5 at 1 mm off the center.[2] On the basal side, the BrM separates the basement membrane of the RPE from the choroidal microvasculature, that is, CC. CC is fenestrated and not surrounded by continuous pericytes or smooth muscle cells. The BrM consists of the inner and outer collagenous layers with an elastic layer between them.[3] The basement membranes of the CC endothelium and the RPE epithelium are classified as part of the BrM. Embedded in the BrM are macromolecules such as proteins and proteoglycans to help in remodeling the extracellular matrix. Because all components of this complex interact with each other, the PR/RPE/BrM/CC complex has been termed the macular neurovascular complex (MNC) in Chapter 1. The central neural function of the MNC is phototransduction by photoreceptors, interneurons, glial cells, and RPE cells. To achieve phototransduction, CC provides fuel and RPE regulates the reciprocal exchange of oxygen, nutrients, biomolecules, and metabolic waste products between the circulation and retina. RPE provides critical support for both PR and the CC because RPE coupling of the activities of neurons and Muller cells to the choroidal blood flow serves as the structural and functional barrier between this part of the central nervous system, that is, the neurosensory retina, and the peripheral choroidal circulation.[4]

Pathobiology of the MNC is associated with AMD development and progression, specifically, drusen formation, RPE hyperpigmentation,[5] RPE atrophy, PR degeneration, BrM thickening, and CC angiogenesis. In attempting to elucidate the underlying pathobiologic mechanisms, increased oxidative stress, mitochondrial destabilization, complement dysregulation-related inflammation, and proangiogenic state have been proposed. However, because AMD development is multifactorial in origin, pinpointing the primary location of morphological and functional defects in MNC is still elusive. There is evidence that the lipid composition change of BrM is the earliest pathobiology of MNC in the context of AMD. This evidence shows that the ratio between neutral lipid and polar phospholipid of BrM is altered with aging, which may also contribute to gradually diffused inner BrM thickening observed in AMD.[5,6] Histological and optical coherence tomography (OCT) images show that atrophy of the CC in the macula, characterized by a decrease in the number and diameter of capillaries, is a critical factor in the AMD development.[7,8] Histological studies revealed that photoreceptor cells are lost early in the disease.[9] Psychophysical testing shows that PR sensitivity losses are as high as 25% in cases of early AMD when visual acuity is normal.[10,11] Most evidence suggests that the primary pathology of AMD occurs in RPE cells, since no significant degenerative change in PR is apparent before overt deterioration of the RPE.[11] Morphologic data also are consistent with the degeneration of PR and thinning of CC being secondary results of the degeneration of RPE cells.[12] Furthermore, because focal RPE hyperpigmentation together with large drusen, the hallmark of AMD, are independent risk factors for the development of advanced AMD, the early RPE hyperpigmentation plays a pathogenic role in AMD progression.[5,7] In spite of numerous studies, the pathogenic sequence leading to AMD development is still in debate. There are at least two reasons explaining this disagreement. First, the variation in clinical manifestations implies that AMD does not follow the same course in all cases. Second, AMD is considered to be a disease of the neurovascular complex. Therefore, all components of this complex interplay when responding to etiologic triggers, resulting in different phenotypes. By mechanistic approach, the sequence of the events for each component may be less critical than how the defect of these components plays a pathophysiologic role in AMD development. In clinical study, the different phenotypes at the same stage of AMD, serving as different subgroups, need to be categorized.

Assuming that the pivotal event of AMD pathobiology occurs in RPE, questions may be raised. What can cause metabolic uncoupling of RPE cells for the disorders of the MNC? And how can the events of other components of MNC interact to cause the neurovascular damage in AMD?

RPE mitochondrial bioenergetic crisis and oxidative stress in AMD

Mitochondria are the fundamental source of energy in RPE, in which ATP is produced through several pathways. The main pathway for ATP production is oxidative phosphorylation (OxPhos). The citric acid cycle and β-oxidation are two additional energy-producing pathways. Unlike other cell types in the retina, RPE mitochondria can utilize fatty acids to produce β-hydroxybutyrate as an alternative energy source.[12–14] Reactive oxygen species (ROS) are by-products of electron transfer and the systematic reduction of oxygen by mitochondria. ROS is important not only because it determines oxidative damage but also because it contributes to retrograde redox signaling from the mitochondria to the cytosol and nucleus.[15] Increasing evidence shows that an accelerated oxidative stress of RPE mitochondria is apparent in postmortem eyes with AMD. The counteraction of ROS initiates compensatory upregulation of specific proteins. For instance, elevated antioxidant enzymes and heat shock proteins in RPE from donors with AMD were indirect evidence for increased oxidative stress. A global proteome analysis of RPE cells found that levels of 12 proteins are altered with AMD and, importantly, most of these proteins are localized to the mitochondria.[14] Those mitochondrial proteins altered in early-stage AMD are proteins with regulatory functions such as stress-induced protein unfolding and aggregation, mitochondrial trafficking and refolding, as well as regulating apoptosis. The proteins related to the regulation of retinoic acid and regeneration of the rhodopsin chromophore were found to be affected in late-stage AMD.[16] Another proteomic analysis of RPE mitochondria confirmed that energy production and mitochondrial protein import and refolding become defective in the eyes with AMD.[17]

Bioenergetic homeostasis of RPE is essential for cellular function; whereas, impaired energy metabolism of RPE mitochondria drives overall retinal damage. In particular, RPE and PRs are typically codependent on glucose utilization. Glucose from the blood is largely unused by the RPE and is transported to PR. PR uses glucose through glycolysis to produce energy and the byproduct lactate. The latter is transported back to the RPE for OxPhos. Thus, they form a codependent ecosystem in using glucose.[14,18] As OxPhos alters in RPE mitochondria, ATP production is reduced, forcing RPE to rely on glycolysis to maintain the cell's energy requirement. Thus, the flow of glucose to the PR is reduced. Consequently, the decreased PR glycolysis could reduce the production of lactate for RPE as an energy source. In other words, suppression of PR glycolysis associated with decreased lactate promotes glucose overutilization by the RPE, starving the PR and leading to neuron degeneration and death.[19,20]

RPE cells of AMD patients exhibit abnormally high amounts of oxidatively modified proteins, lipids, and DNA.[21] Oxidative stress is a state in which either increased levels of ROS are generated or the capacity to reduce ROS impact is insufficient.[22] The generation of ROS has physiologic and pathologic implications for RPE cells. Mitochondrial electron transport chain (mtETC) of RPE is one source of ROS.[23] ROS also may act as second messengers responding to a wide range of cellular functions, for instance, responses to hypoxia by HIF1α pathway.[24] When mtETC malfunctions the amount of ROS may increase substantially.[25] The increased ROS are mainly produced by the I and III complexes of mtETC in association with induced proton leak.[24,26] A small imbalance in mtETC function may lead to a transient accumulation of ROS, which could damage mtDNA, including genes encoding mtETC components. Expression of these damaged genes may lead to the synthesis of functionally deficient proteins of mtETC, further accumulation of ROS, and even more massive damage to mtDNA. As a result, the synthesis of faulty mtETC proteins and further ROS overproduction in repeated cycles may occur.[27] This state is referred to as "mitochondrial vicious cycle," in which an important element is contributing to premature aging and age-associated disease (Fig. 7.1).[25,28]

The role of mtROS and damage to mtDNA of RPE in AMD development begins with the "mitochondrial vicious cycle." As AMD risk factors, oxidative stress and/or mediated inflammation, may induce RPE mtDNA damage and mutations, resulting in an energy deficit and ultimately in cell death. Some cells may adapt to stress conditions and survive it into senescence. The senescent cells can be preferentially associated with RPE degeneration observed in AMD.[29]

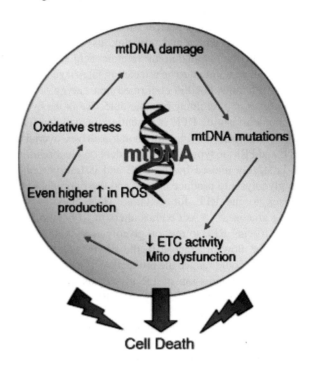

FIGURE 7.1

The mitochondrial "vicious cycle" theory. The theory proposes that oxidative stress and chronic ROS generation increases can be damaging to mtDNA. Much of this damage can be mutagenic giving rise to mtDNA mutations that may accumulate progressively during life. MtDNA mutations, in turn, can be directly responsible for a measurable deficiency in cellular oxidative phosphorylation activity, leading to an enhanced mitochondrial ROS production. Increased ROS generation results in further increases in oxidative stress and an increased rate of mtDNA damage and mutagenesis, thus causing a "vicious cycle" of exponentially increasing oxidative damage and dysfunction, which ultimately culminates in cell death.

Modified from Hiona A, Leeuwenburgh C. The role of mitochondrial DNA mutations in aging and sarcopenia: implications for the mitochondrial vicious cycle theory of aging. Exp Gerontol. *2008;43(1):24–33. https://doi. org/10.1016/j.exger.2007.10.001.*

Hypoxia, oxidative stress and dysfunction of RPE in AMD

Hypoxia occurs when oxygen supply is inadequate to meet demand. A reduced CC density, indicating reduced blood supply, is a critical pathologic characteristic observed in AMD. By using donor eyes with different stages of AMD and normal control eyes, CC density and BrM thickness were quantified histologically. In macula with larger drusen, geographic atrophy, or disciform scarring, the CC density was 63%, 54%, and 43% of normal and the CC diameter was 81%, 73%, and 75% of normal, respectively.[8] These findings demonstrate that the reduced CC oxygen supply occurs in all stages of AMD including the early AMD. The energy-demanding PR and RPE need appropriate oxygen levels for photo- and neuro-transduction. RPE is exposed to extremely high ambient oxygen partial pressures of 70−90 mm Hg.[30] Under physiologic conditions, the oxygen supply to, and demand by, outer retina are at a delicate balance. When CC flow is reduced, the RPE and outer neural retina oxygen supply is insufficient. Thus, when the temporal thickened RPE basal infoldings with underlying BrM aggravates the oxygen barrier, an oxidative-stress related localized hypoxia in both PR and RPE could be established.[31] The early hypoxic event may be contained in a local microenvironment. For instance, a longitudinal OCTA study on early/intermediate AMD corroborated this statement that the CC flow deficit in different regions of the macula correlated with the subsequent development and enlargement of drusen, the hallmark characteristic of AMD. In other words, regions demonstrating new drusen or enlargement of existing drusen showed worsening CC flow deficits as compared to regions without drusen involvement.[32,33]

Hypoxia-inducible factor alpha subunits (HIF-αs) are the transcription factors that mediate responses to hypoxia. Under normal conditions, HIF-αs are constitutively expressed and targeted by von Hippel-Lindau protein (VHL) for ubiquitination and proteasomal degradation. At low oxygen tensions, VHL is inactivated. Thus, this allows HIF-αs to translocate to the nucleus and activate a host of glucose metabolism, erythropoiesis, angiogenesis, and inflammation genes.[34] By using inducible and conditional gene ablation techniques, resulting in perturbation of the VHL/HIF/VEGF pathway in an animal model, hyper-activation of HIF-αs in RPE was achieved.[4] These manipulations altered lipid handling and glucose consumption of RPE cells, leading to reduced nutrient availability for the sensory retina and progressive PR degeneration. Understanding the effects of hypoxia on RPE metabolism, and learning how to control these effects, may provide insights for developing novel therapeutic strategies to treat AMD not only in the late neovascular stage but also in early stages. Hypoxic conditions facilitate the increase of ROS and the process of oxidative stress. The excessive production of ROS causes oxidative damage in RPE including bioenergetic dysfunction and mtDNA damage, which in turn initiates the "mitochondrial vicious cycle" as mentioned earlier (Fig. 7.1).[25,28]

Oxidatively induced mtDNA damage may accumulate and be associated with normal aging and AMD.[23,35] For instance, accumulation of the common 4977 bp deletion in mtDNA (ΔmtDNA 4977) was observed specifically in aging but not in fetal human RPE.[36] Therefore, aging is a risk factor for accumulation of mutations in mtDNA. A comparative study of variation in mtDNA haplogroups in the retinas of AMD patients with non-AMD controls was performed.[37] This study demonstrated that the mt1626T > C and mt73A > G of the J and T haplogroups single-nucleotide polymorphisms (SNPs) occurred more frequently in AMD patients than controls. These polymorphisms are located in the genes encoding NADH dehydrogenase so that this association appears to herald increased ROS production.

As mtDNA lacks both introns and efficient repair systems for its own damage,[38] the extent of damage observed in mtDNA in the retina is greater than in its nuclear counterpart. On the other hand, the mitochondrial genome depends upon the nuclear genome for transcription, translation, replication, and repair. But exact mechanisms for how the two genomes interact with each other are still poorly understood.[38] Overall, the damage in mtDNA could be an important element of AMD pathogenesis, as these genes may underlay RPE dysfunction that is crucial for AMD development.[39]

Role of oxidative stress and inflammation in pathogenesis of AMD

The RPE constantly undergoes oxidative stress, because the retina is one of the highest oxygen-consuming tissues of the human body.[40] High oxygen metabolism, continual exposure to light, high concentrations of polyunsaturated fatty acids, and the increased photo-oxidative stress result in increased ROS production in the retina. ROS overproduction from chronic oxidative stress can exceed the antioxidation capability and lead to modification and damage of carbohydrates, lipids, proteins, and DNA. In fact, an age-related increase in lipofuscin (photo-oxidative stress-induced ROS production in RPE), mtDNA damage of RPE, carboxyethylpyrrole (CEP, an oxidation fragment of docosahexaenoic acid), and malondialdehyde (MDA, products of lipid peroxidation) have been observed in the aging retina.[41] In the retina, PRs are consistently exposed to light and oxygen, and thus are susceptible to oxidative damage. Meanwhile, RPE cells are essential for PR outer segment phagocytosis, and thus critical for PR survival, function and renewal. In principle, RPE degeneration or RPE cell death could cause secondary PR cell death.[21] In AMD, oxidative stress works jointly with other risk factors including aging, smoking, phototoxicity, and genetic factors. The consequences of oxidative stress include sub-RPE and subretinal deposits, RPE/PR cell death, and the resultant inflammatory and immune responses. These processes may aggravate oxidative stress and inflammation, forming a biological vicious cycle leading to AMD development and progression. As evidence for the critical role of oxidative stress in AMD, Age-Related Eye Disease Study 2 has shown that the progression of AMD can be slowed with antioxidant vitamins and zinc supplements.[42] In animal models, the increase in modified oxidative products, such as CEP and MDA, is associated with inflammatory response and AMD-like phenotype.[43,44] For instance, in response to oxidatively damaged lipids, macrophages are activated and accumulated in the subretinal space of mice immunized with CEP, implicating oxidative stress-induced subretinal inflammation in AMD.[21]

AMD is an inflammatory disease. Inflammation is defined as a cellular response to triggers affecting the homeostasis of tissues. Cell-associated and soluble pattern recognition receptors (PRRs), for example, Toll-like receptors (TLRs), inflammasome receptors, and complement components can initiate the cellular responses.[45,46] TLRs are a family of proteins capable of recognizing extra- and intracellular pathogens and initiating innate immune responses.[47] TLRs consist of TL1-TL13 receptors, in which TLR3 and TLR4 are the most interesting to AMD researchers (see Fig. 9.6 in Chapter 9). Both TLR3 and TLR4 are expressed by RPE.[48,49] TLR signaling produces the intracellular receptor NLRP3 and the pro-forms of inflammasome-dependent cytokines IL-1β and IL-18. Cytokine release follows the cleavage of the inflammasome complex assembly-dependent caspase-1.[46] The role of TLR3 in AMD-related pathology remains controversial. The role of TLR4 in AMD development is more recognizable.[50] For instance, TLR4-mediated microglial activation by endogenous photoreceptor proteins in retinal inflammation aggravates retinal cell death. TLR4 participates in photoreceptor outer segments (POS) recognition and phagocytosis, as well as ROS and cytokine production. The impaired phagocytosis of POS under the detrimental photo-oxidative stress causes the accumulation of lipofuscin, which in turn further increases oxidative stress and inflammation.[51] However, the relationship of TLR3 and TLR4 gene polymorphisms with AMD has been studied with inconsistent results (see Chapter 9).[50,52]

The complement system is part of the innate immune system. Complement proteins are mainly synthesized by the liver. Other tissues including tissue macrophages and blood monocytes also produce a significant amount. In addition, there is evidence that complement proteins can be produced locally in the eye, such as in RPE cells.[53] The complement system consists of over 50 proteins and cell surface receptors and is generally divided into three pathways: the classical, the lectin, and the alternative pathways. Although there is evidence that all three complement pathways contribute to the etiology of AMD,[54] alternative pathway (AP) dysfunction, and genetic variants highly predispose individuals to developing AMD.[55,56] Each complement pathway is activated individually, whereas the three pathways converge at the complement component 3 (C3) step and subsequently follow a common pathway (Fig. 9.5 in Chapter 9).[21] The common pathway includes the formation of the C5 convertase, which cleaves C5 to its effector subunits, C5b and the potent anaphylatoxin C5a. C5b together with C6, C7, C8, and C9 form the membrane attack complex (MAC), which can cause pore formation of plasma membrane, resulting in cell lysis (see Fig. 9.5 in Chapter 9).[57] Under physiological conditions, the plasma complement components circulate as inactive precursors. Activation of the complement cascade is effectively controlled by soluble inhibitors such as complement factor H (CFH) and C4-binding protein (C4bp),[58] and membrane-associated regulatory proteins.[59] In AMD patients, higher plasma levels of bioactive fragments, for example, C3a, C3d, Bb, and C5a, have been found, indicating systemic activation of complement pathways plays a pathogenic role.[60−62] A genome-wide association study revealed an association between variants in *CFH* and *CFHR4* and systemic complement activation, in which serum C3d-to-C3 ratio, an indicator of systemic complement activation, was used in AMD patients. Haplotype analysis was performed for eight SNPs across the *CFH/CFHR* locus. The SNP rs6685931 in *CFHR4* and its linked haplotype H1-2 conferred a risk for AMD development, thus could be used to identify candidates among AMD patients who would benefit most from complement-inhibiting therapies.[63] CFH is a key regulator of the alternative pathway (Fig. 9.5 in Chapter 9).[64] CFH is recognized by cell surface membranes and protects host cells from the rapid and progressive destruction of other activated components of the complement system. It may also be synthesized locally, particularly in those tissues that have localized self-turnover mechanisms such as the eye, brain, kidney, liver, and vascular organs.[65] CFH polymorphism (Y402H) is strongly associated with AMD (see Chapter 9). CFH acts as a negative inhibitor regulating the activity of C3-mediated complement AP. Upon activation of AP, factor D (CFD) binds to and cleaves C3-bond factor B (CFB) releasing the N-terminal fragment Ba, resulting in the formation of the C3 convertase of the C3bBb.[66] The half-life of C3bBb is very short ($\sim$90s).[67] Therefore, a stabilization system for C3bBb is required to provide adequate but sustainable host defense. Properdin, a positive regulator secreted by monocytes/macrophages and T lymphocytes,[68] binds C3bBb and proconvertase C3B and C3b to stabilize the C3 convertase.[69] Electron microscopy studies demonstrated that the properdin binding induces structural changes and twists the binding site for CFH.[70] It makes AP C3 convertase more resistant to decay by CFH. Under physiological conditions, a low level of constitutive activation of the alternative pathway is kept under vigilant regulation.[71] Upon activation, as C3b binds covalently to a surface, the bound C3b molecules are rapidly inactivated by complement regulators including CFH.[71] Under pathologic conditions such as in an AMD-like in vitro model, C3b production by RPE cells could trigger C3 activation causing a sustained local chronic activation of the alternative pathway.[72] AMD is primarily a local disorder of the outer retina/choroid complex. A local complement regulatory system exists in this complex. Under normal physiological conditions, RPE cells produce sufficient CFH and protect regional tissues such as RPE cells and BrM from uncontrolled complement attack. Meanwhile, as described earlier, a low level of constitutive activation of the alternative pathway is maintained. Under pathological conditions, the synthesis of CFH in RPE cells is suppressed by proinflammatory cytokines and oxidized POS. Insufficient CFH at the outer retina/choroid complex may lead to excessive complement activation with associated cell and tissue damage. Dysregulation of CFH production at the retinal/choroid interface may play important roles in the development of AMD. However, the molecular mechanistic link between complement dysregulation and AMD pathobiology is still elusive. Recently, two pieces of significant work revealed this link in great depth. In 2015, Toomey et al. used genetically engineered aged $Cfh^{+/-}$ and Cfh^{-fh} mouse models to study the contribution of CFH to AMD etiology.[73] These animals were fed with a high-fat, cholesterol-enriched diet. The production of CFH, C3/C3b, and CFB in tissue lysates and the complement activity in plasma was quantitatively compared between these two models. The visual function of the animals was determined by electroretinography.[73] The decreased levels of CFH of RPE/choroid led to an increase in sub-RPE deposit formation, specifically basal laminar deposits. Notably, sub-RPE deposit formation occurred in both $Cfh^{+/-}$ and Cfh^{-fh} mice, whereas, RPE damage associated with visual function loss only in aged $Cfh^{+/-}$ mice. This study provided data that the underlying mechanism of the deposit accumulation is CFH competition for lipoprotein binding sites in Bruch's membrane. The authors also demonstrated that the amount of sub-RPE deposits is a function of excess complement activation in $Cfh^{+/-}$ mice, but not in Cfh^{-fh} animals. Thus, the formation of sub-RPE deposits is CFH-dependent and regulated via Bruch's membrane lipoprotein binding. Thus, advanced age, high-fat diet, and decreased CFH can induce sub-RPE deposit formation and complement activation. The resultant RPE damage and visual function impairment characterize early AMD.

The pathogenic role of CFH in the regulation of subretinal inflammation was further elucidated by Calippe et al. in 2017.[74] Under normal physiological conditions, the subretinal space is devoid of immune cells, due to the potent immunosuppressive factors produced by the RPE, which eliminate infiltrating leukocytes.[75] It has been known that subretinal mononuclear phagocyte (MP) infiltration causes chronic, nonresolving, age-related inflammation in the eye.[74] Therefore, subretinal MP infiltration may be used as a biomarker of AMD-like inflammation. Notably, CFH deletion in the $Cfh^{-/-}$ model protected the mice from the subretinal accumulation of MP and showed accelerated resolution of inflammation, which probably is caused by uninhibited complement activation followed by exhaustion.[73] The phenotype of $Cfh^{-/-}$ mice (i.e., CFH depletion rather than deficiency) at sub-RPE/subretinal space does not resemble AMD, which is in agreement with the finding of the previous study vide supra.[73] Under steady-state conditions, phagocytes are constantly eliminated in the subretinal space via a homeostatic mechanism involving the interaction of thrombospondin-1 (TSP-1) with integrin-associated TSP-1 receptor (CD47) on subretinal phagocytes. On the other hand, during CFH deficiency, exemplified by the phenotype of *CFH* variant (Y402H), CFH binding to a pattern recognition receptor CR3 can restrain TSP-1 activation with the integrin-associated CD47 receptor. The latter is required for the homeostatic elimination of subretinal phagocytes.[76] The AMD-associated *CFH* (H402) variant markedly increases this inhibitory effect on microglial cell elimination, supporting a causal link to disease etiology (Fig. 7.2).[74] Another important finding of Calippe's work is that plasma CFH is not sufficient to inhibit MP clearance, hence suggesting that locally derived CFH has a significant role in AMD pathogenesis.

Inflammation involves both complement and the inflammasome as two arms of innate immunity. These two arms interact with each other as well.[21,46] Inflammasomes are multiprotein complexes that detect cellular danger and initiate innate

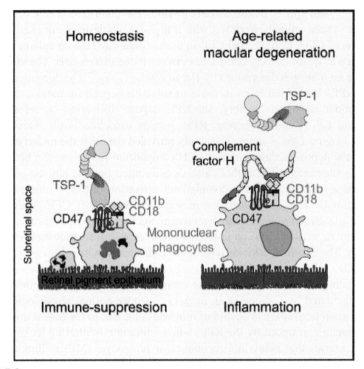

FIGURE 7.2

The pathogenic role of complement factor H in regulation of subretinal inflammation in AMD.

CD11b, integrin CD11b; *CD18*, integrin CD18; *CD47*, integrin CD47; *TSP-1*, thrombospsondin-1.

Modified from the graphical abstract by Calippe B, Augustin S, Beguier F, et al. Complement Factor H Inhibits CD47-Mediated Resolution of Inflammation. Immunity. 2017;46(2):261–272. https://doi.org/10.1016/j. immuni.2017.01.006.

immune defense through activation of IL-1β and IL-18.[77] Inflammasome activation in the RPE was first reported in 2011.[78,79] In patients with geographic atrophy, Alu RNA that abnormally accumulated due to the downregulation of its processing enzyme Dicer triggers NLRP3 inflammasome activation.[79] Alu elements are repetitive retrotransposons belonging to the class of short interspersed nuclear elements and account for a total of more than one million copies in the whole human genome. It has been demonstrated that Alu sequences originate from the retro-transposition of the 7SL RNA.[80,81] The nucleotide-binding and oligomerization domain (NOD)-like Receptor (NLR) family of proteins is a group of PRRs. NLR proteins including NLRP3 are structurally and functionally related to inflammasomes. Among the canonical and noncanonical inflammasome complexes, the NLRP3 inflammasome has been extensively studied (Fig. 7.3).[82–84] NLRP3 inflammasome activation requires

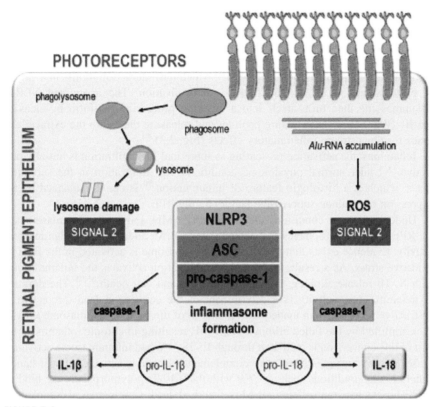

FIGURE 7.3

Inflammasome formation in RPE with effects of NLRP3 inflammasome activation. In the RPE, NLRP3 inflammasome is activated through phagosome-mediated lysosomal damage resulting in IL-1β production and through *Alu* RNA build-up and consequent ROS accumulation, resulting in IL-18 production. NLRP3 (a member of a family of proteins called nucleotide-binding domain and leucine-rich repeat-containing (NLR) proteins), IL-1β, interleukin1β; IL-18, interleukin18; ASC apoptosis-associated speck-like protein; *Alu*-RNA, human Arthro bacterluteus ribonucleic acid sequence; ROS, reactive oxygen species.

Modified from Yamamoto-Rodríguez L, Zarbin MA, Casaroli-Marano RP. New frontiers and clinical implications in the pathophysiology of age-related macular degeneration. Med Clin (Barc). 2020;154(12):496–504. https:// doi.org/10.1016/j.medcli.2020.01.023.

two signals, a "priming signal" and an "activation signal." The "priming signal" pathway relies on the nuclear factor kappa B (NF-κB), upregulating the transcription of NLRP3 and prointerleukin-1β (pro-IL-1β).[85] As pro-IL-1β is not constitutively expressed by RPE, the endogenous level of NLRP3 is not adequate for inflammasome activation, thus the requirement of priming signals is critical.[86] The priming signals for immune cells and RPE cells consist of lipopolysaccharide, tumor necrosis factor-α (TNF-α), nitric oxide, and IL-1α.[86] Upon receiving "activation signals," NLRP3 senses one or multiple intracellular changes such as K^+ efflux,[82] release of lysosomal resident cathepsin B,[87] and/or overproduction of ROS.[88] Once the NLRP3 is activated, it recruits "the apoptosis-associated speck-like protein containing a caspase recruitment domain" (ASC), which has interaction motifs in a variety of proteins, and mediates procaspase-1 autoactivation. The assembled NLRP3 inflammasome then turns itself into a cytokine processing platform by cleaving pro-IL-1β/pro-IL-18 into mature peptides and releasing them into the extracellular space for downstream inflammatory effects (Fig. 7.3).[89]

Inflammasome activation presenting as subretinal MP infiltration is initially protective.[74] Under normal physiologic conditions, MP infiltration in the subretinal space, which is a histologic feature of inflammation,[90] is counterbalanced by the expression of immune-suppressive factors by the RPE.[75]

Under pathologic conditions such as in early AMD, activated inflammasomes in the RPE recruit macrophages that accumulate in BrM, adding more inflammasome activity. Evidence exists that the NLRP3-inflammasome is activated in the RPE by oxidative stress. As a result, lysosomal destabilization activates the inflammasome with IL-1β release, linking to RPE dysfunction and cell death.[86,91] The duration of inflammasome activity is a determinant of the conversion from protective to destructive responses. An inadequate resolution of the acute inflammasome activity is exemplified by the failed elimination of MP, resulting in chronic inflammasome. Part of this conversion is mediated through IL-18.[92] When inflammasome activation causes tissue injury, the alternative complement cascade is activated. For instance, under certain conditions such as *CFH* with the Y402H polymorphism, the binding of CFH to the heparan sulfate in BrM is disturbed, leading to increased complement activation and locally chronic inflammation.[93] In animal models of AMD, CFH was required for the chronic, age-related, subretinal MP accumulation and associated photoreceptor degeneration.[74] In humans, ocular CFH immunoreactivity is stronger in donated AMD tissues,[94] and CFH autoantibodies are protective in AMD.[95] These observations strongly suggest that CFH critically controls inflammation mediated by subretinal MP-accumulation in AMD.

Inflammasomes are cytosolic structures of NLRP3, ASC, and procaspase-1 that bind to the complex molecules regulating the secretion of IL-1β, IL-18, and IL-33 (Fig. 7.4). A recent study showed that sublytic MAC of complement can trigger NLRP3 inflammasome activation.[96] Pore formation by MAC on the cell surface led to increased intracellular and intramitochondrial calcium, resulting in loss of mitochondrial transmembrane potential and triggering of the NLRP3 inflammasome and caspase-1 activation.[97] Based on the data cited earlier, it could be concluded that innate immunity is primarily regulated by mechanisms via complement-inflammasome interaction (Fig. 7.4).

Based on mechanistic studies, complement activation, proinflammatory cytokines, and inflammasome activation have been considered as therapeutic targets for many acute and chronic inflammatory conditions. Drugs inhibiting IL-1, P2X7R, and caspase-1 showed potent inhibition of inflammasome-associated

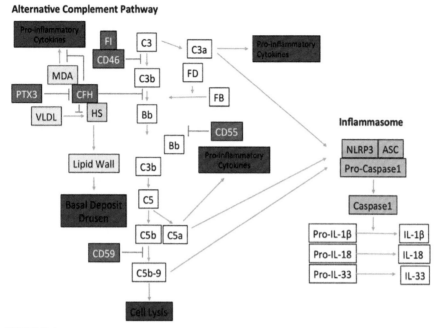

FIGURE 7.4

Diagram of the alternative complement pathway and the inflammasome. Activation of the alternative complement pathway is regulated by factor H (CFH), CD46, CD55, and PTX3. PTX3, by binding CFH, controls the abundance of CFH. Besides its regulation of complement, CFH binds to malondialdehyde (MDA) to control MDA-mediated proinflammatory cytokine production, and heparan sulfates (HS) to compete with very low-density lipoproteins (VLDL) that can become deposited in Bruch's membrane before basal deposit or drusen formation. Complement activation can lead to anaphylatoxins generation of C3a and C5a, which can induce proinflammatory cytokine production, and C5b-9 complex formation, which is regulated by CD59. C3a, C5a, and C5b-9 complexes are implicated in activating the inflammasome. The complex of NLRP3, ASP, and Procaspase1, which upon activation, is cleaved to convert pro-IL-1b, pro-IL-18, and pro-IL-33 into their active forms.

Modified from Datta S, Cano M, Ebrahimi K, Wang L, Handa JT. The impact of oxidative stress and inflammation
on RPE degeneration in non-neovascular AMD. Prog Retin Eye Res. 2017;60:201—218. https://doi.org/10.
1016/j.preteyeres.2017.03.002.

inflammatory diseases.[98,99] P2X7R is a purinergic receptor with downstream signaling coupled to proinflammatory cascades.[98,99] MCC950, a diarylsulfonylures-containing small molecule is able to block both canonical and noncanonical NLRP3 activation. MCC950 specifically inhibits NLRP3-induced ASC oligomerization, attenuating the severity of experimental autoimmune encephalomyelitis, a NLRP3-associated disease.[100] In parallel, inhibition of the alternative complement pathway has been studied for regulating inflammation of AMD. Potent

C5aR antagonists,[101] and the C3 inhibitor compstatin,[102] have been used in various AMD models. Eculizumab (Soliris), a humanized monoclonal antibody that is a complement factor 5 (C5) inhibitor, has been used with great success in treating paroxysmal nocturnal hemoglobinuria and atypical hemolytic uraemic syndrome,[103] suggesting that targeting the complement common pathway might be beneficial in various inflammatory diseases. Regarding dry AMD, there is no effective treatment to reduce its progression yet. To date, several molecules such as eculizumab and other related molecules are being investigated. Although some of them have shown low efficacy in clinical trials,[104] more work needs to be done to validate this proof-of-concept approach (see Chapter 11).

Composition and formation of drusen

In early AMD, the fundamental pathology of the MNC is the subRPE deposits, known as drusen. RPE cells are the origin of numerous components found in drusen. Structural and functional detriments of RPE due to oxidative stress, innate immune-response, and inflammation have an impact on drusen formation. There are two forms of deposits including focal sub-RPE deposits, so-called drusen and diffuse sub-RPE deposits. The characterization of the focal drusen was discussed in depth in previous chapters. The diffuse deposits internal to the RPE basement membrane (BL) and external to the RPE-BL are distinctly defined as basal laminar deposit (BlamD) and basal linear deposit (BLinD), respectively. BlamD contains abundant long-spacing collagen. BLinD contains more membranous material. In addition to conventional sub-RPE-BL drusen, the term subretinal drusenoid deposits (SDDs) was first used by Mimoun et al. in 1990.[105] OCT images showed SDD to be a layer of extracellular deposits between the RPE and photoreceptors.[106] SDD contains some proteins in common with BLinD but differs in lipid composition.[107]

Histologic evidence showed that membranous debris is the major component of soft drusen.[108] The membranous debris derives from large lipoproteins containing apolipoproteins B and E, which are secreted basolaterally by the RPE into BrM. Sub-RPE and BrM lipoproteins have two principal sources, that is, circulating lipoproteins delivering lipophilic essentials and phagocytized outer segments. There is a mechanism for the RPE to offload unneeded lipids to the systemic circulation and avoid lipotoxicity.[109] Circulating lipoproteins are transported from the choroid to the photoreceptors through the RPE. The RPE cells express two types of receptors for lipoprotein uptake including receptors for very low-density lipoprotein cholesterol (VLDL-R) and low-density lipoprotein cholesterol (LDL-R). With these receptors, RPE cells internalize LDL-cholesterol (LDL-C) and less efficiently HDL-C from the choroidal circulation.[110] Polyunsaturated fatty acids, such as DHA and γ-linolenic acid, are also taken up into the RPE from the circulation.[111] Therefore, it is clear that dietary lipids can be taken up by the outer retina. CD36, a fatty acid translocase localized to the inner and outer segments of the rod photoreceptors,[112] facilitates the shedding of disk membranes and RPE phagocytosis.[113] In addition to uptake from the systemic circulation, RPE and photoreceptors, like many mammalian cells, also synthesize their own cholesterol. There is a tight regulation of the intracellular cholesterol concentration via several negative feedback mechanisms.[114] Because lipids are insoluble in water, they are packaged into lipoprotein particles, consisting of an amphipathic lipid monolayer covering a core of hydrophobic lipids.[115] Lipoproteins simulate oil droplets solubilized for transport through aqueous media with a surface of proteins, known as a core-and-surface morphology.[109] Ultrastructural studies using lipid-preserving techniques showed that lipoproteins accumulate with age in human BrM, with the highest concentration in the macular region.[116] Biochemical analysis of BrM extracts showed that they are rich in esterified and unesterified cholesterol. Curcio pointed out that fatty acids in BrM extracts are dominated by linoleate (implicating dietary sources) and not docosahexaenoate (concentrated in photoreceptor outer segments).[109] Meanwhile, OCT imaging documented the volume change of drusen, for example, drusen regression when RPE structure and function are deteriorating.[117]

Histological and SD-OCT studies confirmed that SDDs are subretinal structures.[118] Histochemical studies using oil red O and sterol-specific filipin demonstrated that unesterified cholesterol but not esterified cholesterol was present in SDD, whereas sub-RPE drusen contained both.[107] This difference implies different origins of lipid components in these two types of extracellular deposits, namely SDD versus sub-RPE-BL drusen. The unesterified cholesterol is part of both membranes and lipoproteins, whereas the esterified cholesterol implies in lipoprotein particles. The different lipid compositions in SDD and drusen appear to be related to mineralization pathways and RPE polarized functions.[107,119] In summary, SDDs consist of membranous debris, both unesterified and esterified cholesterol, apolipoprotein E, CFH, and vitronectin.[120] It is important to note that the recent histological studies have clarified that there is no specific physical link between the choroid and SDD appearance as previously suggested.[118] Immunohistochemical staining of regions surrounding SDD has found increased expression of the intermediate filament glial fibrillary acidic protein, a biomarker of glial cells, of Müller cells in a mouse model,[120] indicating a glial response to retinal stress.[121] In a separate in vivo study, irregular and hypertrophied RPE cells and internally migrated RPE cells have been observed in areas adjacent to SDD, suggesting pathogenic roles for RPE degeneration and SDD in AMD development.[120]

In addition to lipids and minerals, the origin of drusen-associated proteins and the aggregated macromolecules in the sub-RPE space have been studied by multiple "discovery-based" approaches, such as proteomics. Lipid chromatography combined with mass spectroscopy (LC MS/MS) has been used to quantitatively analyze proteins in the macular region of the BrM/choroid complex from human postmortem eyes.[122] Compared to normal controls, among 99 altered proteins 56 upregulated and 43 down-regulated were identified. About 60% of the upregulated proteins were immune response and host defense proteins, including many complement proteins and complement-associated proteins such as C3, C5, and CFH. Several damage-associated molecular pattern proteins, initiators of the innate immune response, were among the upregulated proteins. Inflammatory response proteins were detected to be upregulated in multiple stages of AMD progression, supporting the idea that inflammatory processes are involved in both initiating events of AMD and progression to advanced AMD.[122] For instance, 19 proteins were upregulated in early AMD tissues, including 12 proteins elevated >2 SD. Fifteen of these proteins (15/19) were differentially upregulated. Eight of these 15 proteins were associated with inflammatory processes and cellular defense, namely C5, C7, α1-acid glycoprotein 1, α1-antichymotrypsin, α-crystallin A, α-crystallin B, HLA class II histocompatibility antigen DRα, and 4F2 cell-surface antigen heavy chain. Most importantly, HLA class II histocompatibility antigen DRα and C7 were more abundant in early AMD than in late AMD. These findings imply a role for inflammatory processes in initiating events of AMD. Four retinoid processing proteins (RPE-specific 65 kDa protein, cellular retinoic acid-binding protein 1, cellular retinaldehyde binding protein, and interphotoreceptor retinoid-binding protein) were distinctly upregulated in early AMD, suggesting that retinoid metabolism contributes to AMD initiation, likely through mechanisms involving RPE lipofuscin.[123] Advanced glycation endproducts (AGE) receptor 3 (galectin-3), an indicator of the role of AGEs in advanced dry AMD, and other regulatory proteins for extracellular matrix remodeling such as TIMP3 in drusen formation were also found to be upregulated.[123]

Consistent with the study introduced earlier,[122] the proteomic data by Fisher and Ferrington showed that 26 proteins in the neural retina exhibited differential expression with AMD progression.[14] These proteins were mainly involved in microtubule regulation and in protein folding/chaperone activities.[124] A global proteome analysis of the RPE found 12 differentially altered proteins with AMD, which were particularly localized to mitochondria as described earlier.[16] These results indicated that the mitochondria in RPE are potentially the primary location of AMD pathology. Furthermore, RPE mitochondrial proteomics showed a decrease in mitochondrial heat shock protein (mtHSP70), supporting that mitochondrial protein import and refolding as well as energy production defects are associated with AMD.[17] In addition, significantly downregulated proteins accounted for a small fraction (<2%) of the proteins quantified in the macular region in AMD.[122] Proteins decreased in early AMD implicate hematologic malfunctions, reduced ECM integrity, and weakened cellular interactions. The phenomenon that proteins distinctly decrease in advanced dry AMD rather than in neovascular AMD implies the existence of multiple mechanisms of AMD progression.

The quantitative proteomics of macular drusen not only provide the protein compositions of drusen but also the functional classification of druse proteins. The distinctly expressed druse proteins at different stages of AMD delineate multiple pathogenic pathways involved in AMD progression. Furthermore, the quantitative proteomics database provides a discovery-based approach to developing proteomic and genomic prognostic biomarkers of AMD.

Based on the composition of sub-RPE deposits and conventional drusen, drusen formation is summarized in Fig. 7.5.[125] The RPE appears to be centrally involved in sub-RPE deposit and drusen formation. While there are likely various origins of sub-RPE deposit components, the mechanisms triggering retention of lipids and proteins to form

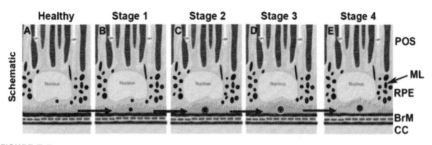

FIGURE 7.5

A model for druse formation. (A—E) is adopted from the schematic diagram proposed for sub-RPE-BL space deposit formation. (A) Healthy eyes show no sub-RPE-BL space deposit formation. (B) At Stage 1, lipid droplets are retained in the sub-RPE-BL space (*black dot*). (C) At Stage 2, mineralization occurs surrounding the lipid droplets (*magenta ring*). (D) At Stage 3, proteins bind to the HAP surfaces (*blue ring*). (E) At Stage 4, proteins and lipids start accumulating around the "seed" (*yellow material*).

Modified from Bergen AA, Arya S, Koster C, et al. On the origin of proteins in human drusen: The meet, greet and stick hypothesis. Prog Retin Eye Res. *2019;70:55—84. https://doi.org/10.1016/j.preteyeres.2018.12.003.*

drusen may be three-fold. The first mechanism is the binding of RPE-produced lipids and lipoproteins to extracellular matrix elements including proteoglycans in BrM, a mechanism similar to plasma lipoproteins binding to arterial intima in atherosclerosis.[126] A second mechanism is the retention of proteins via the formation of large oligomers, a process that is accelerated with mineralization.[127] The third mechanism is the binding of proteins to hydroxyapatite (HAP) spherules, which was recently found in the sub-RPE space and in drusen.[128] Any of these or a combination could be involved. Using HAP-specific fluorescent dyes with confocal microscopic images showed small hollow spherical structures that were visualized within sub-RPE deposits in human cadaveric retinal tissue sections.[128] Protein constituents of drusen, such as β-amyloid, vitronectin, and complement factor H, were localized to the surface of the HAP spherules, either individually or in combination. It was observed that not all investigated drusen proteins appeared to bind to the surface of HAP. However, this finding is a proof that the binding of proteins by HAP is one mechanism integrating lipids and proteins into sub-RPE deposits (illustrated in Fig. 7.5).

Pigmentary abnormalities and RPE migration in dry AMD

The presence of drusen and pigmentary abnormalities (PA) defines early/intermediate AMD.[129] The nature of PA in the retina has been largely uncovered since the advent of SD-OCT. Christenbury et al. reported that SD-OCT hyperreflective foci (HF) in the retina and on the inner surface of drusen spatially correlate with macular hyperpigmentation on color fundus photographs of patients with intermediate AMD.[130,131] Fig. 7.6 is a representative series of fundus photographs and SD-

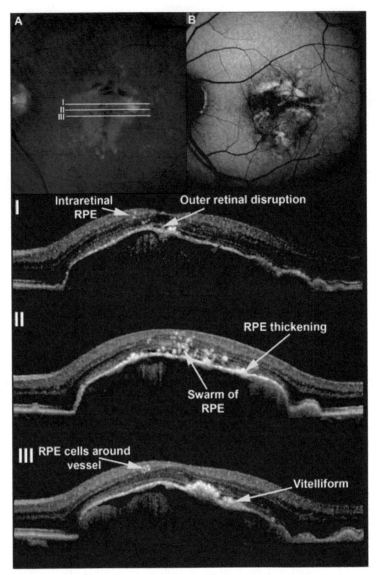

FIGURE 7.6

SD-OCT hyperreflective foci (HF) representing RPE cells migrating from subretinal to intraretinal locations, which correlating to pigmentary changes on fundus photography. (A) Color fundus photo shows a large drusenoid pigment epithelial detachment (PED) in this patient. Pigmentary changes are present on the surface of drusenoid PED, which correlates to sites of increased fundus autofluorescence (B). Areas of OCT scans (I, II, and III) are illustrated in the CFP. A range of RPE-related changes is seen on OCT scans including intraretinal RPE cells and subretinal vitelliform lesions. Note that the ellipsoid zone (*red arrowhead*) is visible on the surface of the pigment epithelial detachment with the exception of the apex, where it is notably absent. In this case, it was possible to distinguish vitelliform lesions from RPE thickening.

Modified from Balaratnasingam C, Messinger JD, Sloan KR, Yannuzzi LA, Freund KB, Curcio CA. Histologic and Optical Coherence Tomographic Correlates in Drusenoid Pigment Epithelium Detachment in Age-Related Macular Degeneration. Ophthalmology. 2017;124(5):644–656. https://doi.org/10.1016/j.ophtha.2016.12. 034.

OCT images of PA in a patient with drusenoid pigment epithelial detachment (PED).[132] Because drusenoid PED is known as a precursor of GA,[108] the SD-OCT findings of hyperreflective foci may characterize the stage of dry AMD before GA, that is, an intermediate stage.[132] Indeed, this study demonstrated that the HF seen by ex vivo SD-OCT of donor eyes with intermediate AMD correlates with RPE migration from subretinal to intraretinal locations as seen on histological sections. The HF by SD-OCT demonstrated different morphologies of PA such as intra-retinal RPE clusters, "swarm of RPE" and RPE around vessels (Fig. 7.6). In parallel, the histologic analysis showed that some expelled RPE organelles represent vitelli-form HF on SD-OCT, which is internal to RPE (Fig. 7.6). Based on longitudinal observation of HF during intermediate AMD, evidence exists that the characteristic HF correlates with various pathologic changes of RPE cells, including RPE hyper-plasia, epithelial-mesenchymal transition, and atrophy. Growing evidence shows that these pathologic changes are secondary to oxidative stress and inflammation.[133,134] Other causes of SD-OCT HF in the retina also have been reported. For instance, during diabetic retinopathy, microglial activation-related HF by SD-OCT was found in the inner retina and extended into the outer retina.[135] Although the presence of HF has been considered as a biomarker for active disease status, the distribution of HF extension and various cellular involvement may reflect distinct features in the context of different diseases. In diabetic retinopathy, the activated microglial cells and macrophages initially ramify at the inner retina, and then migrate to multiple retinal layers, while in intermediate AMD, activated RPE cells migrate from subretinal to inner retinal layers.[133]

Autophagy deficiency, RPE degeneration, and cell death in AMD

Autophagy is a lysosome-mediated degradation process. Dysfunctional autophagy in RPE is associated with increased susceptibility to RPE degeneration, one of the hallmarks of AMD. A key function of RPE cells critical for photoreceptor homeostasis is the phagocytosis, degradation, and recycling of apical POS. This complex process consumes large quantities of oxygen and, together with photo-oxidative stress generated by constant exposure to light, places significant oxidative demands on the RPE. This extensive metabolic activity results in lysosomal accumulation of undigested POS components in the RPE; these oxidized/damaged protein complexes, are the major source of lipofuscin. Once formed, lipofuscin bis-retinoids remain in the RPE for life, as their unique structure makes them resistant to lysosomal degradation.[136] Accumulated lipofuscin components such as the fluorophore A2E inhibit the lysosomal proton pump, thus increasing the lysosomal pH and inhibiting lysosomal hydrolase activity.[137,138] The resultant high levels of intralysosomal lipofuscin make RPE cells more sensitive to lysosomal damage and thus may contribute to the disturbance of the autophagy-lysosomal pathway.[139] Through the autophagy-lysosomal pathway, degradation of cell components occurs inside lysosomes.[140] The autophagy-lysosomal pathways comprise the canonical and the noncanonical pathways, which are differentiated based on the material to be degraded. There are three types of autophagy processes (see Fig. 7.7).[140] In macroautophagy, cytoplasmic components, for example, organelles, are targeted and isolated from the rest of the cell within a double-membraned vesicle known as an autophagosome. The autophagosome fuses with a lysosome, starting waste management. Eventually, the contents of the vesicle (so-called an autolysosome) are degraded and recycled. Chaperone-mediated autophagy recognizes only specific proteins in lysosomes for degradation. A noncanonical pathway unique for POS degradation by RPE combines both phagocytosis and autophagy (Fig. 7.7),[141] efficiently degrading POS via a process called LC3-associated phagocytosis (LAP). Herein, LC3 is referred as microtubule-associated protein light chain 3 (Fig. 7.7).

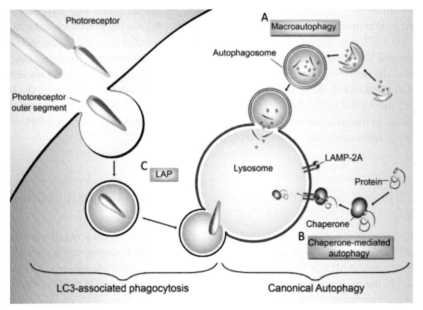

FIGURE 7.7

Canonical autophagy and noncanonical (i.e., LC3-associated) phagocytosis pathways in the retina. (A) Macroautophagy begins with the formation of a double-membrane structure that subsequently forms the autophagosome, which in turn fuses with the lysosome. During chaperone-mediated autophagy (B) chaperones recognize specific proteins, which they transport to the lysosomal membrane, where LAMP-2A mediates the unfolding and translocation of the protein into the lysosomal lumen. (C) LC3-associated phagocytosis (LAP) is a noncanonical pathway through which shed photoreceptor outer segments are ingested, degraded, and recycled.

Modified from Boya P, Esteban-Martínez L, Serrano-Puebla A, Gómez-Sintes R, Villarejo-Zori B. Autophagy in the eye: Development, degeneration, and aging. Prog Retin Eye Res. 2016;55:206–245. https://doi.org/10.1016/j. preteyeres.2016.08.001; Fazeli G, Wehman AM. Safely removing cell debris with LC3-associated phagocytosis. Biol Cell. 2017;109(10):355–363. https://doi.org/10.1111/boc.201700028.

Lipofuscin accumulation, lysosomal alterations, and autophagy deficiency are closely related to RPE function. Autophagy deficiency dramatically increases cell death, whereas stimulation of autophagy has the opposite effect. This suggests that autophagy constitutes a cytoprotective function, because the efficient autophagy-lysosomal pathways could eliminate damaged mitochondria and reduce oxidative stress.[142] Based on these findings, we may be able to locate therapeutic targets for protecting RPE against degeneration. Autophagy is at the crossroad between cell death and survival, improving cell survival through the recycling of metabolic precursors and removing damaged proteins and organelles from the cell. Meanwhile, autophagy modulates inflammatory responses and cell death pathways.[140,143,144] Autophagy can play a role in different forms of regulated cell death, influencing AMD development.[145]

RPE cell death is characterized as an essential late-stage phenomenon of dry AMD,[146] because RPE cell death impairs retinal protective measures and results in progressive photoreceptor degeneration. The mechanism of RPE cell death in AMD has not yet been fully elucidated. Most previous research showed that apoptosis is a major mechanism for RPE cell death in response to oxidative stress in AMD. Recent studies suggest necroptosis, a programmed form of necrosis, as a major mechanism of RPE cell death in response to oxidative stress.[144] Although apoptosis and necrosis have distinct features, they also share common features, such as chromatin condensation, mitochondrial damage, and DNA degradation. The necrotic pathway is summarized in Fig. 7.8.[144] However, no single method is sufficient to unequivocally distinguish between apoptosis and necroptosis. Distinguishing different types of cell death should not be based on either morphological or biochemical criteria alone, but rather by integrating all available data.[147] When apoptosis is inhibited, necrosis may become an alternative route for cell death. The types of cell death appear to be activated flexibly depending on the cell types and cellular context in the retina (Fig. 7.8).[148]

When human RPE cells are cultured in a conditioned medium from cells with an AMD-like phenotype, two types of RPE cells are found. It has been found that unprimed cells exhibited delayed cell lysis, plasma membrane blebbing, cell shrinkage, TUNEL-positive DNA fragmentation, and lack of IL-1β and IL-18 release. In contrast, primed cells demonstrated cell swelling, early cell lysis, TUNEL-positive DNA degradation, caspase-1 activation, and release of IL-1β and IL-18. When comparing cell death in the primed and unprimed cells, it is clear that the unprimed cells experience apoptosis, whereas the primed cells undergo pyroptosis.[149,150] Pyroptosis is a form of regulated cell death driven by inflammasome activation. The priming process requires proinflammatory cytokine release and C5a, a product of alternative complement activation (Figs. 7.4 and 7.9).[21,153] These findings revealed that after priming, the activated inflammasomes alter the predominant cell death mechanism induced by photo-oxidative damage in RPE cells, resulting in a shift from apoptosis to pyroptosis.[145,150] In fact, the presence of caspase-1 during NLRP3 inflammasome activation was found in RPE cells in AMD.[79,145] Most interestingly, increased intravitreal levels of the inflammasome

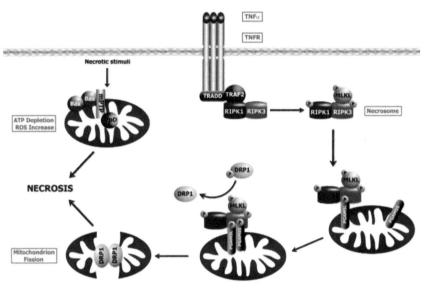

FIGURE 7.8

Overview of the necrotic pathways. Activation of TNF receptor leads to activation of RIP1 and RIP3 kinases when caspase-8 is not present or inactive. Autophosphorylations of RIP1 and RIP3 lead to the formation of necrosome, a complex that initiates the necrotic signaling pathway. Necrosome recruits MLKL protein and assembles signaling complex at the membrane rafts. Recruitment of the PGAM5 marks translocation of the complex to a hydrophilic environment and attachment to the mitochondrial membrane and activation of Drp1 protein that leads to mitochondrial fission and cell death. In the necrosis triggered by calcium overload, the opening of mPTP leads to decrease of mitochondrial membrane potential, collapse of ATP production and release of ROS, and triggering of necrosis in RIP3 dependent manner, although the signaling pathways leading to that event are unknown. *Drp1*, dynamin-related protein 1; *MLKL*, mixed-lineage kinase domain-like pseudokinase; *PGAM5*, phosphoglycerate mutase family member 5; *RIP1 or RIP3 kinases*, receptor-interacting serine/threonine-protein kinase-1 or 3.

Modified from Hanus J, Anderson C, Wang S. RPE necroptosis in response to oxidative stress and in AMD. Ageing Res Rev. 2015;24(Pt B):286–298. https://doi.org/10.1016/j.arr.2015.09.002.

activation products, IL-1β and IL-18, were reported in AMD patients.[151] Taken together, molecular and ultrastructural data suggest that necroptosis and pyroptosis are the predominant mechanisms of RPE death in AMD, while apoptosis may have only a minor contribution.[152]

In recent decades, many novel forms of nonapoptotic regulated cell death have been identified in AMD. For instance, RPE cell death may occur in "pure" and/or "mixed" forms in response to different stresses. The loss of control over cell death contributes to the pathogenesis of AMD.[144,154] It is well known that the suppression of apoptosis by caspase inhibition may reveal necroptotic or pyroptotic

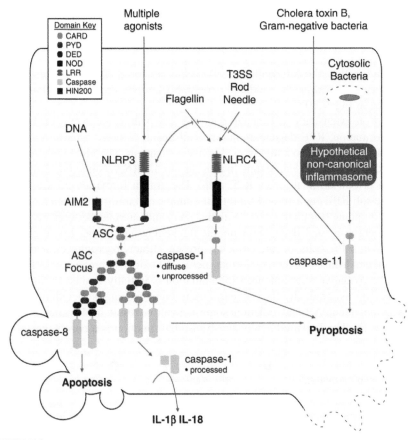

FIGURE 7.9

Canonical and noncanonical inflammasome pathways to cell death and cytokine secretion. Canonical inflammasomes are cytosolic platforms that activate caspase-1 in response to pathogen-associated or danger-associated molecular patterns. Activation of caspase-1 leads to secretion of IL-1β and IL-18, and pyroptosis. Two domain structures for inflammasome initiator proteins are known. (1) NLRs contain a signaling domain (PYD or CARD), a nucleotide-binding oligomerization domain (NOD/NACHT), and a leucine-rich repeat (LRR) domain. (2) AIM2 contains a PYD signaling domain and a DNA-binding HIN-200 domain. AIM2 detects cytosolic DNA. NLRP3 detects multiple agonists such as extracellular ATP, bacterial pore-forming toxins, monosodium urate crystals, and cholesterol crystals. NLRC4 detects cytosolic flagellin or T3SS components that have been injected into the cytosol. The NLR or AIM2 signaling domains (PYD or CARD) bind to ASC by homotypic interactions, triggering the formation of the ASC focus, which recruits procaspase-1, leading to its activation and processing. The ASC focus also recruits procaspase-8, initiating an apoptotic pathway. NLRC4 can additionally interact directly with caspase-1, resulting only in pyroptosis. The platform(s) that activate caspase-11 in response to cytosolic bacteria remain unknown. Caspase-11 triggers pyroptosis directly, and can also activate the canonical NLRP3-ASC-caspase-1 inflammasome pathway leading to IL-1β and IL-18 processing (denoted by the *long curved arrow* to NLRP3).

Modified from Aachoui Y, Sagulenko V, Miao EA, Stacey KJ. Inflammasome-mediated pyroptotic and apoptotic
cell death, and defense against infection. Curr Opin Microbiol. 2013;16(3):319–326. https://doi.org/10.1016/
j.mib.2013.04.004.

pathways.[144,145] Therefore, it is important to assemble a panel of biomarkers and functional tests distinguishing between different forms of cell death in a disease context. Thus, a targeted regulation of cell death may be applicable for controlling AMD.

Taken together, the cell death of AMD is multifactorial. To help understand this complex issue, a pathogenic model of geographic atrophy proposed by Hanus et al. is adapted in Fig. 7.10.[144]

Based on extensive experimental data, the key pathogenic events of AMD are drusen formation, RPE degeneration, and cell death. Notably, photoreceptors and RPE cells are exposed to a highly oxidative environment. The high oxidative exposure of RPE results in accumulating lipofuscin and *Alu* RNA. Numerous components found in drusen originate from RPE cells. The drusen formation in turn leads to increased sub-RPE deposits and subretinal immune cell infiltration such as accumulation of mononuclear phagocytes. With the aging and interplay between genetic and environmental factors, Bruch's membrane thickening and further lipofuscin accumulation in RPE cells occur. Growing drusen attract macrophages and recruit choroidal dendritic cells, thereby further increasing oxidative pressure on RPE cells. While the oxidative stress-induced inflammation is initially limited by innate immune responses, gradually the uncontrolled immune responses including dysregulated complement AP and inflammasome activation result in detrimental effects on RPE cells. The impaired autophagy-lysosomal function is a contributory factor

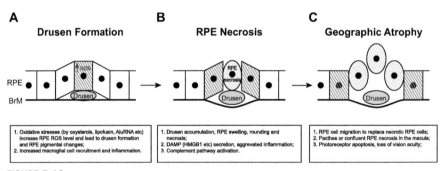

FIGURE 7.10

A model of AMD pathogenesis. RPE cells are exposed to a highly oxidative environment shuffling waste from photoreceptors, and providing trophic support. As the eye ages, cholesterol starts to accumulate on Bruch's membrane, and lipofuscin packets accumulate in RPE cells. Growing drusen attract macrophages and recruit choroidal dendritic cells while drusen accumulate products of lipid peroxidation they start to increase oxidative pressure on RPE cells (A) Damaged RPE cells die from necrosis, contributing to drusen formation, promoting inflammatory response, and promoting damage of the neighboring RPE cells (B) Those events attribute to self-perpetuating RPE cell death events (C).

Modified from Hanus J, Anderson C, Wang S. RPE necroptosis in response to oxidative stress and in AMD. Ageing Res Rev. 2015;24(Pt B):286–298. https://doi.org/10.1016/j.arr.2015.09.002.

to the fate of damaged RPE cells. The damaged RPE cells may undergo regulated cell death via necroptosis and pyroptosis with a minor contribution from apoptosis. In Fig. 7.10, only necroptosis, one of the forms of cell death, is exemplified. Damaged RPE cells are associated with drusen evolution, inflammatory response,[155] and inflammasome-related cytokine release. The damaged RPE cells also promote injury to neighboring RPE cells.[144] Those events attribute to self-perpetuating RPE cell death in the macular. RPE degeneration and cell death, in turn, cause a progressive degeneration of photoreceptors, leading to the irreversible loss of vision in the late stage of dry AMD.

References

1. Strauss O. The retinal pigment epithelium in visual function. *Physiol Rev.* 2005;85(3): 845−881. https://doi.org/10.1152/physrev.00021.2004.
2. Granger CE, Yang Q, Song H, et al. Human retinal pigment epithelium: in vivo cell morphometry, multispectral autofluorescence, and relationship to cone mosaic. *Invest Ophthalmol Vis Sci.* 2018;59(15):5705−5716. https://doi.org/10.1167/iovs.18-24677.
3. Booij JC, Baas DC, Beisekeeva J, Gorgels TGMF, Bergen AAB. The dynamic nature of Bruch's membrane. *Prog Retinal Eye Res.* 2010;29(1):1−18. https://doi.org/10.1016/j.preteyeres.2009.08.003.
4. Kurihara T, Westenskow PD, Gantner ML, et al. Hypoxia-induced metabolic stress in retinal pigment epithelial cells is sufficient to induce photoreceptor degeneration. *Elife.* 2016;5. https://doi.org/10.7554/eLife.14319.
5. Bressler SB, Maguire MG, Bressler NM, Fine SL. Relationship of drusen and abnormalities of the retinal pigment epithelium to the prognosis of neovascular macular degeneration. The macular photocoagulation study group. *Arch Ophthalmol.* 1990;108(10): 1442−1447. https://doi.org/10.1001/archopht.1990.01070120090035.
6. Pauleikhoff D, Zuels S, Sheraidah GS, Marshall J, Wessing A, Bird AC. Correlation between biochemical composition and fluorescein binding of deposits in Bruch's membrane. *Ophthalmology.* 1992;99(10):1548−1553. https://doi.org/10.1016/s0161-6420(92)31768-3.
7. Mullins RF, Johnson MN, Faidley EA, Skeie JM, Huang J. Choriocapillaris vascular dropout related to density of drusen in human eyes with early age-related macular degeneration. *Invest Ophthalmol Vis Sci.* 2011;52(3):1606−1612. https://doi.org/10.1167/iovs.10-6476.
8. Ramrattan RS, van der Schaft TL, Mooy CM, de Bruijn WC, Mulder PG, de Jong PT. Morphometric analysis of Bruch's membrane, the choriocapillaris, and the choroid in aging. *Invest Ophthalmol Vis Sci.* 1994;35(6):2857−2864.
9. Bird A. Role of retinal pigment epithelium in age-related macular disease: a systematic review. *Br J Ophthalmol.* September, 2020;19. https://doi.org/10.1136/bjophthalmol-2020-317447.
10. Dimitrov PN, Robman LD, Varsamidis M, et al. Visual function tests as potential biomarkers in age-related macular degeneration. *Invest Ophthalmol Vis Sci.* 2011;52(13): 9457−9469. https://doi.org/10.1167/iovs.10-7043.

11. Bird AC, Phillips RL, Hageman GS. Geographic atrophy: a histopathological assessment. *JAMA Ophthalmol.* 2014;132(3):338−345. https://doi.org/10.1001/jamaophthalmol.2013.5799.

12. Young RW. Pathophysiology of age-related macular degeneration. *Surv Ophthalmol.* 1987;31(5):291−306. https://doi.org/10.1016/0039-6257(87)90115-9.

13. Adijanto J, Du J, Moffat C, Seifert EL, Hurle JB, Philp NJ. The retinal pigment epithelium utilizes fatty acids for ketogenesis. *J Biol Chem.* 2014;289(30):20570−20582. https://doi.org/10.1074/jbc.M114.565457.

14. Fisher CR, Ferrington DA. Perspective on AMD pathobiology: a bioenergetic crisis in the RPE. *Invest Ophthalmol Vis Sci.* 2018;59(4):AMD41. https://doi.org/10.1167/iovs.18-24289.

15. Murphy MP. How mitochondria produce reactive oxygen species. *Biochem J.* 2009; 417(1):1−13. https://doi.org/10.1042/BJ20081386.

16. Nordgaard CL, Berg KM, Kapphahn RJ, et al. Proteomics of the retinal pigment epithelium reveals altered protein expression at progressive stages of age-related macular degeneration. *Invest Ophthalmol Vis Sci.* 2006;47(3):815−822. https://doi.org/10.1167/iovs.05-0976.

17. Nordgaard CL, Karunadharma PP, Feng X, Olsen TW, Ferrington DA. Mitochondrial proteomics of the retinal pigment epithelium at progressive stages of age-related macular degeneration. *Invest Ophthalmol Vis Sci.* 2008;49(7):2848−2855. https://doi.org/10.1167/iovs.07-1352.

18. Kanow MA, Giarmarco MM, Jankowski CS, et al. Biochemical adaptations of the retina and retinal pigment epithelium support a metabolic ecosystem in the vertebrate eye. *Elife.* 2017;6. https://doi.org/10.7554/eLife.28899.

19. Dunaief JL, Dentchev T, Ying G-S, Milam AH. The role of apoptosis in age-related macular degeneration. *Arch Ophthalmol.* 2002;120(11):1435−1442. https://doi.org/10.1001/archopht.120.11.1435.

20. Curcio CA, Medeiros NE, Millican CL. Photoreceptor loss in age-related macular degeneration. *Invest Ophthalmol Vis Sci.* 1996;37(7):1236−1249.

21. Datta S, Cano M, Ebrahimi K, Wang L, Handa JT. The impact of oxidative stress and inflammation on RPE degeneration in non-neovascular AMD. *Prog Retin Eye Res.* 2017;60:201−218. https://doi.org/10.1016/j.preteyeres.2017.03.002.

22. Pizzino G, Irrera N, Cucinotta M, et al. Oxidative stress: harms and benefits for human health. *Oxid Med Cell Longev.* 2017;2017:8416763. https://doi.org/10.1155/2017/8416763.

23. Kaarniranta K, Pawlowska E, Szczepanska J, Jablkowska A, Blasiak J. Role of mitochondrial DNA damage in ROS-mediated pathogenesis of age-related macular degeneration (AMD). *Int J Mol Sci.* 2019;20(10). https://doi.org/10.3390/ijms20102374.

24. Guzy RD, Hoyos B, Robin E, et al. Mitochondrial complex III is required for hypoxia-induced ROS production and cellular oxygen sensing. *Cell Metabolism.* 2005;1(6): 401−408. https://doi.org/10.1016/j.cmet.2005.05.001.

25. Hiona A, Leeuwenburgh C. The role of mitochondrial DNA mutations in aging and sarcopenia: implications for the mitochondrial vicious cycle theory of aging. *Exp Gerontol.* 2008;43(1):24−33. https://doi.org/10.1016/j.exger.2007.10.001.

26. Nanayakkara GK, Wang H, Yang X. Proton leak regulates mitochondrial reactive oxygen species generation in endothelial cell activation and inflammation - a novel concept. *Arch Biochem Biophys.* 2019;662:68−74. https://doi.org/10.1016/j.abb.2018.12.002.

27. Cline SD. Mitochondrial DNA damage and its consequences for mitochondrial gene expression. *Biochim Biophys Acta.* 2012;1819(9-10):979−991. https://doi.org/10.1016/j.bbagrm.2012.06.002.

28. Kauppila TES, Kauppila JHK, Larsson N-G. Mammalian mitochondria and aging: an update. *Cell Metab.* 2017;25(1):57−71. https://doi.org/10.1016/j.cmet.2016.09.017.

29. Blasiak J, Piechota M, Pawlowska E, Szatkowska M, Sikora E, Kaarniranta K. Cellular senescence in age-related macular degeneration: can autophagy and DNA damage response play a role? *Oxid Med Cell Longev.* 2017;2017:5293258. https://doi.org/10.1155/2017/5293258.

30. Winkler BS, Boulton ME, Gottsch JD, Sternberg P. Oxidative damage and age-related macular degeneration. *Mol Vis.* 1999;5:32.

31. Dieguez HH, Romeo HE, Alaimo A, et al. Oxidative stress damage circumscribed to the central temporal retinal pigment epithelium in early experimental non-exudative age-related macular degeneration. *Free Radic Biol Med.* 2019;131:72−80. https://doi.org/10.1016/j.freeradbiomed.2018.11.035.

32. Nassisi M, Tepelus T, Nittala MG, Sadda SR. Choriocapillaris flow impairment predicts the development and enlargement of drusen. *Graefes Arch Clin Exp Ophthalmol.* 2019;257(10):2079−2085. https://doi.org/10.1007/s00417-019-04403-1.

33. Borrelli E, Shi Y, Uji A, et al. Topographic analysis of the choriocapillaris in intermediate age-related macular degeneration. *Am J Ophthalmol.* 2018;196:34−43. https://doi.org/10.1016/j.ajo.2018.08.014.

34. De Bels D, Corazza F, Balestra C. Oxygen sensing, homeostasis, and disease. *N Engl J Med.* 2011;365(19):1845. https://doi.org/10.1056/NEJMc1110602. author reply 1846.

35. Chinnery PF, Samuels DC, Elson J, Turnbull DM. Accumulation of mitochondrial DNA mutations in ageing, cancer, and mitochondrial disease: is there a common mechanism? *Lancet.* 2002;360(9342):1323−1325. https://doi.org/10.1016/S0140-6736(02)11310-9.

36. Barreau E, Brossas JY, Courtois Y, Tréton JA. Accumulation of mitochondrial DNA deletions in human retina during aging. *Invest Ophthalmol Vis Sci.* 1996;37(2):384−391.

37. Jones MM, Manwaring N, Wang JJ, Rochtchina E, Mitchell P, Sue CM. Mitochondrial DNA haplogroups and age-related maculopathy. *Arch Ophthalmol.* 2007;125(9):1235−1240. https://doi.org/10.1001/archopht.125.9.1235.

38. Penta JS, Johnson FM, Wachsman JT, Copeland WC. Mitochondrial DNA in human malignancy. *Mutat Res.* 2001;488(2):119−133. https://doi.org/10.1016/s1383-5742(01)00053-9.

39. Kenney MC, Atilano SR, Boyer D, et al. Characterization of retinal and blood mitochondrial DNA from age-related macular degeneration patients. *Invest Ophthalmol Vis Sci.* 2010;51(8):4289−4297. https://doi.org/10.1167/iovs.09-4778.

40. Yu D-Y, Cringle SJ. Retinal degeneration and local oxygen metabolism. *Exp Eye Res.* 2005;80(6):745−751. https://doi.org/10.1016/j.exer.2005.01.018.

41. Jarrett SG, Boulton ME. Consequences of oxidative stress in age-related macular degeneration. *Mol Aspects Med.* 2012;33(4):399−417. https://doi.org/10.1016/j.mam.2012.03.009.

42. Age-Related Eye Disease Study 2 Research Group. Lutein + zeaxanthin and omega-3 fatty acids for age-related macular degeneration: the age-related eye disease study 2 (AREDS2) randomized clinical trial. *JAMA.* 2013;309(19):2005−2015. https://doi.org/10.1001/jama.2013.4997.

43. Hollyfield JG, Bonilha VL, Rayborn ME, et al. Oxidative damage-induced inflammation initiates age-related macular degeneration. *Nat Med.* 2008;14(2):194−198. https://doi.org/10.1038/nm1709.

44. Suzuki M, Kamei M, Itabe H, et al. Oxidized phospholipids in the macula increase with age and in eyes with age-related macular degeneration. *Mol Vis.* 2007;13:772−778.

45. Masters SL, De Nardo D. Innate immunity. *Curr Opin Immunol.* 2014;26:v−vi. https://doi.org/10.1016/j.coi.2013.12.006.

46. Kauppinen A, Paterno JJ, Blasiak J, Salminen A, Kaarniranta K. Inflammation and its role in age-related macular degeneration. *Cell Mol Life Sci.* 2016;73(9):1765−1786. https://doi.org/10.1007/s00018-016-2147-8.

47. Kawai T, Akira S. The role of pattern-recognition receptors in innate immunity: update on Toll-like receptors. *Nat Immunol.* 2010;11(5):373−384. https://doi.org/10.1038/ni.1863.

48. Elner SG, Petty HR, Elner VM, et al. TLR4 mediates human retinal pigment epithelial endotoxin binding and cytokine expression. *Trans Am Ophthalmol Soc.* 2005;103:126−135. discussion 135-137.

49. Kumar MV, Nagineni CN, Chin MS, Hooks JJ, Detrick B. Innate immunity in the retina: Toll-like receptor (TLR) signaling in human retinal pigment epithelial cells. *J Neuroimmunol.* 2004;153(1-2):7−15. https://doi.org/10.1016/j.jneuroim.2004.04.018.

50. Kaarniranta K, Koskela A, Felszeghy S, Kivinen N, Salminen A, Kauppinen A. Fatty acids and oxidized lipoproteins contribute to autophagy and innate immunity responses upon the degeneration of retinal pigment epithelium and development of age-related macular degeneration. *Biochimie.* 2019;159:49−54. https://doi.org/10.1016/j.biochi.2018.07.010.

51. Parmar VM, Parmar T, Arai E, Perusek L, Maeda A. A2E-associated cell death and inflammation in retinal pigmented epithelial cells from human induced pluripotent stem cells. *Stem Cell Res.* 2018;27:95−104. https://doi.org/10.1016/j.scr.2018.01.014.

52. Despriet DDG, Bergen AAB, Merriam JE, et al. Comprehensive analysis of the candidate genes CCL2, CCR2, and TLR4 in age-related macular degeneration. *Invest Ophthalmol Vis Sci.* 2008;49(1):364−371. https://doi.org/10.1167/iovs.07-0656.

53. Fernandez-Godino R, Garland DL, Pierce EA. A local complement response by RPE causes early-stage macular degeneration. *Hum Mol Genet.* 2015;24(19):5555−5569. https://doi.org/10.1093/hmg/ddv287.

54. Rohrer B, Coughlin B, Kunchithapautham K, et al. The alternative pathway is required, but not alone sufficient, for retinal pathology in mouse laser-induced choroidal neovascularization. *Mol Immunol.* 2011;48(6-7):e1−e8. https://doi.org/10.1016/j.molimm.2010.12.016.

55. Schramm EC, Clark SJ, Triebwasser MP, Raychaudhuri S, Seddon JM, Atkinson JP. Genetic variants in the complement system predisposing to age-related macular degeneration: a review. *Mol Immunol.* 2014;61(2):118−125. https://doi.org/10.1016/j.molimm.2014.06.032.

56. Karki RG, Powers J, Mainolfi N, et al. Design, synthesis, and preclinical characterization of selective factor D inhibitors targeting the alternative complement pathway. *J Med Chem.* 2019;62(9):4656−4668. https://doi.org/10.1021/acs.jmedchem.9b00271.

57. Sharp TH, Koster AJ, Gros P. Heterogeneous MAC initiator and pore structures in a lipid bilayer by phase-plate cryo-electron tomography. *Cell Rep.* 2016;15(1):1−8. https://doi.org/10.1016/j.celrep.2016.03.002.

58. Ferreira VP, Pangburn MK, Cortés C. Complement control protein factor H: the good, the bad, and the inadequate. *Mol Immunol.* 2010;47(13):2187—2197. https://doi.org/10.1016/j.molimm.2010.05.007.

59. Bergseth G, Ludviksen JK, Kirschfink M, Giclas PC, Nilsson B, Mollnes TE. An international serum standard for application in assays to detect human complement activation products. *Mol Immunol.* 2013;56(3):232—239. https://doi.org/10.1016/j.molimm.2013.05.221.

60. Scholl HPN, Issa PC, Walier M, et al. Systemic complement activation in age-related macular degenerationToland AE, ed. *PLoS One.* 2008;3(7):e2593. https://doi.org/10.1371/journal.pone.0002593.

61. Reynolds R, Hartnett ME, Atkinson JP, Giclas PC, Rosner B, Seddon JM. Plasma complement components and activation fragments: associations with age-related macular degeneration genotypes and phenotypes. *Invest Ophthalmol Vis Sci.* 2009;50(12):5818. https://doi.org/10.1167/iovs.09-3928.

62. Lechner J, Chen M, Hogg RE, et al. Higher plasma levels of complement C3a, C4a and C5a increase the risk of subretinal fibrosis in neovascular age-related macular degeneration: complement activation in AMD. *Immun Ageing.* 2016;13(1):4. https://doi.org/10.1186/s12979-016-0060-5.

63. Lorés-Motta L, Paun CC, Corominas J, et al. Genome-wide association study reveals variants in CFH and CFHR4 associated with systemic complement activation: implications in age-related macular degeneration. *Ophthalmology.* 2018;125(7):1064—1074. https://doi.org/10.1016/j.ophtha.2017.12.023.

64. Donoso LA, Vrabec T, Kuivaniemi H. The role of complement factor H in age-related macular degeneration: a review. *Survey Ophthalmol.* 2010;55(3):227—246. https://doi.org/10.1016/j.survophthal.2009.11.001.

65. Mandal MNA, Ayyagari R. Complement factor H: spatial and temporal expression and localization in the eye. *Invest Ophthalmol Vis Sci.* 2006;47(9):4091—4097. https://doi.org/10.1167/iovs.05-1655.

66. Milder FJ, Gomes L, Schouten A, et al. Factor B structure provides insights into activation of the central protease of the complement system. *Nat Struct Mol Biol.* 2007;14(3):224—228. https://doi.org/10.1038/nsmb1210.

67. Pangburn MK, Müller-Eberhard HJ. The C3 convertase of the alternative pathway of human complement. Enzymic properties of the bimolecular proteinase. *Biochem J.* 1986;235(3):723—730. https://doi.org/10.1042/bj2350723.

68. Schwaeble W, Dippold WG, Schäfer MK, et al. Properdin, a positive regulator of complement activation, is expressed in human T cell lines and peripheral blood T cells. *J Immunol.* 1993;151(5):2521—2528.

69. Hourcade DE. The role of properdin in the assembly of the alternative pathway C3 convertases of complement. *J Biol Chem.* 2006;281(4):2128—2132. https://doi.org/10.1074/jbc.M508928200.

70. Kajander T, Lehtinen MJ, Hyvarinen S, et al. Dual interaction of factor H with C3d and glycosaminoglycans in host-nonhost discrimination by complement. *Proc Nat Academy Sci.* 2011;108(7):2897—2902. https://doi.org/10.1073/pnas.1017087108.

71. Pangburn MK, Schreiber RD, Müller-Eberhard HJ. Formation of the initial C3 convertase of the alternative complement pathway. Acquisition of C3b-like activities by spontaneous hydrolysis of the putative thioester in native C3. *J Experiment Med.* 1981;154(3):856—867. https://doi.org/10.1084/jem.154.3.856.

72. Fernandez-Godino R, Bujakowska KM, Pierce EA. Changes in extracellular matrix cause RPE cells to make basal deposits and activate the alternative complement pathway. *Human Mol Gene.* 2018;27(1):147−159. https://doi.org/10.1093/hmg/ddx392.

73. Toomey CB, Kelly U, Saban DR, Bowes Rickman C. Regulation of age-related macular degeneration-like pathology by complement factor H. *Proc Natl Acad Sci USA.* 2015;112(23):E3040−3049. https://doi.org/10.1073/pnas.1424391112.

74. Calippe B, Augustin S, Beguier F, et al. Complement factor H inhibits CD47-mediated resolution of inflammation. *Immunity.* 2017;46(2):261−272. https://doi.org/10.1016/j.immuni.2017.01.006.

75. Levy O, Calippe B, Lavalette S, et al. Apolipoprotein E promotes subretinal mononuclear phagocyte survival and chronic inflammation in age-related macular degeneration. *EMBO Mol Med.* 2015;7(2):211−226. https://doi.org/10.15252/emmm.201404524.

76. Hajishengallis G, Reis ES, Mastellos DC, Ricklin D, Lambris JD. Novel mechanisms and functions of complement. *Nat Immunol.* 2017;18(12):1288−1298. https://doi.org/10.1038/ni.3858.

77. Martinon F, Burns K, Tschopp J. The Inflammasome. *Mol Cell.* 2002;10(2):417−426. https://doi.org/10.1016/S1097-2765(02)00599-3.

78. Kaneko H, Dridi S, Tarallo V, et al. DICER1 deficit induces Alu RNA toxicity in age-related macular degeneration. *Nature.* 2011;471(7338):325−330. https://doi.org/10.1038/nature09830.

79. Tarallo V, Hirano Y, Gelfand BD, et al. DICER1 loss and Alu RNA induce age-related macular degeneration via the NLRP3 inflammasome and MyD88. *Cell.* 2012;149(4):847−859. https://doi.org/10.1016/j.cell.2012.03.036.

80. Schmid CW, Deininger PL. Sequence organization of the human genome. *Cell.* 1975;6(3):345−358. https://doi.org/10.1016/0092-8674(75)90184-1.

81. Berger A, Strub K. Multiple roles of Alu-related noncoding RNAs. *Prog Mol Subcell Biol.* 2011;51:119−146. https://doi.org/10.1007/978-3-642-16502-3_6.

82. Muñoz-Planillo R, Kuffa P, Martínez-Colón G, Smith BL, Rajendiran TM, Núñez G. K^+ efflux is the common trigger of NLRP3 inflammasome activation by bacterial toxins and particulate matter. *Immunity.* 2013;38(6):1142−1153. https://doi.org/10.1016/j.immuni.2013.05.016.

83. Lawlor KE, Vince JE. Ambiguities in NLRP3 inflammasome regulation: is there a role for mitochondria? *Biochim Biophys Acta.* 2014;1840(4):1433−1440. https://doi.org/10.1016/j.bbagen.2013.08.014.

84. Yamamoto-Rodríguez L, Zarbin MA, Casaroli-Marano RP. New frontiers and clinical implications in the pathophysiology of age-related macular degeneration. *Med Clin.* 2020;154(12):496−504. https://doi.org/10.1016/j.medcli.2020.01.023.

85. Sutterwala FS, Haasken S, Cassel SL. Mechanism of NLRP3 inflammasome activation. *Ann N Y Acad Sci.* 2014;1319:82−95. https://doi.org/10.1111/nyas.12458.

86. Tseng WA, Thein T, Kinnunen K, et al. NLRP3 inflammasome activation in retinal pigment epithelial cells by lysosomal destabilization: implications for age-related macular degeneration. *Invest Ophthalmol Vis Sci.* 2013;54(1):110−120. https://doi.org/10.1167/iovs.12-10655.

87. Hornung V, Bauernfeind F, Halle A, et al. Silica crystals and aluminum salts activate the NALP3 inflammasome through phagosomal destabilization. *Nat Immunol.* 2008;9(8):847−856. https://doi.org/10.1038/ni.1631.

88. Zhou R, Yazdi AS, Menu P, Tschopp J. A role for mitochondria in NLRP3 inflammasome activation. *Nature*. 2011;469(7329):221−225. https://doi.org/10.1038/nature09663.

89. Gao J, Liu RT, Cao S, et al. NLRP3 inflammasome: activation and regulation in age-related macular degeneration. *Media Inflammat*. 2015;2015:1−11. https://doi.org/10.1155/2015/690243.

90. Bosset S, Bonnet-Duquennoy M, Barré P, et al. Photoageing shows histological features of chronic skin inflammation without clinical and molecular abnormalities. *Br J Dermatol*. 2003;149(4):826−835. https://doi.org/10.1046/j.1365-2133.2003.05456.x.

91. Kauppinen A, Niskanen H, Suuronen T, Kinnunen K, Salminen A, Kaarniranta K. Oxidative stress activates NLRP3 inflammasomes in ARPE-19 cells—implications for age-related macular degeneration (AMD). *Immunol Lett*. 2012;147(1-2):29−33. https://doi.org/10.1016/j.imlet.2012.05.005.

92. Reuter BK, Pizarro TT. Commentary: the role of the IL-18 system and other members of the IL-1R/TLR superfamily in innate mucosal immunity and the pathogenesis of inflammatory bowel disease: friend or foe? *Eur J Immunol*. 2004;34(9):2347−2355. https://doi.org/10.1002/eji.200425351.

93. Langford-Smith A, Keenan TDL, Clark SJ, Bishop PN, Day AJ. The role of complement in age-related macular degeneration: heparan sulphate, a ZIP code for complement factor H? *J Innate Immun*. 2014;6(4):407−416. https://doi.org/10.1159/000356513.

94. Hageman GS, Anderson DH, Johnson LV, et al. A common haplotype in the complement regulatory gene factor H (HF1/CFH) predisposes individuals to age-related macular degeneration. *Proc Natl Acad Sci USA*. 2005;102(20):7227−7232. https://doi.org/10.1073/pnas.0501536102.

95. Dhillon B, Wright AF, Tufail A, et al. Complement factor h autoantibodies and age-related macular degeneration. *Invest Ophthalmol Vis Sci*. 2010;51(11):5858−5863. https://doi.org/10.1167/iovs.09-5124.

96. Triantafilou K, Hughes TR, Triantafilou M, Morgan BP. The complement membrane attack complex triggers intracellular Ca^{2+} fluxes leading to NLRP3 inflammasome activation. *J Cell Sci*. 2013;126(Pt 13):2903−2913. https://doi.org/10.1242/jcs.124388.

97. Triantafilou M, Hughes TR, Morgan BP, Triantafilou K. Complementing the inflammasome. *Immunology*. 2016;147(2):152−164. https://doi.org/10.1111/imm.12556.

98. Arulkumaran N, Unwin RJ, Tam FW. A potential therapeutic role for P2X7 receptor (P2X7R) antagonists in the treatment of inflammatory diseases. *Expert Opin Investigat Drug*. 2011;20(7):897−915. https://doi.org/10.1517/13543784.2011.578068.

99. Mangan MSJ, Olhava EJ, Roush WR, Seidel HM, Glick GD, Latz E. Targeting the NLRP3 inflammasome in inflammatory diseases. *Nat Rev Drug Discov*. 2018;17(8):588−606. https://doi.org/10.1038/nrd.2018.97.

100. Coll RC, Robertson AAB, Chae JJ, et al. A small-molecule inhibitor of the NLRP3 inflammasome for the treatment of inflammatory diseases. *Nat Med*. 2015;21(3):248−255. https://doi.org/10.1038/nm.3806.

101. Parsons N, Annamalai B, Obert E, Schnabolk G, Tomlinson S, Rohrer B. Inhibition of the alternative complement pathway accelerates repair processes in the murine model of choroidal neovascularization. *Mol Immunol*. 2019;108:8−12. https://doi.org/10.1016/j.molimm.2019.02.001.

102. Chi Z-L, Yoshida T, Lambris JD, Iwata T. Suppression of drusen formation by compstatin, a peptide inhibitor of complement C3 activation, on cynomolgus monkey with

early-onset macular degeneration. *Adv Exp Med Biol*. 2010;703:127−135. https://doi.org/10.1007/978-1-4419-5635-4_9.

103. Schrezenmeier H, Höchsmann B. Eculizumab opens a new era of treatment for paroxysmal nocturnal hemoglobinuria. *Expert Rev Hematol*. 2009;2(1):7−16. https://doi.org/10.1586/17474086.2.1.7.

104. Gil-Martínez M, Santos-Ramos P, Fernández-Rodríguez M, et al. Pharmacological advances in the treatment of age-related macular degeneration. *Curr Med Chem*. 2020; 27(4):583−598. https://doi.org/10.2174/0929867326666190726121711.

105. Mimoun G, Soubrane G, Coscas G. Macular drusen. *J Fr Ophtalmol*. 1990;13(10): 511−530.

106. Zhang Y, Wang X, Sadda SR, et al. Lifecycles of individual subretinal drusenoid deposits and evolution of outer retinal atrophy in age-related macular degeneration. *Ophthalmol Retina*. 2020;4(3):274−283. https://doi.org/10.1016/j.oret.2019.10.012.

107. Spaide RF, Ooto S, Curcio CA. Subretinal drusenoid deposits AKA pseudodrusen. *Surv Ophthalmol*. 2018;63(6):782−815. https://doi.org/10.1016/j.survophthal.2018.05.005.

108. Sarks JP, Sarks SH, Killingsworth MC. Evolution of geographic atrophy of the retinal pigment epithelium. *Eye*. 1988;2(Pt 5):552−577. https://doi.org/10.1038/eye.1988.106.

109. Curcio CA. Antecedents of soft drusen, the specific deposits of age-related macular degeneration, in the biology of human macula. *Invest Ophthalmol Vis Sci*. 2018; 59(4):AMD182−AMD194. https://doi.org/10.1167/iovs.18-24883.

110. Elner VM. Retinal pigment epithelial acid lipase activity and lipoprotein receptors: effects of dietary omega-3 fatty acids. *Trans Am Ophthalmol Soc*. 2002;100:301−338.

111. Schnebelen C, Viau S, Grégoire S, et al. Nutrition for the eye: different susceptibility of the retina and the lacrimal gland to dietary omega-6 and omega-3 polyunsaturated fatty acid incorporation. *Ophthalmic Res*. 2009;41(4):216−224. https://doi.org/10.1159/000217726.

112. Calvo D, Gómez-Coronado D, Suárez Y, Lasunción MA, Vega MA. Human CD36 is a high affinity receptor for the native lipoproteins HDL, LDL, and VLDL. *J Lipid Res*. 1998;39(4):777−788.

113. Ryeom SW, Sparrow JR, Silverstein RL. CD36 participates in the phagocytosis of rod outer segments by retinal pigment epithelium. *J Cell Sci*. 1996;109(Pt 2):387−395.

114. Buhaescu I, Izzedine H. Mevalonate pathway: a review of clinical and therapeutical implications. *Clin Biochem*. 2007;40(9-10):575−584. https://doi.org/10.1016/j.clinbiochem.2007.03.016.

115. Brunham LR, Hayden MR. Human genetics of HDL: insight into particle metabolism and function. *Prog Lipid Res*. 2015;58:14−25. https://doi.org/10.1016/j.plipres.2015.01.001.

116. Guyton JR, Klemp KF. Ultrastructural discrimination of lipid droplets and vesicles in atherosclerosis: value of osmium-thiocarbohydrazide-osmium and tannic acid-paraphenylenediamine techniques. *J Histochem Cytochem*. 1988;36(10):1319−1328. https://doi.org/10.1177/36.10.2458408.

117. Balaratnasingam C, Yannuzzi LA, Curcio CA, et al. Associations between retinal pigment epithelium and drusen volume changes during the lifecycle of large drusenoid pigment epithelial detachments. *Invest Ophthalmol Vis Sci*. 2016;57(13):5479−5489. https://doi.org/10.1167/iovs.16-19816.

118. Zweifel SA, Spaide RF, Curcio CA, Malek G, Imamura Y. Reticular pseudodrusen are subretinal drusenoid deposits. *Ophthalmology*. 2010;117(2):303−312. https://doi.org/10.1016/j.ophtha.2009.07.014. e1.

119. Baek J-H, Lim D, Park KH, et al. Quantitative proteomic analysis of aqueous humor from patients with drusen and reticular pseudodrusen in age-related macular degeneration. *BMC Ophthalmol.* 2018;18(1):289. https://doi.org/10.1186/s12886-018-0941-9.

120. Greferath U, Guymer RH, Vessey KA, Brassington K, Fletcher EL. Correlation of histologic features with in vivo imaging of reticular pseudodrusen. *Ophthalmology.* 2016;123(6):1320−1331. https://doi.org/10.1016/j.ophtha.2016.02.009.

121. Vessey KA, Wilkinson-Berka JL, Fletcher EL. Characterization of retinal function and glial cell response in a mouse model of oxygen-induced retinopathy. *J Comp Neurol.* 2011;519(3):506−527. https://doi.org/10.1002/cne.22530.

122. Yuan X, Gu X, Crabb JS, et al. Quantitative proteomics: comparison of the macular Bruch membrane/choroid complex from age-related macular degeneration and normal eyes. *Mol Cell Proteom.* 2010;9(6):1031−1046. https://doi.org/10.1074/mcp.M900523-MCP200.

123. Crabb JW. The proteomics of drusen. *Cold Spring Harb Perspect Med.* 2014;4(7): a017194. https://doi.org/10.1101/cshperspect.a017194.

124. Ethen CM, Reilly C, Feng X, Olsen TW, Ferrington DA. The proteome of central and peripheral retina with progression of age-related macular degeneration. *Invest Ophthalmol Vis Sci.* 2006;47(6):2280−2290. https://doi.org/10.1167/iovs.05-1395.

125. Bergen AA, Arya S, Koster C, et al. On the origin of proteins in human drusen: The meet, greet and stick hypothesis. *Prog Retin Eye Res.* 2019;70:55−84. https://doi.org/10.1016/j.preteyeres.2018.12.003.

126. Tabas I, Williams KJ, Borén J. Subendothelial lipoprotein retention as the initiating process in atherosclerosis: update and therapeutic implications. *Circulation.* 2007;116(16):1832−1844. https://doi.org/10.1161/CIRCULATIONAHA.106.676890.

127. Lengyel I, Flinn JM, Peto T, et al. High concentration of zinc in sub-retinal pigment epithelial deposits. *Exp Eye Res.* 2007;84(4):772−780. https://doi.org/10.1016/j.exer.2006.12.015.

128. Thompson RB, Reffatto V, Bundy JG, et al. Identification of hydroxyapatite spherules provides new insight into subretinal pigment epithelial deposit formation in the aging eye. *Proc Natl Acad Sci USA.* 2015;112(5):1565−1570. https://doi.org/10.1073/pnas.1413347112.

129. Ferris FL, Wilkinson CP, Bird A, et al. Clinical classification of age-related macular degeneration. *Ophthalmology.* 2013;120(4):844−851. https://doi.org/10.1016/j.ophtha.2012.10.036.

130. Folgar FA, Chow JH, Farsiu S, et al. Spatial correlation between hyperpigmentary changes on color fundus photography and hyperreflective foci on SDOCT in intermediate AMD. *Invest Ophthalmol Vis Sci.* 2012;53(8):4626−4633. https://doi.org/10.1167/iovs.12-9813.

131. Leuschen JN, Schuman SG, Winter KP, et al. Spectral-domain optical coherence tomography characteristics of intermediate age-related macular degeneration. *Ophthalmology.* 2013;120(1):140−150. https://doi.org/10.1016/j.ophtha.2012.07.004.

132. Balaratnasingam C, Messinger JD, Sloan KR, Yannuzzi LA, Freund KB, Curcio CA. Histologic and optical coherence tomographic correlates in drusenoid pigment epithelium detachment in age-related macular degeneration. *Ophthalmology.* 2017;124(5):644−656. https://doi.org/10.1016/j.ophtha.2016.12.034.

133. Christenbury JG, Folgar FA, O'Connell RV, Chiu SJ, Farsiu S, Toth CA. Progression of intermediate age-related macular degeneration with proliferation and inner retinal

migration of hyperreflective foci. *Ophthalmology*. 2013;120(5):1038−1045. https://doi.org/10.1016/j.ophtha.2012.10.018.

134. Curcio CA, Zanzottera EC, Ach T, Balaratnasingam C, Freund KB. Activated retinal pigment epithelium, an optical coherence tomography biomarker for progression in age-related macular degeneration. *Invest Ophthalmol Vis Sci*. 2017;58(6):BIO211−BIO226. https://doi.org/10.1167/iovs.17-21872.

135. Kang J-W, Chung H, Chan Kim H. Correlation of optical coherence tomographic hyper-reflective foci with visual outcomes in different patterns of diabetic macular edema. *Retina*. 2016;36(9):1630−1639. https://doi.org/10.1097/IAE.0000000000000995.

136. Eldred GE, Lasky MR. Retinal age pigments generated by self-assembling lysosomo-tropic detergents. *Nature*. 1993;361(6414):724−726. https://doi.org/10.1038/361724a0.

137. Bergmann M, Schütt F, Holz FG, Kopitz J. Inhibition of the ATP-driven proton pump in RPE lysosomes by the major lipofuscin fluorophore A2-E may contribute to the pathogenesis of age-related macular degeneration. *FASEB J*. 2004;18(3):562−564. https://doi.org/10.1096/fj.03-0289fje.

138. Krohne TU, Stratmann NK, Kopitz J, Holz FG. Effects of lipid peroxidation products on lipofuscinogenesis and autophagy in human retinal pigment epithelial cells. *Exp Eye Res*. 2010;90(3):465−471. https://doi.org/10.1016/j.exer.2009.12.011.

139. Gómez-Sintes R, Ledesma MD, Boya P. Lysosomal cell death mechanisms in aging. *Age Res Rev*. 2016;32:150−168. https://doi.org/10.1016/j.arr.2016.02.009.

140. Boya P, Esteban-Martínez L, Serrano-Puebla A, Gómez-Sintes R, Villarejo-Zori B. Autophagy in the eye: development, degeneration, and aging. *Prog Retin Eye Res*. 2016;55:206−245. https://doi.org/10.1016/j.preteyeres.2016.08.001.

141. Fazeli G, Wehman AM. Safely removing cell debris with LC3-associated phagocytosis. *Biol Cell*. 2017;109(10):355−363. https://doi.org/10.1111/boc.201700028.

142. Bonet-Ponce L, Saez-Atienzar S, da Casa C, et al. On the mechanism underlying ethanol-induced mitochondrial dynamic disruption and autophagy response. *Biochim Biophys Acta*. 2015;1852(7):1400−1409. https://doi.org/10.1016/j.bbadis.2015.03.006.

143. Kaarniranta K, Sinha D, Blasiak J, et al. Autophagy and heterophagy dysregulation leads to retinal pigment epithelium dysfunction and development of age-related macular degeneration. *Autophagy*. 2013;9(7):973−984. https://doi.org/10.4161/auto.24546.

144. Hanus J, Anderson C, Wang S. RPE necroptosis in response to oxidative stress and in AMD. *Age Res Rev*. 2015;24(Pt B):286−298. https://doi.org/10.1016/j.arr.2015.09.002.

145. Kaarniranta K, Tokarz P, Koskela A, Paterno J, Blasiak J. Autophagy regulates death of retinal pigment epithelium cells in age-related macular degeneration. *Cell Biol Toxicol*. 2017;33(2):113−128. https://doi.org/10.1007/s10565-016-9371-8.

146. Jang K-H, Do Y-J, Son D, Son E, Choi J-S, Kim E. AIF-independent parthanatos in the pathogenesis of dry age-related macular degeneration. *Cell Death Dis*. 2018;8(1). https://doi.org/10.1038/cddis.2016.437. e2526-e2526.

147. Krysko DV, Vanden Berghe T, D'Herde K, Vandenabeele P. Apoptosis and necrosis: Detection, discrimination and phagocytosis. *Methods*. 2008;44(3):205−221. https://doi.org/10.1016/j.ymeth.2007.12.001.

148. Trichonas G, Murakami Y, Thanos A, et al. Receptor interacting protein kinases mediate retinal detachment-induced photoreceptor necrosis and compensate for inhibition of apoptosis. *Proc Natl Acad Sci USA*. 2010;107(50):21695−21700. https://doi.org/10.1073/pnas.1009179107.

149. Brandstetter C, Holz FG, Krohne TU. Complement component C5a primes retinal pigment epithelial cells for inflammasome activation by lipofuscin-mediated photooxidative damage. *J Biol Chem*. 2015;290(52):31189−31198. https://doi.org/10.1074/jbc.M115.671180.

150. Brandstetter C, Patt J, Holz FG, Krohne TU. Inflammasome priming increases retinal pigment epithelial cell susceptibility to lipofuscin phototoxicity by changing the cell death mechanism from apoptosis to pyroptosis. *J Photochem Photobiol B: Biol*. 2016;161:177−183. https://doi.org/10.1016/j.jphotobiol.2016.05.018.

151. Zhao M, Bai Y, Xie W, et al. Interleukin-1β level is increased in vitreous of patients with neovascular age-related macular degeneration (nAMD) and polypoidal choroidal vasculopathy (PCV)Wen R, ed. *PLoS One*. 2015;10(5):e0125150. https://doi.org/10.1371/journal.pone.0125150.

152. Ardeljan CP, Ardeljan D, Abu-Asab M, Chan C-C. Inflammation and cell death in age-related macular degeneration: an immunopathological and ultrastructural model. *J Clin Med*. 2014;3(4):1542−1560. https://doi.org/10.3390/jcm3041542.

153. Aachoui Y, Sagulenko V, Miao EA, Stacey KJ. Inflammasome-mediated pyroptotic and apoptotic cell death, and defense against infection. *Curr Opin Microbiol*. 2013;16(3):319−326. https://doi.org/10.1016/j.mib.2013.04.004.

154. Linkermann A, Stockwell BR, Krautwald S, Anders H-J. Regulated cell death and inflammation: an auto-amplification loop causes organ failure. *Nat Rev Immunol*. 2014;14(11):759−767. https://doi.org/10.1038/nri3743.

155. Qin S, Rodrigues GA. Progress and perspectives on the role of RPE cell inflammatory responses in the development of age-related macular degeneration. *J Inflamm Res*. 2008;1:49−65. https://doi.org/10.2147/jir.s4354.

Pathogenesis of neovascular age-related macular degeneration

Angiogenesis and CNV formation

Angiogenesis is the process of new vessel formation from preexisting ones.[1] Under physiological and developmental conditions, angiogenesis is tightly regulated by a coordinated balance between pro- and antiangiogenic factors. Alterations in this fine-tuned balance could possibly lead to the increased production of proangiogenic mediators and the loss of inhibitory factors. For instance, neovascular AMD (nAMD) is characterized by the loss of this balance associated with choriocapillaris endothelial cell (CEC) dysfunction, leading to pathologic angiogenesis forming choroidal neovascularization (CNV).[2] CNV breaks through Bruch's membrane into the sub-RPE space and/or the subretinal space, leading to exudation, hemorrhage, retinal edema, pigment epithelial detachment, and fibrosis, which can cause severe irreversible vision loss. Within the last 15 years, anti-VEGF therapy has revolutionized the nAMD treatment paradigm. Intravitreal injection of VEGF inhibitors can prevent vision loss and even improve vision in patients with nAMD. But, nAMD still accounts for 90% of AMD-related vision loss.[3] As CNV plays a central pathogenic role in nAMD, the underlying mechanisms of CNV formation need to be fully elucidated. Furthermore, a comprehensive approach targeting angiogenic control is required to improve outcomes of nAMD treatment. Because the function of several proangiogenic mediators is cross regulated, selecting an upstream and targeting multiple cascades are the promising strategies for nAMD therapy. This chapter emphasizes understanding key initiating factors for angiogenic signaling pathways and focuses on the mechanism of multiple cell—cell interaction in CEC migration and proliferation.[4]

NADPH oxidase-derived ROS and angiogenesis

In vascular endothelial cells (ECs), nicotinamide adenine dinucleotide phosphate oxidase (NADPH oxidase) is the major source of superoxide (O_2^-) and reactive oxygen species (ROS).[5] Structurally, NADPH oxidase is a membrane-bound enzyme complex consisting of catalytic subunits (Nox1, Nox2, and Nox4), p22phox, p47phox, p67phox, and a small signaling G protein (GTPase Rac1).[5,6]

Functionally, NADPH oxidase-derived ROS is a double-edged sword. Excessive amounts of ROS have deleterious effects on cell membranes, while physiological concentrations of ROS are essential to host defense as signaling molecules. Thus, whether the function of the EC-generated ROS is physiologic or pathologic depends on concentration.[7] Therefore, nonspecifically suppressing NADPH oxidase-derived ROS may present safety concerns.[8] However, dietary antioxidants and zinc that can block down-stream oxidative damage caused by ROS for patients with early AMD can slow the progression to nAMD, though modestly.[9]

In the NADPH oxidase enzyme complex (Nox), Nox2 is an essential component.[10] Nox2 expression and Nox2-dependent ROS production are increased by oxidative stress, angiotensin II, VEGF, and angiopoietin-2 in ECs.[11] Nox4 is most abundantly expressed in ECs, and is involved in O_2^- production.[5] NADPH oxidases are highly compartmentalized in subcellular locations. The specific location may contribute to localized ROS production and activated specific redox signaling pathways.[12] Without stimulation, Nox2 and its regulatory proteins as well as Nox4 exist in an intracellular perinuclear compartment, especially endoplasmic reticulum that is associated with actin cytoskeleton.[13] Nox4 also localizes to the nucleus in human ECs, which participates in oxidative stress-responsive gene expression.[14] Rac1 is a subunit for some Nox isoforms that aggregate to activate NADPH oxidase. Nox2 and Rac1 accumulate at the site of new leading edge in actively migrating ECs.[15] Furthermore, in ECs, the death receptor activation causes clustering of cholesterol-enriched domains in the cell membrane (lipid raft), where Nox2, p47phox, and Rac1 are recruited to increase ROS and to form redox signaling platforms (Fig. 8.1).[16,20] The resultant increase in ROS production promotes cytoskeletal reorganization and directs EC migration. For example, in an in vitro model of EC migration in response to injury, Nox2 activity and actin-binding ability were monitored. When ROS production of ECs is increased at the margin of an injured area, Nox2 also translocates to the leading edge, where it colocalizes and associates with the actin-binding activity, indicating cytoskeletal reorganization in migrating ECs.[15]

In the context of the AMD microenvironment, extracellular stimuli for CECs such as hypoxia/ischemia promote ROS and VEGF production. Through ligand-receptor dimerization, external VEGF binds to two tyrosine kinase receptors, VEGF receptor-1 (VEGFR1, Flt-1) and VEGFR2 in ECs (Figs. 8.1 and 8.4).[20,58] The mitogenic and chemotactic effects of VEGF in ECs are mediated mainly through VEGFR2.[17] Phosphorylation of VEGFR2 leads to activation and translocation of the small GTPase Rac1 to the plasma membrane, thus stimulating the Nox2-based NADPH oxidase in ECs. The ROS derived from NADPH oxidase may oxidize and inactivates protein tyrosine phosphatases (PTP) that negatively regulate VEGFR2by promoting its autophosphorylation (Figs. 8.1 and 8.4).[20,58] ROS derived from NADPH oxidases plays a critical role in growth factor-induced switch from a quiescent to an angiogenic phenotype in ECs.[18] The resultant activation of down-stream redox signaling events links to EC proliferation and migration.[5,19] This is a feed-forward ROS-induced ROS-release loop coordinated by the endogenous NADPH oxidase/mtROS axis. By this mechanism, sustained activation of the

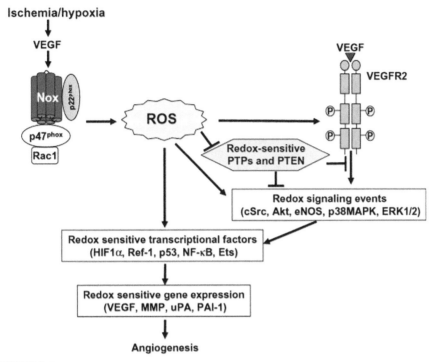

FIGURE 8.1

Role of ROS derived from NADPH oxidase (Nox) in VEGF signaling linked to induction of transcription factors and genes involved in angiogenesis. Ischemia/hypoxia stimulates the induction of VEGF that stimulates NADPH oxidase to produce ROS, thereby inducing oxidative inactivation of protein tyrosine phosphatases (PTPs) and phosphatase and tensin homolog (PTEN) to promote VEGFR2 autophosphorylation and downstream redox signaling events or directly activating redox signaling kinases. These events are converged and integrated to induce various redox-sensitive transcriptional factors and gene expression, which are involved in angiogenesis.

Modified from Ushio-Fukai M, Nakamura Y. Reactive oxygen species and angiogenesis: NADPH oxidase as target for cancer therapy. Cancer Lett. 2008;266(1):37—52. https://doi.org/10.1016/j.canlet.2008.02.044.

VEGFR2 angiogenesis signaling pathway is generated (Figs. 8.1 and 8.2).[20,30] Here, mtROS represents mitochondria-derived ROS, which is also an important source of endogenous ROS production. Therefore, VEGF-induced and NADPH oxidase-derived ROS link to actin at the leading edge of injury, which promotes cytoskeletal reorganization and endothelial migration (Fig. 8.1).[20]

Cell—cell and cell—matrix interactions in CNV formation

The central processes in CNV formation are CEC migration and proliferation. Multiple cellular components at the macular region and systemically recruited immune

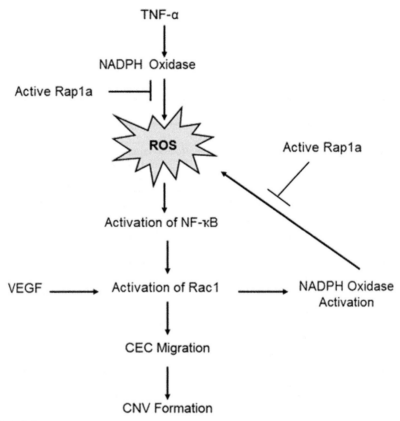

FIGURE 8.2

TNFα signaling pathway and feed-forward loop in inflammation- and oxidative stress-regulated CEC migration and choroidal neovascularization (CNV) formation. *ROS*, reactive oxygen species; *TNF*, tumor necrosis factor; *VEGF*, vascular endothelial growth factor. *Rap1a*, a member of the family of Ras-related proteins.

Modified from Wang H, Fotheringham L, Wittchen ES, Hartnett ME. Rap1 GTPase inhibits tumor necrosis factor-α-induced choroidal endothelial migration via NADPH oxidase- and NF-κB-dependent activation of Rac1. Am J Pathol. 2015;185(12):3316–3325. https://doi.org/10.1016/j.ajpath.2015.08.017.

cells interact and participate in CNV formation. The cellular components include photoreceptors (PR), RPE, BrM (i.e., extracellular matrix), macrophages (derived from circulation and resident microglia), CEC, and pericytes. Presumably, the triggering event of CNV formation occurs in RPE. Under oxidative stress, PR and RPE produce VEGF, initiating the VEGF signaling pathway in CECs.[21,22] The interaction of RPE and CECs has been elucidated by cell culture studies. Under oxidative-stress, there is increased release of exosomes containing VEGFR-1 and VEGFR-2 to the extracellular matrix (ECM). Exosomes are small membranous vesicles released into the ECM by many cell types, including RPE cells. The biophysically compatible form of membranous vesicles makes exosomes essential for cell-to-cell communication.[23] When RPE-derived exosomes interact with neighboring CECs, they can incorporate VEGF receptors into the new cell membrane.[24] RPE also produces other proangiogenic cytokines such as monocyte colonization protein and IL8, further influencing neighboring cells.[25] Although the cellular sources of AMD-related mononuclear phagocytes are not completely clear, they probably include systemically recruited monocytes, resident microglia, and choroidal macrophages/dendritic cells.[26] The inflammatory role of macrophages in AMD progression has been long recognized (see Chapter 7). For example, drusen regression and RPE clumping coordinate the process of macrophage activation for clearance of subretina/sub-RPE inflammatory debris.[27] By using coculture technique, the macrophage-RPE interaction has been studied. Activated macrophages can induce morphological and functional changes of RPE cells, including altered inflammatory gene expression.[28] There is evidence that macrophage-RPE interaction may occur via TNFα signaling from activated macrophages (Fig. 8.2).[30] TNFα can suppress the RPE expression of the *OTX2* gene. The protein encoded by this gene is orthodenticle homeobox 2 (OTX2) controlling essential, homeostatic RPE genes.[29] In addition, macrophages express TNFα, which stimulates proinflammatory cytokines produced by RPE as well as NADPH oxidase-derived ROS. Studies using laser-induced CNV animal model showed that TNFα-mediated Rac1 activation is under the control of NF-kB activation that is a classical signaling pathway involved in TNF α-mediated inflammation. Therefore, TNF α-mediated signaling transduction enters a "feed-forward loop" as described earlier, promoting inflammation- and oxidative stress-regulated CEC migration (Fig. 8.2).[30,31]

Histopathological studies detailed the involvement of inflammatory cells in CNV. It has been confirmed that an increase in subretinal macrophage infiltration enhances CNV formation,[32,33] while the elimination of macrophages decreases CNV.[34] The first animal model of experimental CNV was developed by Ryan et al. in nonhuman primates.[35] This model created a BrM rupture by laser, which induced a local inflammatory response resulting in angiogenesis. This model revealed an angiogenic contribution of BrM, a specific ECM between RPE and CEC, to CNV formation. In our previous work on ECM, a critical role of BrM in CEC survival was demonstrated. When cultured CECs were seeded onto the pre-prepared RPE-ECM, CEC survival was supported and regulated by insoluble component molecules of the RPE-ECM and soluble growth factors that bind to the ECM.[36] Both CECs and macrophages produce matrix metalloproteinases (MMPs), which enable the CNV to digest and penetrate tissue planes. The MMPs are inhibited by tissue inhibitors of metalloproteinases (TIMPs) produced by RPE.[37] In addition, macrophages express tissue factor, a protein involved with fibrinogenesis leading to a fibrin scaffold facilitating CNV growth.[25] In a study on postmortem eyes with AMD, Grossniklaus et al. provided morphological evidence that macrophages concentrate at areas of CEC ingrowth through the BrM.[38,39] The macrophage infiltration was also found at the margins of the defects of BrM.[40] After CEC ingrowth through BrM, that is, RPE/CEC-ECM, making contact with RPE, the activated CECs may migrate across the RPE into the neurosensory retina.[41] Before CEC transmigration, the molecular interactions between CECs and RPE or CEC and RPE-ECM begin with their physical contact. First, physically RPE-ECM is an indispensable component making this cell–cell interaction possible. Second, the obtained data showed that the physical contact between CECs and RPE results in an increase in the activity of the GTPase Rac1 within the CECs. This increase is dependent on upstream activation of PI 3-K/Akt1 pathway.[42]

In addition to complex cell–cell interactions, CNV formation is a dynamic event,[2,39] depending on a balance of growth promoters and inhibitors over time. RPE cells, as a major source of ocular angio-regulatory proteins, contribute to the angiogenetic balance by the production of positive and negative regulatory factors including VEGF,[21,22] thrombospondin-1 (TSP1), and pigment epithelium-derived factor (PEDF). TSP1 is a homo-trimeric matricellular protein produced by various cell types including RPE cells,[43] and as a major component of the BrM.[44] It plays a critical role in the regulation of vascular homeostasis, immunity, and wound healing.[45] A number of studies have demonstrated roles for PEDF in the modulation of vascular leakage and vessel growth in AMD.[46] A cohort study with multivariate analyses showed a consistent decrease in PEDF in plasma from dry AMD patients. Decreased RPE production of PEDF and TSP1 as endogenous inhibitors of angiogenesis produces a proangiogenic state in nAMD.[47] Among the wet AMD patients, a strong positive correlation between VEGF and PEDF concentrations was observed.[48] These findings suggest: first, a suppressed level of PEDF is a risk factor for dry AMD and second, PEDF plays a compensatory role counterbalancing VEGF surge in wet AMD.[47]

After VEGF-driven sprouting angiogenesis, a process of new blood vessel maturation may follow.[49] This process is completed by the combined effects of both VEGF and platelet-derived growth factor (PDGF). PDGF comprises a family of five polypeptides including PDGF-BB, the predominant isoform in ocular tissues signaling via the receptor tyrosine kinase PDGFR ββ.[50] If VEGF levels fall, ECs undergo apoptosis. If VEGF levels remain high, vessel maturation is achieved by recruiting of vascular wall cells, such as pericytes (Fig. 8.3). The recruitment of pericytes is PDGF dependent.[49] The vessel maturation induces a prosurvival signal in ECs. When both VEGF and PDGF are inhibited, it may facilitate an antagonistic effect on new blood vessel formation.[51] It has been demonstrated in CNV animal models that a PDGF receptor β positive (PDGFRβ (+)) scaffold is formed and new vessels infiltrate this scaffold to initiate CNV. Thus, when proliferating PDGFRβ (+) cells were suppressed, CNV formation was attenuated.[51] It has been observed that in the natural course of CNV involution, at some point, the balance shifts toward antimigratory, antiangiogenic, and antiproteolytic activity. At this stage, by RPE the angiogenic/proteolytic/migratory cytokine production decreases, whereas TGFβ and TIMP3 production upregulate. In this stage, the CNV may become a collagenized fibrotic scar. It is possible that hemorrhagic RPE detachment contributes to the development of a disciform scar at macula. An end stage of nAMD pursues.[2,52,53]

The signaling pathways involving in CEC migration and CNV formation are summarized in Fig. 8.3.

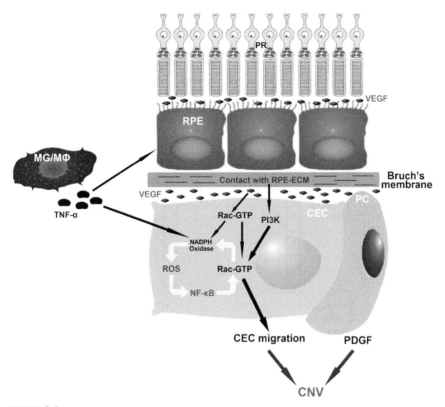

FIGURE 8.3

CNV formation via cell–cell and cell-extracellular matrix (ECM) interactions with a "feed-forward loop" mechanism. Hypoxia and oxidative stress promote VEGF production by photoreceptors (PR) and RPE cells. TNFα released by activated microglia/macrophage (MG/MΦ) causes overproduction of VEGF by RPE cells and activation of NADPH oxidase of CECs. VEGF attracts and activates CECs via activation of Rac-GTP and NADPH oxidase. NADPH oxidase-generated ROS triggers Rac-GTP via NFkB signaling, which further activates NADPH oxidase, thus setting up a feed-forward loop (in white circle). Thus, activated CECs migrate and proliferate to form CNV. In parallel, the contact-induced migration of CECs undergoes a Rac-GTP and PI 3-K-dependent signaling pathway. As a result, CECs transmigrate across RPE-ECM and RPE monolayer. During the process of CEC migration and proliferation, pericyte-derived PDGF is critical in CNV maturation.

VEGF and beyond

VEGFs are central regulators of physiological and pathological angiogenesis.[54] In humans, the VEGF family consists of five secreted protein ligands—VEGF-A, B, C, D, and placental growth factor (PlGF). The five ligands have different binding affinities for three tyrosine kinase receptors: VEGFR1, 2, and 3.[55] VEGF-A, B, and PlGF bind to VEGFR1, VEGF-A binds to VEGFR2, and VEGF-C and -D bind to VEGFR3.[56] Of the VEGF ligands, the role of VEGF-A signaling in vascular ECs has been most extensively studied (Fig. 8.4). VEGF-A interacts with VEGFR2 (Flk1) and VEGFR1 (Flt1), which regulate endothelial responses, such as the

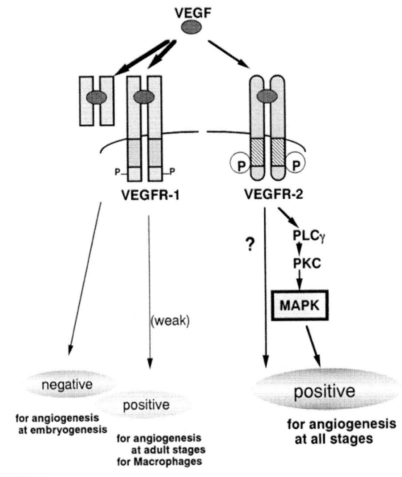

FIGURE 8.4

A model for VEGF signaling pathway from two main VEGFRs (Flt-1 and KDR/Flk-1). VEGFR-1 (Flt-1) has functions in either a negative or positive manner depending on the biological system, cell types, or developmental stages (see the context above). In this figure, *small p,* weak auto-phosphorylation; *large P,* strong auto-phosphorylation; *PLCγ,* phospholipase C gamma; *PKC,* protein kinase C; *MAPK,* mitogen-activated protein kinase.

Modified from Shibuya M. Structure and dual function of vascular endothelial growth factor receptor-1 (Flt-1). Int J Biochem Cell Biol. *2001;33(4):409–420. https://doi.org/10.1016/s1357-2725(01)00026-7.*

proliferation and migration of ECs, vascular permeability, and induction of tip cell filopodia, that is, slender cytoplasmic projections from the nascent sprout.[57] Flt1 is a high-affinity receptor for VEGF-A, but it undergoes only weak tyrosine auto-phosphorylation in response to the ligand (Fig. 8.4).[58] A soluble form (sFlt1) synthesized by ECs is capable of binding VEGF-A, thereby inhibiting the proangiogenic functions of the ligand.[59,60]

During angiogenesis, hypoxia-activated ECs start a new blood vessel sprout from the existing damaged vessel. A single specialized EC, called a tip cell, instructing many adjacent stalk cells to follow, guides vessel sprouting toward growth factor gradients, for example, gradients of VEGF and angiopoietin. The balance between tip and stalk cells is regulated by endothelial Notch signaling through the Notch ligand Delta-like 4 (Dll4) expressed in tip cells. In stalk cells, Dll4 signals activate Notch downstream targets and reduce VEGF receptor expression levels, thereby, in turn, suppresses a tip cell (Fig. 8.5). By using loss-of-function and gain-of-function mouse models, Benedito et al. studied the role of Jag1 in retinal angiogenesis.[61] This study suggests that Jag1, a ligand that interacts with Dll4-mediated Notch signaling, negatively regulates Notch activity and antagonizes Dll4-mediated Notch activation. Jag1 is expressed in stalk cells but is absent or minimally expressed in tip cells. In contrast, Dll4 is strongly expressed in tip cells, but only at lower levels in stalk cells (Fig. 8.5). Fringe proteins, named β3-N-acetylglucosaminyltransferases, modulate Notch activity by modifying O-fucose residues on epidermal growth factor-like (EGF) repeats of Notch (Fig. 8.5).[62,63]

The angiopoietins (Ang-1 and Ang-2) are growth factors that play a key role in vessel homeostasis, angiogenesis, and vascular permeability. Both ligands interact with the Tie-2 transmembrane receptor tyrosine kinase. Tie-2 is preferentially expressed on endothelial cells. Loss- and gain-of-function experiments have demonstrated the critical contributions of the angiopoietin/Tie-2 system in vascular development and vascular diseases (Fig. 8.6).[64–66,79] Ang-1/Tie2 binding regulates the PI 3-Kinase/Akt signal transduction pathway.[67,68] Ang-2 is a weaker agonist when competing with Ang-1 for binding and reducing phosphorylation of Tie2. Thus Ang-2 is considered to present a natural Ang-1/Tie2 inhibitor.[69] In other words, Ang-2 has been characterized as a weak Tie-2 agonist that competitively inhibits Ang-1/Tie2 signaling.[70] Structural studies have identified an agonistic domain in Ang-1 that is capable of converting chimeric ligand of Ang-2 such as Ang-2-TAG, into a full agonist,[71] indicating the close structural relationship between Ang-1 and Ang-2. Overall data suggest that Ang-1 protects from pathological angiogenesis and drives toward a quiescent, mature vessel formation,[72] whereas Ang-2 promotes vascular leakage and abnormally activated vessels (Fig. 8.6).[73,74,79] Ang-2 also amplifies proapoptotic signals in pericytes under stresses such as proinflammatory cytokines,[75,76] contributing to the destabilization of vessels. Regula et al. studied the interplay of VEGF-A and angiopoietins in an in vitro model of EC barrier breakdown.[74] The data showed that VEGF-A increases the amount of Ang-2, whereas Ang-1 reduces the secretion of Ang-2. EC barrier breakdown is mainly done by VEGF-A. When adding anti-Ang-2 together with VEGF-A, barrier

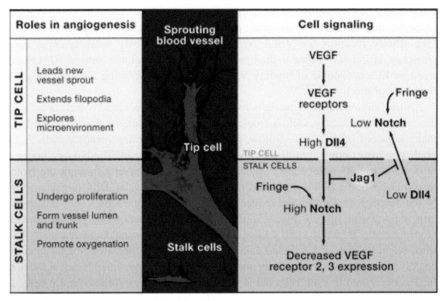

FIGURE 8.5

Tip and stalk cell selection in sprouting angiogenesis. VEGF produced by hypoxic cells activates endothelial cells to form a new blood vessel sprout. A sprouting blood vessel is composed of one tip cell and many stalk cells. VEGF induces expression of Delta-like 4 (Dll4) in the tip cell, which signals to stalk cells to activate Notch downstream targets and to reduce VEGF receptor expression levels, thereby suppressing tip cell. In the stalk cell, the glycosyltransferase Fringe modifies Notch receptors to enhance Notch signaling induced by Dll4 from the tip cell, further reducing stalk cell VEGF receptor (VEGFR) levels and perhaps inducing quiescence. However, Jagged-1 (Jag1) in the stalk cell can antagonize Dll4-Notch signaling to maintain an activated stalk cell phenotype that is responsive to VEGF, thereby promoting angiogenesis. Stalk cells also express low levels of Dll4. Fringe could allow for Jag1 to inhibit possible Dll4-mediated signaling between stalk cells or from stalk cells to the tip cell. In tip cells lacking Fringe, Jag1 might promote angiogenesis by signaling directly to Notch to induce VEGFR3 expression.

Modified from Suchting S, Eichmann A. Jagged gives endothelial tip cells an edge. Cell. 2009;137(6): 988–990. https://doi.org/10.1016/j.cell.2009.05.024.

breakdown was alleviated. This suggests that VEGF-A, at least in part, signals via Ang-2 to trigger EC barrier breakdown (Fig. 8.6).[74,79] The function of Ang-2 for new blood vessel formation is VEGF-A concentration-dependent. For example, in a genetically modified mouse model with ischemic retinopathy, Ang-2 accelerates new vessel formation in response to high VEGF-A levels; however, if VEGF-A levels are low, Ang2 promotes regression of NV.[77] Recently, the role of Angiopoietin/Tie2 pathways in choriocapillaris (CC) sprouting was further elucidated by the work of Kim et al.[78] In their experiment, transgenic mouse models depleting Tie2 or Ang-1 were used. Impaired Ang-1/Tie2 signaling leads to CC loss, indicating

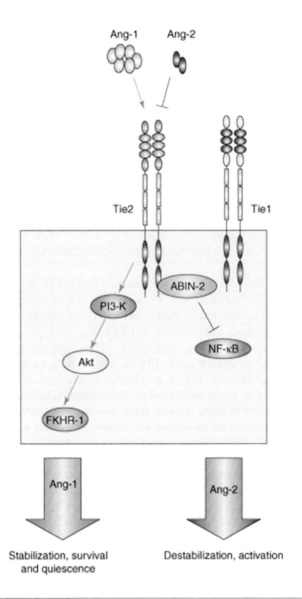

FIGURE 8.6

Angiopoietin-1 and angiopoietin-2 signaling in regulating the quiescent and activated endothelial-cell phenotype. The Tie2 ligand Ang-1 binds to Tie2 and induces its autophosphorylation. Ang-1-mediated PI 3-kinase activation results in the phosphorylation and activation of Akt. Akt signaling controls the quiescent endothelial-cell phenotype and promotes endothelial-cell (yellow box) survival. Moreover, Akt phosphorylates and inactivates FKHR-1(a transcription factor of Forkhead family). Consequently, endothelial Ang-2 expression is inhibited. Phosphorylated Tie2 also interacts with ABIN-2 (A20-binding inhibitor of NF-kB 2) and prevents NF-kB signaling, thereby suppressing the expression of inflammation-associated molecules. Ang-2 release from endothelial storage pools and binding to Tie2 interferes negatively with Ang-1-mediated Tie2 signaling and results in destabilization, thereby rendering the endothelium responsive to stimulation by inflammatory and angiogenic cytokines. Abbreviation: *PI3K,* PI 3-kinase.

Modified from Fiedler U, Augustin HG. Angiopoietins: a link between angiogenesis and inflammation. Trends Immunol. *2006;27(12):552–558. https://doi.org/10.1016/j.it.2006.10.004.*

Ang-1/Tie2 signaling is essential to CC survival. When CNV was induced by laser photocoagulation in these mice, Tie2 depletion worsens CNV formation and suppresses the ability of CC to regenerate around the CNV lesions. When a dual functioning antibody, that is, anti-Ang-2-binding and anti-Tie2-activating antibody, was applied, suppression of CNV and promotion of CC regeneration was observed, suggesting a beneficial role of the Angiopoietin/Tie2 pathway in alleviating hypoxia and oxidative stress in the context of CNV.[78]

The angiopoietin receptor Tie2 is also regulated by a phosphatase, vascular endothelial protein tyrosine phosphatase (VE-PTP).[80] VE-PTP is associated with Tie2 and deactivates it via dephosphorylation (Fig. 8.7).[79] Therefore, biochemically VE-PTP acts like Ang-2 when binding to Tie2.[81] Like Ang-2 too, VE-PTP is increased in hypoxic retina.[77]

In addition to angiogenesis, vasculogenesis, a process of de novo blood vessel formation appears to contribute to CNV formation. Adults maintain a reservoir of bone marrow (BM) hematopoietic stem cells (HSCs) that may be mobilized to reach damaged choriocapillaris as precursors of CECs (Fig. 8.7).[77,82] Functional VEGF receptor-1 is expressed in repopulating HSCs.[83] Hematopoietic bone marrow cells provide endothelial progenitor cells (EPCs). Evidence exists that the chemokine stromal-cell-derived factor-1 (SDF-1, also known as CXCL12, is expressed by hypoxic tissues. SDF-1 is a specific ligand of the receptor CXCR4, which is widely expressed by mobile BM cells. It has a major role in the recruitment and retention of CXCR4[+] BM cells to the proangiogenic niches, supporting revascularization of ischemic tissue.[84,85] The underlying mechanisms by which SDF-1 activates EPCs have recently been discovered.[86] Circulating SDF-1 is translocated from the plasma to the BM. After SDF-1 enters the BM microenvironment, it induces the activation of matrix metalloproteinase-9 (MMP-9) and the release of soluble kit-ligand (sKitL). Subsequently, sKitL induces the release of more SDF-1, enhancing mobilization of the CXCR4[+] and c-Kit[+] cells to the circulation.[87] Once established in the circulation, CXCR4[+] BM cells preferably incorporate into ischemic microenvironments via specific adhesion molecules.[88] SDF-1 expressed and presented by EPCs, at the site of injury, probably has an important role in triggering EPC arrest and resettlement into the neo-angiogenic niches (Fig. 8.7).[77,89]

The causal role of angiogenesis in nAMD is depicted in Fig. 8.7.[77] Key initiating triggers such as NADPH oxidase- and mitochondria-derived ROS have been identified. In parallel, key regulators of pro- and antiangiogenic balance, such as VEGF, PDGF, angiopoietins, and extracellular matrix molecules have been extensively studied. These studies have facilitated the development of therapeutic agents that target the underlying pathological angiogenesis. Among these, VEGF serves as a central player for the formation of CNV through its promotion of endothelial cell survival and migration, elevated vascular permeability, and ocular inflammation. The emerging strategies regulating VEGF signaling pathway and beyond will be used to develop a paradigm of the next generation of antiangiogenic drugs in nAMD.

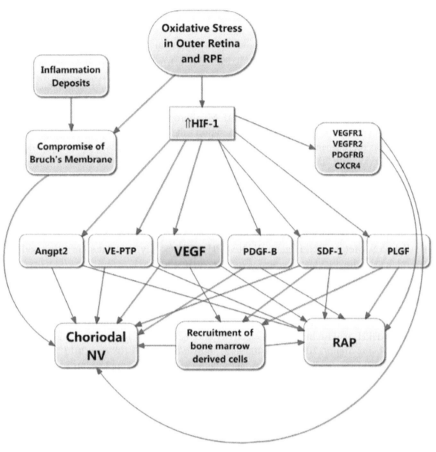

FIGURE 8.7

Molecular pathogenesis of choroidal neovascularization (CNV). This schematic highlights several important molecular signals involved in CNV. Oxidative stress in the retinal pigmented epithelium (RPE) and photoreceptors causes increased levels of HIF-1, which upregulates vasoactive gene products including Ang-2 (Angpt2), VE-PTP, VEGF, PDGF-β, SDF-1, and PlGF. Retinal angiomatous proliferation (RAP) occurs if VEGF levels in photoreceptors are sufficiently high to cause a gradient that reaches the deep capillary bed of the retina where there is a constitutive expression of Ang-2 (Angpt2). Choroidal NV occurs if there is the elevation of VEGF and Ang-2 combined with perturbation of Bruch's membrane and the RPE. The other HIF-1-responsive gene products fuel the process similar to the situation in retinal NV.

Modified from Campochiaro PA. Molecular pathogenesis of retinal and choroidal vascular diseases. Prog Retin Eye Res. *2015;49:67–81. https://doi.org/10.1016/j.preteyeres.2015.06.002.*

References

1. Alizadeh E, Mammadzada P, André H. The different facades of retinal and choroidal endothelial cells in response to hypoxia. *IJMS*. 2018;19(12):3846. https://doi.org/10.3390/ijms19123846.
2. Grossniklaus HE, Green WR. Choroidal neovascularization. *Am J Ophthalmol*. 2004; 137(3):496−503. https://doi.org/10.1016/j.ajo.2003.09.042.
3. Little K, Ma JH, Yang N, Chen M, Xu H. Myofibroblasts in macular fibrosis secondary to neovascular age-related macular degeneration - the potential sources and molecular cues for their recruitment and activation. *EBioMedicine*. 2018;38:283−291. https://doi.org/10.1016/j.ebiom.2018.11.029.
4. Gau D, Veon W, Capasso TL, et al. Pharmacological intervention of MKL/SRF signaling by CCG-1423 impedes endothelial cell migration and angiogenesis. *Angiogenesis*. 2017; 20(4):663−672. https://doi.org/10.1007/s10456-017-9560-y.
5. Ushio-Fukai M. VEGF signaling through NADPH oxidase-derived ROS. *Antioxid Redox Signal*. 2007;9(6):731−739. https://doi.org/10.1089/ars.2007.1556.
6. Sahoo S, Meijles DN, Pagano PJ. NADPH oxidases: key modulators in aging and age-related cardiovascular diseases? *Clin Sci*. 2016;130(5):317−335. https://doi.org/10.1042/CS20150087.
7. Brieger K, Schiavone S, Miller FJ, Krause K-H. Reactive oxygen species: from health to disease. *Swiss Med Wkly*. 2012;142:w13659. https://doi.org/10.4414/smw.2012.13659.
8. Altenhöfer S, Radermacher KA, Kleikers PWM, Wingler K, Schmidt HHHW. Evolution of NADPH oxidase inhibitors: selectivity and mechanisms for target engagement. *Antioxid Redox Signal*. 2015;23(5):406−427. https://doi.org/10.1089/ars.2013.5814.
9. Evans JR, Lawrenson JG. Antioxidant vitamin and mineral supplements for slowing the progression of age-related macular degeneration. *Cochrane Database Syst Rev*. 2017;7: CD000254. https://doi.org/10.1002/14651858.CD000254.pub4.
10. Görlach A, Brandes RP, Nguyen K, Amidi M, Dehghani F, Busse R. A gp91phox containing NADPH oxidase selectively expressed in endothelial cells is a major source of oxygen radical generation in the arterial wall. *Circ Res*. 2000;87(1):26−32. https://doi.org/10.1161/01.res.87.1.26.
11. Ushio-Fukai M. Redox signaling in angiogenesis: role of NADPH oxidase. *Cardiovasc Res*. 2006;71(2):226−235. https://doi.org/10.1016/j.cardiores.2006.04.015.
12. Terada LS. Specificity in reactive oxidant signaling: think globally, act locally. *J Cell Biol*. 2006;174(5):615−623. https://doi.org/10.1083/jcb.200605036.
13. Ambasta RK, Kumar P, Griendling KK, Schmidt HHHW, Busse R, Brandes RP. Direct interaction of the novel Nox proteins with p22phox is required for the formation of a functionally active NADPH oxidase. *J Biol Chem*. 2004;279(44):45935−45941. https://doi.org/10.1074/jbc.M406486200.
14. Van Buul JD, Fernandez-Borja M, Anthony EC, Hordijk PL. Expression and localization of NOX2 and NOX4 in primary human endothelial cells. *Antioxid Redox Signal*. 2005; 7(3-4):308−317. https://doi.org/10.1089/ars.2005.7.308.
15. Ikeda S, Yamaoka-Tojo M, Hilenski L, et al. IQGAP1 regulates reactive oxygen species-dependent endothelial cell migration through interacting with Nox2. *Arterioscler Thromb Vasc Biol*. 2005;25(11):2295−2300. https://doi.org/10.1161/01.ATV.0000187472.55437.af.
16. Zhang AY, Yi F, Zhang G, Gulbins E, Li P-L. Lipid raft clustering and redox signaling platform formation in coronary arterial endothelial cells. *Hypertension*. 2006;47(1): 74−80. https://doi.org/10.1161/10.1161/01.HYP.0000196727.53300.62.

17. Simons M, Gordon E, Claesson-Welsh L. Mechanisms and regulation of endothelial VEGF receptor signalling. *Nat Rev Mol Cell Biol.* 2016;17(10):611−625. https://doi.org/10.1038/nrm.2016.87.

18. Kim Y-M, Kim S-J, Tatsunami R, Yamamura H, Fukai T, Ushio-Fukai M. ROS-induced ROS release orchestrated by Nox4, Nox2, and mitochondria in VEGF signaling and angiogenesis. *Am J Physiol, Cell Physiol.* 2017;312(6):C749−C764. https://doi.org/10.1152/ajpcell.00346.2016.

19. Oshikawa J, Kim S-J, Furuta E, et al. Novel role of p66Shc in ROS-dependent VEGF signaling and angiogenesis in endothelial cells. *Am J Physiol Heart Circ Physiol.* 2012;302(3):H724−732. https://doi.org/10.1152/ajpheart.00739.2011.

20. Ushio-Fukai M, Nakamura Y. Reactive oxygen species and angiogenesis: NADPH oxidase as target for cancer therapy. *Cancer Lett.* 2008;266(1):37−52. https://doi.org/10.1016/j.canlet.2008.02.044.

21. Lopez PF, Sippy BD, Lambert HM, Thach AB, Hinton DR. Transdifferentiated retinal pigment epithelial cells are immunoreactive for vascular endothelial growth factor in surgically excised age-related macular degeneration-related choroidal neovascular membranes. *Invest Ophthalmol Vis Sci.* 1996;37(5):855−868.

22. Vallée A, Lecarpentier Y, Guillevin R, Vallée J-N. Aerobic glycolysis hypothesis through WNT/beta-catenin pathway in exudative age-related macular degeneration. *J Mol Neurosci.* 2017;62(3−4):368−379. https://doi.org/10.1007/s12031-017-0947-4.

23. Atienzar-Aroca S, Flores-Bellver M, Serrano-Heras G, et al. Oxidative stress in retinal pigment epithelium cells increases exosome secretion and promotes angiogenesis in endothelial cells. *J Cell Mol Med.* 2016;20(8):1457−1466. https://doi.org/10.1111/jcmm.12834.

24. Stoorvogel W, Kleijmeer MJ, Geuze HJ, Raposo G. The biogenesis and functions of exosomes. *Traffic.* 2002;3(5):321−330. https://doi.org/10.1034/j.1600-0854.2002.30502.x.

25. Grossniklaus HE, Ling JX, Wallace TM, et al. Macrophage and retinal pigment epithelium expression of angiogenic cytokines in choroidal neovascularization. *Mol Vis.* 2002; 8:119−126.

26. Silverman SM, Wong WT. Microglia in the retina: roles in development, maturity, and disease. *Annu Rev Vis Sci.* 2018;4:45−77. https://doi.org/10.1146/annurev-vision-091517-034425.

27. Ma W, Zhang Y, Gao C, Fariss RN, Tam J, Wong WT. Monocyte infiltration and proliferation reestablish myeloid cell homeostasis in the mouse retina following retinal pigment epithelial cell injury. *Sci Rep.* 2017;7(1):8433. https://doi.org/10.1038/s41598-017-08702-7.

28. Ma W, Zhao L, Fontainhas AM, Fariss RN, Wong WT. Microglia in the mouse retina alter the structure and function of retinal pigmented epithelial cells: a potential cellular interaction relevant to AMD. Koch K-W, ed. *PLoS One.* 2009;4(11):e7945. https://doi.org/10.1371/journal.pone.0007945

29. Mathis T, Housset M, Eandi C, et al. Activated monocytes resist elimination by retinal pigment epithelium and downregulate their OTX2 expression via TNF-α. *Aging Cell.* 2017;16(1):173−182. https://doi.org/10.1111/acel.12540.

30. Wang H, Fotheringham L, Wittchen ES, Hartnett ME. Rap1 GTPase inhibits tumor necrosis factor-α-induced choroidal endothelial migration via NADPH oxidase- and NF-κB-dependent activation of Rac1. *Am J Pathol.* 2015;185(12):3316−3325. https://doi.org/10.1016/j.ajpath.2015.08.017.

31. Wittchen ES, Nishimura E, McCloskey M, et al. Rap1 GTPase activation and barrier enhancement in rpe inhibits choroidal neovascularization in vivo. *PLoS One*. 2013; 8(9):e73070. https://doi.org/10.1371/journal.pone.0073070.

32. Combadière C, Feumi C, Raoul W, et al. CX3CR1-dependent subretinal microglia cell accumulation is associated with cardinal features of age-related macular degeneration. *J Clin Invest*. 2007;117(10):2920—2928. https://doi.org/10.1172/JCI31692.

33. Oh H, Takagi H, Takagi C, et al. The potential angiogenic role of macrophages in the formation of choroidal neovascular membranes. *Invest Ophthalmol Vis Sci*. 1999; 40(9):1891—1898.

34. Espinosa-Heidmann DG, Suner IJ, Hernandez EP, Monroy D, Csaky KG, Cousins SW. Macrophage depletion diminishes lesion size and severity in experimental choroidal neovascularization. *Invest Ophthalmol Vis Sci*. 2003;44(8):3586—3592. https://doi.org/ 10.1167/iovs.03-0038.

35. Ryan SJ. The development of an experimental model of subretinal neovascularization in disciform macular degeneration. *Trans Am Ophthalmol Soc*. 1979;77:707—745.

36. Liu X, Ye X, Yanoff M, Li W. Extracellular matrix of retinal pigment epithelium regulates choriocapillaris endothelial survival in vitro. *Exp Eye Res*. 1997;65(1):117—126. https://doi.org/10.1006/exer.1997.0317.

37. Steen B, Sejersen S, Berglin L, Seregard S, Kvanta A. Matrix metalloproteinases and metalloproteinase inhibitors in choroidal neovascular membranes. *Invest Ophthalmol Vis Sci*. 1998;39(11):2194—2200.

38. Grossniklaus HE, Cingle KA, Yoon YD, Ketkar N, L'Hernault N, Brown S. Correlation of histologic 2-dimensional reconstruction and confocal scanning laser microscopic imaging of choroidal neovascularization in eyes with age-related maculopathy. *Arch Ophthalmol*. 2000;118(5):625—629. https://doi.org/10.1001/archopht.118.5.625.

39. Grossniklaus HE, Martinez JA, Brown VB, et al. Immunohistochemical and histochemical properties of surgically excised subretinal neovascular membranes in age-related macular degeneration. *Am J Ophthalmol*. 1992;114(4):464—472. https://doi.org/ 10.1016/s0002-9394(14)71859-8.

40. Dastgheib K, Green WR. Granulomatous reaction to Bruch's membrane in age-related macular degeneration. *Arch Ophthalmol*. 1994;112(6):813—818. https://doi.org/ 10.1001/archopht.1994.01090180111045.

41. Stevens TS, Bressler NM, Maguire MG, et al. Occult choroidal neovascularization in age-related macular degeneration. A natural history study. *Arch Ophthalmol*. 1997; 115(3):345—350. https://doi.org/10.1001/archopht.1997.01100150347006.

42. Peterson LJ, Wittchen ES, Geisen P, Burridge K, Hartnett ME. Heterotypic RPE-choroidal endothelial cell contact increases choroidal endothelial cell transmigration via PI 3-kinase and Rac1. *Exp Eye Res*. 2007;84(4):737—744. https://doi.org/10.1016/ j.exer.2006.12.012.

43. Adams JC, Lawler J. The thrombospondins. *Int J Biochem Cell Biol*. 2004;36(6): 961—968. https://doi.org/10.1016/j.biocel.2004.01.004.

44. Uno K, Bhutto IA, McLeod DS, Merges C, Lutty GA. Impaired expression of thrombospondin-1 in eyes with age related macular degeneration. *Br J Ophthalmol*. 2006;90(1):48—54. https://doi.org/10.1136/bjo.2005.074005.

45. Masli S, Sheibani N, Cursiefen C, Zieske J. Matricellular protein thrombospondins: influence on ocular angiogenesis, wound healing and immuneregulation. *Curr Eye Res*. 2014;39(8):759—774. https://doi.org/10.3109/02713683.2013.877936.

46. Farnoodian M, Wang S, Dietz J, Nickells RW, Sorenson CM, Sheibani N. Negative regulators of angiogenesis: important targets for treatment of exudative AMD. *Clin Sci.* 2017;131(15):1763−1780. https://doi.org/10.1042/CS20170066.

47. Farnoodian M, Kinter JB, Yadranji Aghdam S, Zaitoun I, Sorenson CM, Sheibani N. Expression of pigment epithelium-derived factor and thrombospondin-1 regulate proliferation and migration of retinal pigment epithelial cells. *Physiol Rep.* 2015;3(1). https://doi.org/10.14814/phy2.12266.

48. Machalińska A, Safranow K, Mozolewska-Piotrowska K, Dziedziejko V, Karczewicz D. PEDF and VEGF plasma level alterations in patients with dry form of age-related degeneration−a possible link to the development of the disease. *Klin Oczna.* 2012; 114(2):115−120.

49. Benjamin LE, Hemo I, Keshet E. A plasticity window for blood vessel remodelling is defined by pericyte coverage of the preformed endothelial network and is regulated by PDGF-B and VEGF. *Development.* 1998;125(9):1591−1598.

50. Klinghoffer RA, Duckworth B, Valius M, Cantley L, Kazlauskas A. Platelet-derived growth factor-dependent activation of phosphatidylinositol 3-kinase is regulated by receptor binding of SH2-domain-containing proteins which influence ras activity. *Mol Cell Biol.* 1996;16(10):5905−5914. https://doi.org/10.1128/mcb.16.10.5905.

51. Siedlecki J, Wertheimer C, Wolf A, et al. Combined VEGF and PDGF inhibition for neovascular AMD: anti-angiogenic properties of axitinib on human endothelial cells and pericytes in vitro. *Graefes Arch Clin Exp Ophthalmol.* 2017;255(5):963−972. https://doi.org/10.1007/s00417-017-3595-z.

52. Holloway TB, Verhoeff FH. Disc-like degeneration of the macula with microscopic report concerning a tumor-like mass in the macular region. *Trans Am Ophthalmol Soc.* 1928;26:206−228.

53. Gass JD. Pathogenesis of disciform detachment of the neuroepithelium. *Am J Ophthalmol.* 1967;63(3):1−139.

54. Karaman S, Leppänen V-M, Alitalo K. Vascular endothelial growth factor signaling in development and disease. *Development.* 2018;145(14). https://doi.org/10.1242/dev.151019.

55. Takahashi H, Shibuya M. The vascular endothelial growth factor (VEGF)/VEGF receptor system and its role under physiological and pathological conditions. *Clin Sci.* 2005; 109(3):227−241. https://doi.org/10.1042/CS20040370.

56. Matsumoto K, Ema M. Roles of VEGF-A signalling in development, regeneration, and tumours. *J Biochem.* 2014;156(1):1−10. https://doi.org/10.1093/jb/mvu031.

57. Blanco R, Gerhardt H. VEGF and Notch in tip and stalk cell selection. *Cold Spring Harb Perspect Med.* 2013;3(1):a006569. https://doi.org/10.1101/cshperspect.a006569.

58. Shibuya M. Structure and dual function of vascular endothelial growth factor receptor-1 (Flt-1). *Int J Biochem Cell Biol.* 2001;33(4):409−420. https://doi.org/10.1016/s1357-2725(01)00026-7.

59. Ambati BK, Nozaki M, Singh N, et al. Corneal avascularity is due to soluble VEGF receptor-1. *Nature.* 2006;443(7114):993−997. https://doi.org/10.1038/nature05249.

60. Miller JW. Beyond VEGF-the Weisenfeld lecture. *Invest Ophthalmol Vis Sci.* 2016; 57(15):6911−6918. https://doi.org/10.1167/iovs.16-21201.

61. Benedito R, Roca C, Sörensen I, et al. The notch ligands Dll4 and Jagged1 have opposing effects on angiogenesis. *Cell.* 2009;137(6):1124−1135. https://doi.org/10.1016/j.cell.2009.03.025.

62. Suchting S, Eichmann A. Jagged gives endothelial tip cells an edge. *Cell*. 2009;137(6): 988−990. https://doi.org/10.1016/j.cell.2009.05.024.

63. Haupt F, Krishnasamy K, Napp LC, et al. Retinal myeloid cells regulate tip cell selection and vascular branching morphogenesis via notch ligand delta-like 1. *Sci Rep*. 2019;9(1): 9798. https://doi.org/10.1038/s41598-019-46308-3.

64. Puri MC, Rossant J, Alitalo K, Bernstein A, Partanen J. The receptor tyrosine kinase TIE is required for integrity and survival of vascular endothelial cells. *EMBO J*. 1995;14(23): 5884−5891.

65. Asahara T, Chen D, Takahashi T, et al. Tie2 receptor ligands, angiopoietin-1 and angiopoietin-2, modulate VEGF-induced postnatal neovascularization. *Circ Res*. 1998; 83(3):233−240. https://doi.org/10.1161/01.res.83.3.233.

66. Augustin HG, Koh GY, Thurston G, Alitalo K. Control of vascular morphogenesis and homeostasis through the angiopoietin-Tie system. *Nat Rev Mol Cell Biol*. 2009;10(3): 165−177. https://doi.org/10.1038/nrm2639.

67. Davis S, Aldrich TH, Jones PF, et al. Isolation of angiopoietin-1, a ligand for the TIE2 receptor, by secretion-trap expression cloning. *Cell*. 1996;87(7):1161−1169. https:// doi.org/10.1016/S0092-8674(00)81812-7.

68. Kim I, Kim HG, So JN, Kim JH, Kwak HJ, Koh GY. Angiopoietin-1 regulates endothelial cell survival through the phosphatidylinositol 3'-Kinase/Akt signal transduction pathway. *Circ Res*. 2000;86(1):24−29. https://doi.org/10.1161/01.res.86.1.24.

69. Kim I, Kim JH, Moon SO, Kwak HJ, Kim NG, Koh GY. Angiopoietin-2 at high concentration can enhance endothelial cell survival through the phosphatidylinositol 3'-kinase/ Akt signal transduction pathway. *Oncogene*. 2000;19(39):4549−4552. https://doi.org/ 10.1038/sj.onc.1203800.

70. Saharinen P, Eklund L, Miettinen J, et al. Angiopoietins assemble distinct Tie2 signalling complexes in endothelial cell-cell and cell-matrix contacts. *Nat Cell Biol*. 2008;10(5): 527−537. https://doi.org/10.1038/ncb1715.

71. Yu X, Seegar TCM, Dalton AC, et al. Structural basis for angiopoietin-1-mediated signaling initiation. *Proc Natl Acad Sci USA*. 2013;110(18):7205−7210. https:// doi.org/10.1073/pnas.1216890110.

72. Lee J, Park D-Y, Park DY, et al. Angiopoietin-1 suppresses choroidal neovascularization and vascular leakage. *Invest Ophthalmol Vis Sci*. 2014;55(4):2191−2199. https://doi.org/ 10.1167/iovs.14-13897.

73. Ziegler T, Horstkotte J, Schwab C, et al. Angiopoietin 2 mediates microvascular and hemodynamic alterations in sepsis. *J Clin Invest*. 2013. https://doi.org/10.1172/ JCI66549.

74. Regula JT, Lundh von Leithner P, Foxton R, et al. Targeting key angiogenic pathways with a bispecific CrossMAb optimized for neovascular eye diseases. *EMBO Mol Med*. 2016;8(11):1265−1288. https://doi.org/10.15252/emmm.201505889.

75. Cai J, Kehoe O, Smith GM, Hykin P, Boulton ME. The angiopoietin/Tie-2 system regulates pericyte survival and recruitment in diabetic retinopathy. *Invest Ophthalmol Vis Sci*. 2008;49(5):2163−2171. https://doi.org/10.1167/iovs.07-1206.

76. Park SW, Yun J-H, Kim JH, Kim K-W, Cho C-H, Kim JH. Angiopoietin 2 induces pericyte apoptosis via α3β1 integrin signaling in diabetic retinopathy. *Diabetes*. 2014;63(9): 3057−3068. https://doi.org/10.2337/db13-1942.

77. Campochiaro PA. Molecular pathogenesis of retinal and choroidal vascular diseases. *Prog Retin Eye Res*. 2015;49:67−81. https://doi.org/10.1016/j.preteyeres.2015.06.002.

78. Kim J, Park JR, Choi J, et al. Tie2 activation promotes choriocapillary regeneration for alleviating neovascular age-related macular degeneration. *Sci Adv.* 2019;5(2):eaau6732. https://doi.org/10.1126/sciadv.aau6732.

79. Fiedler U, Augustin HG. Angiopoietins: a link between angiogenesis and inflammation. *Trends Immunol.* 2006;27(12):552−558. https://doi.org/10.1016/j.it.2006.10.004.

80. Fachinger G, Deutsch U, Risau W. Functional interaction of vascular endothelial-protein-tyrosine phosphatase with the angiopoietin receptor Tie-2. *Oncogene.* 1999; 18(43):5948−5953. https://doi.org/10.1038/sj.onc.1202992.

81. Yacyshyn OK, Lai PFH, Forse K, Teichert-Kuliszewska K, Jurasz P, Stewart DJ. Tyrosine phosphatase beta regulates angiopoietin-Tie2 signaling in human endothelial cells. *Angiogenesis.* 2009;12(1):25−33. https://doi.org/10.1007/s10456-008-9126-0.

82. Grant MB, May WS, Caballero S, et al. Adult hematopoietic stem cells provide functional hemangioblast activity during retinal neovascularization. *Nat Med.* 2002;8(6): 607−612. https://doi.org/10.1038/nm0602-607.

83. Hattori K, Heissig B, Wu Y, et al. Placental growth factor reconstitutes hematopoiesis by recruiting VEGFR1(+) stem cells from bone-marrow microenvironment. *Nat Med.* 2002;8(8):841−849. https://doi.org/10.1038/nm740.

84. Ceradini DJ, Kulkarni AR, Callaghan MJ, et al. Progenitor cell trafficking is regulated by hypoxic gradients through HIF-1 induction of SDF-1. *Nat Med.* 2004;10(8):858−864. https://doi.org/10.1038/nm1075.

85. Petit I, Jin D, Rafii S. The SDF-1−CXCR4 signaling pathway: a molecular hub modulating neo-angiogenesis. *Trends Immunol.* 2007;28(7):299−307. https://doi.org/10.1016/j.it.2007.05.007.

86. Dar A, Goichberg P, Shinder V, et al. Chemokine receptor CXCR4-dependent internalization and resecretion of functional chemokine SDF-1 by bone marrow endothelial and stromal cells. *Nat Immunol.* 2005;6(10):1038−1046. https://doi.org/10.1038/ni1251.

87. Heissig B, Hattori K, Dias S, et al. Recruitment of stem and progenitor cells from the bone marrow niche requires MMP-9 mediated release of kit-ligand. *Cell.* 2002;109(5): 625−637. https://doi.org/10.1016/s0092-8674(02)00754-7.

88. Vajkoczy P, Blum S, Lamparter M, et al. Multistep nature of microvascular recruitment of ex vivo-expanded embryonic endothelial progenitor cells during tumor angiogenesis. *J Exp Med.* 2003;197(12):1755−1765. https://doi.org/10.1084/jem.20021659.

89. Yao L, Salvucci O, Cardones AR, et al. Selective expression of stromal-derived factor-1 in the capillary vascular endothelium plays a role in Kaposi sarcoma pathogenesis. *Blood.* 2003;102(12):3900−3905. https://doi.org/10.1182/blood-2003-02-0641.

Genetics of age-related macular degeneration

Mendelian diseases and complex diseases

The contribution of genetics to human disease has been long recognized. The genetic bases of the diseases may be monogenic or complex in origin. In monogenic Mendelian diseases, a mutation in a single gene transmitted in families predominantly leads to devastating phenotypic outcomes. Therefore, they are termed as simple genetic diseases.[1,2] Mendelian diseases, typically rare and very infrequently encountered at physicians' offices, are exemplified by monogenic macular dystrophies, which include autosomal dominant disorders such as Best disease, North Carolina macular dystrophy, Sorsby macular dystrophy, malattia leventinese/Doyne' honeycomb dystrophy, pattern dystrophy, late-onset retinal degeneration, and autosomal recessive disorders such as Stargardt disease and mitochondrial diseases.[3]

In addition to monogenic diseases, other diseases develop from a combination of multiple genetic and environmental factors. They are considered as complex genetic diseases. Common complex diseases frequently seen in the real clinical practice, include diabetes and age-related macular degeneration (AMD) (Fig. 9.1).[2]

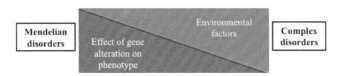

FIGURE 9.1

The contribution of genetics and the environment in Mendelian and in complex diseases. Complex diseases derive from a combination of multiple heritable and environmental factors. Gene alterations normally lead to disease phenotypes but the effect of genetic factors may be modulated by environmental influences. Environmental components may also accumulate over lifetime and change the equilibrium toward disease, with or without the presence of genetic mutations.

Modified from Marques SCF, Oliveira CR, Pereira CMF, Outeiro TF. Epigenetics in neurodegeneration: a new layer of complexity. Prog Neuro-Psychopharmacol Biol Psychiatry. 2011;35(2):348–355. https://doi.org/10.1016/j.pnpbp.2010.08.008.

Heritability of AMD

The importance of heritability of AMD was revealed by twin studies. Meyers et al. reported a cohort study in which 134 twin pairs were recruited from 1986 to 1994. Monozygosity and dizygosity of these twins were confirmed by genetic tests.[4] The criteria for AMD diagnosis included the different size, type, and number of drusen, well-demarcated geographic atrophy (GA), and any neovascular changes, which are consistent with clinical classifications. Based on these criteria, a statistical Fisher's test was used to determine whether the concordance of AMD differed significantly between monozygotic and dizygotic pairs. The results showed that fundus features and vision loss are strikingly similar in monozygotic twins with AMD but not in dizygotic twins.[4]

In another twin study in 2009, 42 twin pairs with normal visual acuity, matching restricted criteria that exclude clinical AMD were recruited.[5] This cohort comprises age-matched 21 pairs of monozygotic twins and 21 pairs of dizygosity. A series of psychophysical and electroretinographic tests were performed. All color and flicker threshold and cone absolute threshold were significantly higher in the monozygotic pairs than that of the dizygotic pairs. Rod absolute threshold and rod and cone recovery rate were essentially similar for both monozygotic and dizygotic twin pairs. These findings indicated that cone thresholds and flicker thresholds are strongly determined by genetics, whereas, rod thresholds and adaptive abilities may be influenced more by environmental factors. This twin study demonstrated that genetic and environmental factors contribute differently to neuronal processes in the retina, which may influence the disease risk and diseases severity in various stages of AMD.

Molecular genetics of AMD
Methods of molecular genetics of AMD

AMD is a spectrum of macular disease with heterogeneous disease manifestations and varied disease severity. Heritability in complex genetic diseases cannot be defined by the methodology through which identifying Mendelian disease genes has been successfully applied. In 2001, the Human Genome Project was completed. It provided a necessary map of the human genome and the crucial information in which polymorphism data had been collected over the years (http://www.ncbi.nlm.nih.gov/projects/SNP/index.htm) and the database of resequencing project (http://hapmap.ncbi.nlm.nih.gov/) was established. From 2000 to 2005, genome-wide association studies (GWAS) were developed to identify genetic variants responsible for disease risk. Typical GWAS obey the concept of using phenotype-first, in which the participants are classified by their clinical manifestation(s), not by genotype-first approach. And then a large collection of DNA samples of well-phenotyped subjects is collected and analyzed. This is a case-control DNA collection. In GWAS for AMD, the people with AMD (cases) and age- and gender-matched people without AMD (controls) are recruited for the comparative study of DNA sequence. Designing large longitudinal cohort studies provides many advantages for GWAS, in which not only disease phenotypes but also quantitative phenotypes, for example stratifying drusen size, type, and number of subjects in the case group, can be analyzed. The longitudinal design of such cohort studies may also provide a gold standard in "case definition" in epidemiology, by which the incidence rate, not prevalence rate, can be determined.

The genomic variation in GWAS is represented by single nucleotide polymorphisms (SNPs). SNP is the basic unit of genetic variation that refers to single base-pair changes in the DNA sequence of an individual's genome. The method of GWAS is evolving rapidly. The first GWAS was done with only 100,000 SNPs. Two companies, Affymetrix and Illumina, have produced increasingly dense and more optimal arrays containing up to several millions of SNPs. Genotyping with arrays is based on oligonucleotides specific for a small area (approx. 50 base pairs) surrounding the targeted SNPs. Before GWAS analysis, a modified step called "imputation" was performed. This modification is a process of "guessing the genotype" of adjacent SNPs from the actual SNP obtained by the arrays. The basis of "guessing the genotype" is the existence of the database of HapMap reference genotype, which was derived from few hundred samples. Currently, the reference population has increased in sample size and ethnic diversity. This step allows many more SNPs to be analyzed.

GWAS rely on the phenomenon of linkage disequilibrium, wherein SNPs are not inherited individually but instead are in linkage disequilibrium blocks, with many nearby SNPs being highly associated. This enables the selection of one SNP (the tag SNP) that represents up to 50,000 surrounding base pairs.[6] Through the high-throughput technique, for example, HapMap project that is gradually replaced by the National Center for Biotechnology Information (NCBI) Genomes Project (http://www.1000genomes.org/), genotyping sets of 500,000−1,000,000 tag SNPs can cover approximately 80% of all common SNPs in the genome.[7]

As whole genome sequencing technologies are rapidly improving and becoming less expensive, they will replace the current genotyping technologies. Whole genome sequencing approaches can make up the deficiency in the information obtained separately through genotyping arrays and exome sequencing. Through genotyping arrays such as the products made by Affymetrix and Illumina, GWAS largely evaluated common variants but missed rare variants. Exome analysis may miss many GWAS variants because DNA variations outside the exons can affect gene activity and protein production. The use of a whole-genome sequencing approach defines a genetic architecture characterized by GWAS loci that include the relevant gene, and rare variants of large effect.[8]

In molecular genetics, GWAS has revolutionized the technology delineating the extent of genetic variants in different individuals. It allows us to see if any variant is associated with a trait of disease with complex etiology. Based on GWAS, AMD has been characterized as having polygenic and multifactorial inheritance, wherein heritability is determined by the joint action of multiple genes and their interaction with environmental factors (Fig. 9.2).[9]

Interpretation of GWAS statistical significance and genetic effects

GWAS has been considered as a standard method for candidate gene discovery. It has been accepted that GWAS would provide an effective and unbiased approach

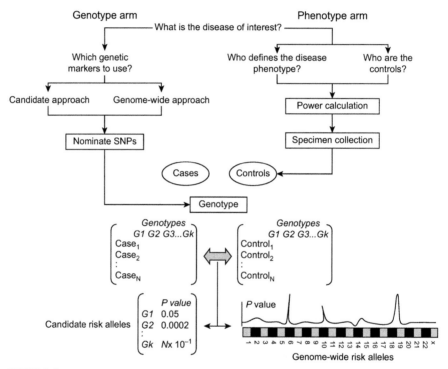

FIGURE 9.2

Schematic illustration of genome-wide association studies (GWAS). The genetic association studies have two arms: a phenotype arm based on the clinically defined features of the common disease and a genotype arm. The genotyping arm, as it pertains to contemporary association studies, starts with the decisive nomination of markers, in particular, single-nucleotide polymorphisms (SNPs). If one assumes a more agnostic approach, then a "genome-wide association study" that systematically surveys representative SNPs across all chromosomes would be appropriate. These initial putative risk alleles are then further filtered by statistical adjustments for multiple hypothesis testing. In GWAS, SNPs can be tabulated by *P*-value if limited in number or displayed across the entire genome.

Modified from Tsao H, Florez JC. Introduction to genetic association studies. J Invest Dermatol. 2007;127(10): 2283–2287. https://doi.org/10.1038/sj.jid.5701054.

to revealing the risk alleles for genetically complex non-Mendelian disorders. In fact, the success in GWAS is contingent on detecting the association of SNPs with candidate gene variants statistically. There are two requirements in GWAS. First, the SNPs must capture the linkage disequilibrium in case and control samples; second, the gene variant needs to have a sufficient frequency for detection.

Utilizing the results of GWAS is to combine studies via a meta-analysis. Meta-analysis is a well-established and validated statistical approach for combining evidence across any number of independent studies, as long as each of the studies shares the same research hypothesis. The results used in meta-analyses can be represented by an "effect size." The effect size is a statistical concept that measures the strength of the relationship between two variables on a numeric scale. Traditional approaches include *Fisher's* method of combining *P*-values; some researchers have used this method or a weighted version in GWAS. The Manhattan plot showing the *P*-values from *Fisher's* test is exemplified in Fig. 9.3.[10] These *P*-value approaches have disadvantages, when they cannot provide an overall estimate of the effect size.[11] Therefore, GWAS researchers have also used odds ratios as a measure of the genetic risk effect.

The genetics of early-stage and late-stage AMD

AMD is a spectrum central-retina disease that evolves in stages of varied severities (Fig. 1.1 of Chapter 1). The classification of AMD is broadly characterized into early and late-stage AMD. Although early-stage AMD has heterogeneous manifestations, it is not associated with visual impairment. Since early AMD usually is asymptomatic, it is observed less frequently in retinal clinics. Both GA and neovascular AMD may be categorized as one disease status termed late-stage or advanced stage AMD, because the poor visual outcome of both disease entities is the same. The detailed classification of AMD based on clinical manifestations, multimodal imaging, and histological findings is given in Chapter 3.

Before the era of GWAS, the heritability of early and late AMD was estimated using twin studies. Seddon et al. reported a large cohort twin study of AMD.[12] This study includes all levels of AMD, including the early, intermediate stages and the advanced stages of AMD in twins. In their cohort, the heritability of overall AMD was estimated to be 46%. Heritability was significant for intermediate AMD (67%) and advanced AMD (71%), respectively.[12] In another twin study, the heritability of early AMD was estimated to be 35%−55%.[13] The findings of twin studies revealed that the heritability of early AMD is lower than that of late AMD.

Signaling the era of GWAS, a breakthrough in the molecular genetics of AMD emerged when novel and replicated loci on chromosome 1q31, in late-stage AMD individuals, was found by genome-wide family-based linkage studies.[14]

Moving forward, four genome-wide single-nucleotide polymorphic association studies with AMD case-control cohorts discovered the association of a variant (Y402H) in the complement factor H (*CFH*) gene with late-stage AMD in

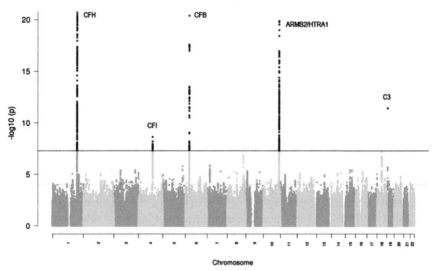

FIGURE 9.3

Manhattan plots for genome-wide association analyses of the discovery cohort comparing subjects with choroidal neovascularization to subjects without AMD. The y-axes of the plots are truncated at 1×10^{-20}. $-\log10(P)$ = negative logarithm (base 10) of the single nucleotide polymorphism's P-value; *ARMS2/HTRA1* = age-related maculopathy susceptibility 2/HtrA serine peptidase 1; *CFH*, complement factor H; *CFB*, complement factor B; *C3*, complement component 3; *CFI*, complement factor I. *CFH, CFI, CFB, ARMS2/HTRA1*, and *C3* all had P-values less than the genome-wide significance threshold of 5×10^{-8}.

Modified from Sobrin L, Ripke S, Yu Y, et al. Heritability and genome-wide association study to assess genetic differences between advanced age-related macular degeneration subtypes. Ophthalmology. *2012;119(9): 1874–1885. https://doi.org/10.1016/j.ophtha.2012.03.014.*

2005.[15-18] The variant observed is an SNP where thymine substitutes for cytosine at nucleotide 1277 in exon 9, with a resulting tyrosine-to histidine change in amino acid position 402, that is, Y402H of the protein. The *CFH* gene, located on chromosome 1q25-31 region, regulates a protein that inhibits the activation of the complement pathway. Another strong signal was observed in the *ARMS2/HTRA1* locus on 10q26.[19] Other studies identified AMD risk variants in *C3* and *CFB* as shown in Manhattan plots of Fig. 9.3.[10,20]

A recent meta-analysis of large case-control studies implicated a total of 19 risk loci in AMD.[21] Most importantly, the estimated odds ratios (ORs, representing genetic effect) per adverse allele in late-stage AMD, for *CFH* risk alleles and *ARMS2* risk alleles exceed 2.0, which is high among complex diseases.[22] Since these variants explain a large proportion of its heritability, the data not only imply the discovery of causative genes, but also highlight the possible underlying biologic pathways involved in the late-stage AMD.[21]

In contrast, based on recent meta-analysis data from five GWAS at the *CFH* and *ARMS2/HTRA1* loci, which had high genetic effects on late-stage AMD, these risk loci had much lower genetic effects, that is, *CFH* SNP rs1329424 (OR = 1.41) and the *ARMS2/HTRA1* SNP rs3793917 (OR = 1.43), on early-stage AMD.[23] Furthermore, by using a similar sample size to assess genetic association with early-stage AMD in a number of GWAS that had assessed the associations with late-stage AMD, no significant variants were found besides *CFH* and *ARMS2* variants at a lower risk. This implies that the genetic contribution to early-stage AMD either is small, or there is a reason to question whether large effect loci unique to early-stage AMD exist.[23] However, it is notable that the risk variants in *CFH* and *ARMS2* display the same trend of genetic effects for early and late-stage AMD. This implies that the different stages of AMD share some common and also possess distinct genetic architecture.

Although the difference in genetic effects on late-stage and early-stage AMD is currently unknown,[24] different approaches to search risk-associated gene variants in early stages of AMD should be explored further. It is crucial to understand the underlying mechanisms in various subgroups of early AMD because that may provide insights into a preventive strategy for incident AMD, which is discussed in Chapter 12.

Complement pathway genes and AMD

Identifying AMD risk variants in complement factor H (*CFH*), complement component C3 (*C3*), complement component C7 (*C7*), complement component C2 (*C2*)/complement factor B (*CFB*), and complement factor I (*CFI*) indicates that activation of complement pathways, particularly the alternative pathway, involved in AMD pathogenesis.[16,20,25]

A well-designed case-control GWAS identified and confirmed that *CFH* gene is strongly associated with late-stage AMD.[18] First of all, phenotypes of the case subjects comprise large drusen, a hallmark of AMD, combining clinical evidence of late-stage AMD, that is, GA and/or neovascular AMD. Second, the statistically significant two SNPs are obtained with the following feature, $P < 4.8 \times 10^{-7}$ that is, 0.05 divided by 103,611 = 4.8×10^{-7} among 103,611 tested SNPs on 22 autosomal chromosomes. Third, these two SNPs (rs380390 and rs10272438) lie in an intron of the gene for *CFH* located on chromosome 1q31. Fourth, although these two SNPs are noncoding, analysis of linkage disequilibrium throughout this chromosomal region revealed that the two SNPs lie in a 500-kb region of high linkage disequilibrium. Fifth, using the International HapMap database to look at linkage-disequilibrium blocks, these two associated SNPs lie in a block that is 41 kb long and entirely contained within the *CFH* gene. The variant observed is an SNP where thymine substitutes for cytosine at nucleotide 1277 in exon 9, with a resulting tyrosine-to histidine change in amino acid position 402, that is, Y402H of the protein. The Tyr402His amino acid substitution was the first CFH variant shown to be strongly associated with AMD in the Caucasian population.[15-18] The Tyr402His variant appears to be much more frequent in people from Caucasian and African descent (allele frequency of approximately 35%) than in Hispanics and Asians (allele frequencies of approximately 17% and 7%, respectively).[26] The Tyr402His variant shows marginal association with AMD in Asians. Apart from Tyr402His, several other *CFH* polymorphisms and haplotypes have been reported to confer an increased risk of AMD, both in Caucasians and Asians.[27] Several other haplotypes of *CFH* and adjacent regions, one of them containing a deletion of *CFHR1* and *CFHR3*,[28] actually lower the risk of AMD.[29] In Fig. 9.4, the structure and function of *CFH* related proteins, named the regulators of complement activation, that are encoded by a gene cluster on chromosome 1q32, are demonstrated by Boon et al.[27]

In addition to the Y402H variant in *CFH*, 20 out of 84 polymorphisms that are around this locus also showed a strong association with AMD. These 20 polymorphisms were defined as four common haplotypes. Two of them increased

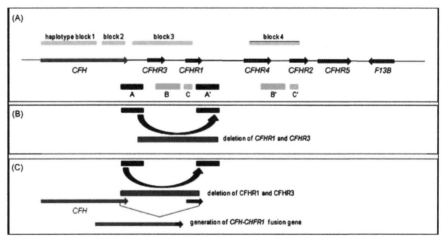

FIGURE 9.4

The *CFH* region of the regulator of complement activation (RCA) gene cluster on chromosome 1q32. (A) Genomic organization of the *CFH* and *CFHR1–5* genes. The region contains four haplotype blocks (orange). Three large duplicated regions are present in the cluster (A and A', B and B', C and C'). (B) Nonhomologous recombination between the 3' ends of the duplicated regions A and A' leads to a deletion of the *CFHR1* and *CFHR3* genes. This rearrangement is relatively common in African and European populations, and decreases the risk of AMD. (C) Nonhomologous recombination between the 5' ends of the duplicated regions A and A' leads to a deletion of the *CFHR1* and *CFHR3* genes, and to the generation of a *CFH-CFHR1* fusion gene. The fusion gene consists of the first 21 exons of *CFH* and the last two exons of *CFHR1*.

Modified from Boon CJF, van de Kar NC, Klevering BJ, et al. The spectrum of phenotypes caused by variants in the CFH gene. Mol Immunol. 2009;46(8–9):1573–1594. https://doi.org/10.1016/j.molimm.2009.02.013.

susceptibility and two others were protective against AMD. As multiple studies showed, for complex diseases protective alleles may be as important as risk alleles because there is potential to derive highly effective, genomically based medicines.[30]

The *CFH* gene regulates the production of a protein that normally inhibits the activation of complement. It blocks the activation of C3—C3b and degrades C3b (Fig. 9.5).[31] The resultant upregulation of the inflammatory response and uncontrolled membrane attack complex formation may damage the retinal pigment epithelium (RPE), contributing to pathogenesis and progression of AMD. Although multiple studies support this hypothesis, the specific functional significance of the *CFH* Y402H polymorphism in the development of AMD remains elusive.

Based on a recent meta-analysis, the association of *C3* genetic polymorphisms with late-stage AMD is confirmed. Two nonsynonymous SNPs were demonstrated to have an increased pathogenic effect on advanced AMD (rs2230199, allelic model: OR = 1.49; homozygote model: OR = 2.33; rs1047286, allelic model: OR = 1.45, homozygote model: OR = 2.06).[32] C3 is the central molecule of the complement cascade that includes the classical, alternative, and lectin pathways (Fig. 9.5).[31] *C3* gene is located on chromosome 19p13 (Fig. 9.3) and exhibits nine common genetic SNPs. Cleavage of C3 into C3a and C3b is the central step in complement activation. In the alternative pathway, C3 activation is under the control of CFB, a key pathway component, and CFH, a potent negative regulator.[33,34] Both CFB and CFH are expressed by RPE cells.[33,35,36] The interaction between C3 and CFH is supported by the finding that C3b is a major physiological ligand of CFH (Fig. 9.5).[31,37]

Other complement pathway gene variants may contribute to AMD etiology. Candidate gene analysis revealed protective alleles within the *C2/CFB* locus on chromosome 6p21.3.[38,39] C2 is a serum glycoprotein that functions as part of the classical pathway (Fig. 9.5). Activated C1 cleaves C2 into C2a and C2b. The serine proteinase C2a then combines with complement factor 4b to create the C3 or C5 convertase. Variation in *CFB* and *C2* genes involved in the initiation of the alternative complement cascade and activation of the classic component pathway is associated with the risk of AMD. Haplotype analyses of SNPs in *CFB* and *C2* identify a statistically significant common risk haplotype (H1, OR = 1.32) and two weak protective haplotypes (H7, OR = 0.45 and H10, OR = 0.36, respectively) among Caucasians.[38] While a case-control study showed that *C2/CFB* variants play protective roles in the development of AMD and polypoidal choroidal vasculopathy, a clinical variant of neovascular AMD in Japanese.[40] These data expand and refine our understanding of the complement genetic risk factors for AMD.

Genetic variants of other factors in the complement pathways, complement component 7 (C7) and complement factor I (Fig. 9.5), have also been implicated through candidate gene association studies with AMD. By using an existing GWAS dataset, *C7* was identified as potentially associated with subtypes of AMD. The statistical scores for the *C7* SNP were not significant at the genome level but were significant at the pathway level, suggesting that studying at the pathway level can be beneficial for identifying SNP signals that could be lost at the

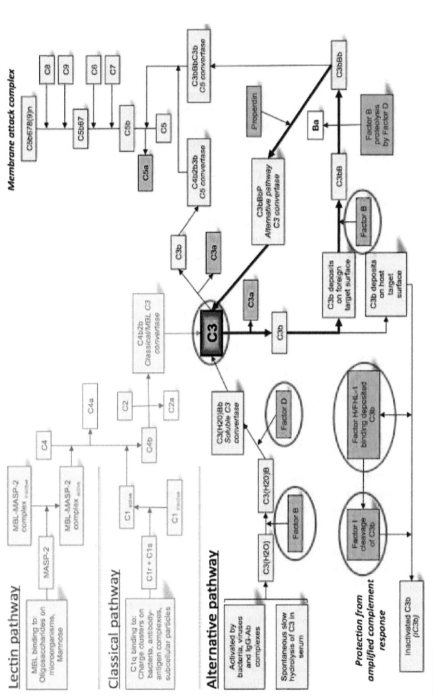

FIGURE 9.5

The role of complement pathways in pathogenesis of AMD. Flow diagram showing the three pathways of complement activation, that is, lectin, classical or alternative pathways. All three pathways of activation converge on the complement protein C3 (*red box*) and its breakdown into C3b, which itself feeds into the amplification loop (highlighted by *thick black arrows*). This in turn generates a number of anaphylatoxins such as C3a and C5a (*pink boxes*) and ultimately results in the deposition of the terminal membrane attack complex (MAC). Complement activation can be fine-tuned on a surface through the action of various complement factors (*blue boxes*), where activation can be inhibited (factor H, FHL-1, factor I) or encouraged (factor B, factor D, properdin). A number of genetic alterations have been associated with AMD risk and most of these affect genes of the alternative pathways of complement (highlighted with *red circles*).

Modified from McHarg S, Clark SJ, Day AJ, Bishop PN. Age-related macular degeneration and the role of the complement system. Mol Immunol. 2015;67(1):43–50. https://doi.org/10.1016/j.molimm.2015.02.032.

genome-wide level.[41] This study identified a protective haplotype for *C7* (rs2876849) for the neovascular AMD subtype.

In a case-control association study, targeted sequencing of the *CFI* gene across the coding region and splice sites of the canonical *CFI* transcript was performed in AMD patients.[42] Twenty rare coding nonsynonymous variants, including the previously reported G119R allele,[42] were identified. Due to their rarity, the variants will never generate genome-wide statistical significance. This study showed that multiple rare and ultra-rare alleles in *CFI* appear to contribute to AMD pathogenesis. CFI, a serine protease is involved in the inactivation of C3b and the subsequent inhibition of the amplification of the alternative pathway response (Fig. 9.5). Biochemical evidence shows that the function of CFI may be reduced when it is bound to β-amyloid that is a major constituent of AMD-related druse.[43]

To date, the role of the complement system in the pathogenesis of AMD has been proposed and studied extensively. This is because several complement components have been detected in AMD-related drusen,[44] and at higher plasma levels of C3a, C3d, Bb, and C5a in AMD patients.[45] Most importantly, polymorphisms in several complement genes (*CFH, CFB, C2, C3, C7,* and *CFI*) are genetic risk factors of AMD as described earlier. Mechanistically, CFH may inhibit CD47-mediated resolution of subretinal inflammation and this inhibitory effect could be enhanced by the AMD associated *CFH* (H402) variant.[31,46]

A recent study using postmortem donor eyes provided evidence that the alternative complement pathway is activated in AMD eyes.[47] The donor eyes were categorized by having no or minimal drusen (controls) and large drusen with advanced AMD. C3, CFB, and CFD, which are correlated with activity of the alternative complement pathway, were predominantly localized to the choroidal vasculature and Bruch's membrane (BrM/C) and were elevated in BrM/C extracts of advanced AMD eyes as compared to control. A significant increase in CFB activation was found in the vitreous of advanced AMD eyes as compared with controls. Based on the complement gene scores, calculated with odds ratios for SNPs in the complement pathway, the risk variants consist of complement factor H (*CFH*), *C3, C2,* and *CFB*. These genetic variants expressed by the degree of gene scores were correlated with alternative pathway complement activation in vitreous of advanced AMD eyes.[47]

Inflammation and immune-related genes

Genetic linkage and genome-wide association studies have identified AMD susceptibility alleles in multiple complement genes as described earlier. Innate immunity appears to play a key role in the pathogenesis of AMD. Therefore, other inflammatory genes have been evaluated for possible association with AMD, including Toll-like receptors (*TLRs*), C-motif chemokine receptor type 2 (*CCR-2*) and *CCR*-like gene, interleukins, and human leukocyte antigens (*HLA*).[48,49] Toll-like receptor genes encode proteins that are principal sensors of infection. The proteins are a type of pattern-recognition receptors that initiate an appropriate inflammatory response to foreign pathogens such as bacteria, fungi, and viruses. To date, more than 10 TLR family members have been identified in humans. All TLRs consist of an amino-terminal domain, characterized by multiple leucine-rich repeats, and a carboxy-terminal Toll/interleukin-1 receptor (TIR) domain that interacts with TIR-containing adaptors. Nucleic acid-sensing TLRs (TLR3, TLR7, TLR8, and TLR9) are localized within endosomal compartments, whereas the other TLRs reside at the plasma membrane (Fig. 9.6).[49,50,51,52]

To examine the overall genetic basis of AMD, a genome-wide scan in extended families ascertained with late-stage AMD was performed. The extended genome-wide scan showed that susceptibility loci lie on chromosome 1q, 3p, 9q, and 10q.[14,53] TLR4 gene becomes interesting because this gene is located at genetic locus 9q32-33, which has been associated with AMD. However, the relationship of TLR4 gene polymorphisms with AMD has been studied with inconsistent results.[48]

Polymorphisms in *TLR2, TLR3,* and *TLR7* also have been investigated for associations with AMD. In a case-control study, the genotyping of polymorphisms *TLR2* (*TLR2*-Arg753Gln: rs5743708) was determined using real-time PCR. *TLR2* Arg753Gln genotype had approximately four times greater risk of AMD compared with the control genotype (OR = 3.88; $P = .001$), suggesting that *TLR2* polymorphism contributes to the pathogenesis of AMD.[54]

One case-control study and two replication analyses showed that *TLR3* L412F variant at rs3775291 locus was protective against GA but had no association with CNV.[55] However, the risk association of the SNP changes of *TLR3* gene at rs3775291 locus was found differently in multiple other populations. For instance, no significant association in genotype and allele frequency of *TLR3* gene at rs3775291 locus was found in AMD patients as compared to control in North India.[56]

In one report, coding SNPs in *TLR7* (rs179008) were not associated with AMD.[57] The current data imply that the genetic influence of *TLR* variants appears to have no major impact on AMD risk. Therefore further replication efforts may be needed to establish the contributions of these genes.

As histopathology studies showed that drusen, the hallmark of AMD, contain complement components, complement regulators, immunoglobulins, and anaphyla-toxins, the indication is that local inflammation and immunologic response are associated with the development of AMD.[58] Therefore, an association of the common gene variants of multiple inflammatory factors with AMD has been studied. In a population-based case-control study, subjects were genotyped for common sequence variations in the C-motif Chemokine Receptor 2 (*CCR2*), C-motif Chemokine Ligand 2 (*CCL2*), and *TLR4* genes.[48] In this study, analysis of single nucleotide polymorphisms (SNPs) in *CCL2* and *CCR2* genes did not demonstrate an association with AMD. For *CCL2*, one haplotype containing the minor allele of *C35C* was significantly associated with AMD, but this result was not sustained after adjustment for multiple testing. In this study, RPE cells were harvested from postmortem eyes with AMD. Expression analysis did not demonstrate altered RNA expression of

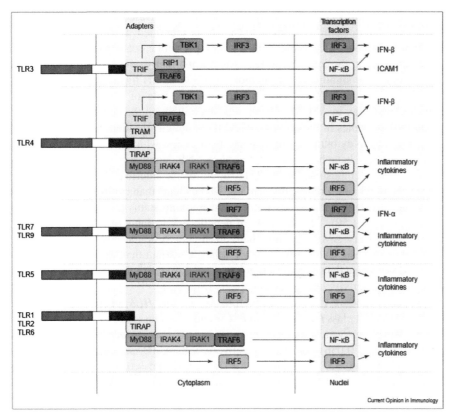

FIGURE 9.6

Schematic illustration of Toll-like receptor (TLR) -signaling pathways. All TLRs except for TLR3 share the MyD88-dependent pathway that activates NF-kB and subsequently induces genes encoding inflammatory cytokines. IRAK1, IRAK4, and TRAF6 are located downstream of MyD88. TIRAP is involved in the MyD88-dependent pathway downstream of TLR2 and TLR4. TRIF is utilized in the TLR3-and TLR4-mediated activation of IRF3 and the subsequent induction of expression of IRF3-dependent genes such as that coding for IFN-b. TRAM is specifically involved in IRF3 activation inTLR4 signaling. TBK1 (together with IKKi) is responsible for the activation of IRF3 downstream of TRIF in TLR3-and TLR4 signaling. TRIF utilizesRIP1 and TRAF6 to activate NF-kB. IRF7 associates with MyD88, IRAK1, and TRAF6, and mediates TLR7-and TLR9-induced IFN-aproduction.IRF5 also associates with MyD88 and TRAF6 to induce genes encoding inflammatory cytokines.

Modified from Kawai T, Akira S. Pathogen recognition with Toll-like receptors. Curr Opin Immunol. 2005;17(4):
338–344. http://doi.org/10.1016/j.coi.2005.02.007.

CCL2 and *CCR2* in these RPE cells. A recent study using bioinformatics strategy focused on chemokine receptors and their pathways and their genetic association with AMD.[59] In this study, RNA sequencing data demonstrated differentially expressed genes, SNPs, indels (insertion and deletions), and simple sequence repeats between the healthy controls and AMD donor samples. Based on these differentially expressed genes, pathway enrichment analysis identified dysfunctional pathways including chemokine signaling pathways, complement cascade pathways, and cytokine signaling in the immune system. Most importantly, allele-specific expression was found to be significant for chemokine (C−C motif) ligand (*CCL*) 2, 3, 4, 13, 19, 21; *CCR1* and *CCR5*, etc.[59] Therefore, the role of chemokine receptors' signaling pathway in AMD has been indicated, although the common genetic variation in these genes in the etiology of AMD is not clearly identified to date.

Variations in cytokine expression and their genes, which may modulate susceptibility to AMD, have been studied. Based on SNP genotyping data, a case (AMD)-control study demonstrated that -251A allele of the interleukin 8 (IL8) promoter gene polymorphism is more prevalent in AMD patients than control after adjustment with age, sex, body mass index (BMI), and smoking status ($P = .043$, OR = 1.23, 95% CI = 1.0−1.50).[60] In the study of genetic risk variants of *CFH* Y402H polymorphisms of dry AMD patients, there are higher systemic levels of IL-6, IL-18, and tumor necrosis factor-α in those with the CC variant than that of other variants ($P < .01$).[61] These data suggest a regulatory role of genetic factors in proinflammatory cytokine activity in dry AMD patients (Fig. 9.7).[62,63]

To determine if genetic polymorphisms in the *HLA* genes are associated with AMD, *HLA* class *I−A, I−B*, and *I−Cw* and *HLA* class *II DRB1* and *DQB1* principal allele groups were genotyped in a case-control cohort study.[64] Allele *Cw*0701 ($P = .004$, Pc = 0.036) correlated positively with AMD, whereas alleles *B*4001 ($P = .003$, Pc = 0.027) and *DRB1*1301($P = .001$, Pc = 0.009) were negatively associated. These *HLA* associations were independent of any linkage disequilibrium. Immunohistochemistry demonstrated differential HLA class I expression in choriocapillaris endothelial cells. These findings indicate that *HLA* polymorphisms influence the development of AMD, possibly via modulating choroidal immune function.

Other replicated loci with high genetic effect on AMD

Chromosome 1q31 and 10q26 are the most frequently replicated loci that show strong association with advanced AMD.[65] Variants identified by SNP genotyping within C1q31, which imply biologic relevance of complement factor H, have been recognized as the first major AMD-susceptibility allele. Multiple studies revealed that the 10q26 region harbors a second major genetic locus of AMD susceptibility.[65] Three genes, *PLEKHA1, LOC387715/ARMS2* (age-related maculopathy susceptibility 2), and *HTRA1/PRSS11*(high-temperature requirement factorA1), overlap at C10q26 (Fig. 9.8).[66,67]

Using regional SNP genotyping within C10q26, variants in the *PLEKHA1, LOC387715/ARMS2*, and *HTRA1* locus were identified as showing strong associations with late AMD.[19,65] Based on the analysis of ORs and population attributable risks for these associations, the magnitude of the associations of these genes at

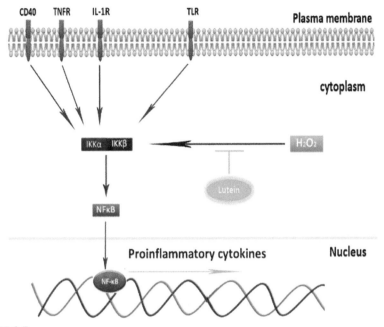

FIGURE 9.7

The regulation of intracellular inflammation with proinflammatory cytokines. The final pathway of NF-kB activation induced by various triggers such as the TNF receptor (TNFR), the IL-1 receptor (IL-1R), Toll-like receptors (TLRs), and the CD40 molecule. Triggering these receptors leads to the activation of NADPH oxidase, which in turn induces higher intracellular levels of H_2O_2. Activation of the IkB kinase (IKK) complex is mediated via H_2O_2 and scavenging via lutein as an example will prevent IkB degradation, nuclear translocation of NF-kB, and DNA binding of NF-kB thereby blocking the proinflammatory cytokine response.

Modified from Kijlstra A, Tian Y, Kelly ER, Berendschot TTJM. Lutein: more than just a filter for blue light. Prog Retin Eye Res. *2012;31(4):303–315. http://doi.org/10.1016/j.preteyeres.2012.03.002.*

10q26 was comparable to that calculated for *CHF* gene, and their associations appear to act independently.[19]

Individual SNPs under the chromosome 10 linkage peak were highly significantly associated with risk of AMD ($P < 10^{-20}$). Particularly, by using multimarker haplotype tests, one such haplotype was markedly associated with risk of AMD ($P < 10^{-56}$), and is also strongly correlated with several SNPs including rs10490924 ($r^2 = 0.79$), the same SNP that has shown maximal association with risks of late AMD in other studies.[65] Subsequently, rs10490924 was genotyped and showed that this is the most associated SNP or haplotype in the region of *LOC387715*.[29] All nonsynonymous SNPs in this critical region were genotyped, yielding a highly significant association ($P < .00001$) between *PLEKHA1/LOC387715* and AMD. The association of either a single or a double copy of the

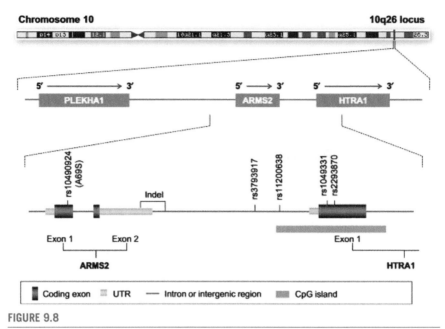

FIGURE 9.8

An overview of the 10q26 locus, showing the three genes, *PLEKHA1, ARMS2,* and *HTRA1*, most significantly associated variants to AMD risk.

Modified from Wang G. Chromosome 10q26 locus and age-related macular degeneration: a progress update. Exp Eye Res. *2014;119:1–7. https://doi.org/10.1016/j.exer.2013.11.009.*

high-risk allele within the *PLEKHA1/LOC387715* locus accounts for an odds ratio of 5.0 (95% confidence interval 3.2–7.9) for AMD and a population attributable risk as high as 57%.[19,65]

The discovery of the genetic association of *LOC387715/ARMS2* loci with late AMD strongly suggested that there is a *LOC387715/ARMS2* gene-related specific biologic pathway underlying AMD development. *LOC387715/ARMS2* encodes a 12 kDa mitochondrial associated protein that has been found in neural retinal tissue and RPE cells. Kanda and coauthors expressed human retinal *LOC387715/ARMS2* cDNA translated via an expression vector in African green monkey kidney fibroblast cells.[67] The expressed protein is a 12-kDa protein, which colocalizes to mitochondrial markers at the mitochondrial outer membrane with immunoblot analysis. The rs10490924 SNP results in the substitution of serine-for-alanine at position 69 (A69S) and may cause misfolding of the associated protein. In addition to the possible dysfunction of the mitochondrial outer membrane protein, the susceptibility of mitochondrial DNA to oxidative damage and the limitations of its base repair system have prompted linkage of a second biologic pathway, the oxidative stress pathway, with the development of AMD. A recent study demonstrated that ARMS2 protein is localized to the mitochondrial outer membrane in the human retina, further supporting a possible role for oxidative stress in AMD.[67]

Based on GWAS in a Caucasian case-control cohort and a Chinese population case-control cohort, a variant in *HTRA1* gene is considered to be a major contributor to AMD.[68,69] This consideration was supported by the knowledge of the expression and function of *HTRA1* gene in the immune system as well as its expression in the retina.[70] The *HTRA1* (high-temperature requirement factorA1) gene is a member of the mammalian HTRA serine protease gene family. The protein is expressed by many cells such as human mast cells and is an inhibitor of transforming growth factor-beta (TGFβ) family members. *HTRA1* is one of four *HTRA* genes involved in cell growth, apoptosis, and inflammatory reactions. Its expression in human fibroblasts is age-dependent.[71] HTRA1 protein is a key modulator of degradation of proteoglycans in the extracellular matrix. It has been suggested that HTRA1 protein plays a role in extracellular matrix remodeling of Bruch's membrane and RPE, which subsequently contributes to drusen formation, neovascularization, and RPE atrophy in AMD eyes.[72] The regulation of *HTRA1* gene expression levels may be influenced by variants in its promotor region. The SNP rs11200638 is located within a conserved genomic region upstream of human *HTRA1* genes. In a GWAS, the influence of SNP rs11200638 on the *HTRA1* promoter was studied with human ARPE19 (retinal pigment epithelium cell line) and HeLaS3 cells. The study suggests that the sequence change associated with SNP rs11200638 enhances the transcription of *HTRA1*.[69] To further evaluate the effects of SNP rs11200638 on *HTRA1* promoter activity, the wild type *HTRA1* promoter with different lengths and the mutant sequence carrying the AMD-risk allele at the SNP rs11200638 were constructed and then transfected into different cell lines. A quantitative RT-PCR analysis generated a controversial result, which shows that there is no significant change in *HTRA1* expression between AMD retinas and controls.[67] However, a recent bioinformatics study showed that some genes in chromosome 10q26 may be responsible for risk for AMD. SNPs in 10q26 that influence the expression of only *PLEKHA1* or *ARMS2* are not associated with risk for AMD, while most SNPs that influence the expression of *HTRA1* are associated with risk for AMD.[73]

Regarding common alleles with high effect in *ARMS2* and *HTRA1* associated with AMD (Fig. 9.8), both variants lie together within 200 kB in the 10q26 region and are well known to be in almost complete linkage disequilibrium. Therefore, statistical genetic analysis alone is not sufficient to distinguish which of these two genes is responsible. The *ARMS2* gene product is expressed in the retina and RPE and is associated with mitochondria and thus may affect oxidative stress. However, the *HTRA1* gene product may influence matrix metalloproteinases, TGFβ, and the inflammatory response within the macula (Fig. 9.8).[66,74]

Mitochondrial genes and AMD

Mitochondrial damage and dysfunction are associated with aging and the development of neurodegenerative diseases, including AMD.[75] Mitochondrial DNA (mtDNA) damage and a decreased capacity for repair have been consistently documented.[75] RPE mitochondrial bioenergetic events and oxidative stress in AMD are referred to Chapter 7. Ultrastructural evidence in human eyes showed an age-related decline in the number and mitochondrial integrity in the RPE, and a larger decline in RPE with AMD.[76] The cumulative data demonstrated the susceptibility of mtDNA to oxidative stress, which may contribute to the pathogenesis of AMD. However, from a genetics perspective, there has not been strong evidence to confirm this theory regarding mitochondria and AMD.

In searching the mtDNA changes in AMD, moderate genetic effects of mtDNA variants on AMD have been found.[77] In a case-control study, the restriction fragment length polymorphism analysis was used to compare mtDNA variations and determine mtDNA haplogroups in either early or late AMD.[77] After adjusting for age, sex, and smoking status, mtDNA haplogroup H, the most prevalent haplogroup for European populations, was found to be protective against AMD, with (early and late) AMD (OR = 0.75), with early AMD (OR = 0.75), and with large soft drusen (OR = 0.7). Analysis of retinal mtDNA from AMD eyes as compared to controls showed that AMD mtDNA had higher levels of oxidative damage, as evidenced by 8-OHdG staining, a marker of oxidative DNA damage, and a higher frequency of SNPs.[78,79] Based on these data, it is reasonable to say that the genetic effects of mitochondrial contributions in the etiology of AMD require further study.[80]

Potential extrinsic and intrinsic triggers of AMD-related inflammation

Molecular genetic studies have not yet identified the molecules that trigger the activation of the alternative complement pathway in PR/RPE/BrM/CC complex. If there are such molecules, they might be introduced into the eye by exogenous pathogens and related byproducts, or they could be generated endogenously as part of normal physiologic processes. To reveal these triggers, the approach of human-based molecular genetic studies (linkage or association methods with families and/or case-control cohorts) has been used.

Cigarette smoking appears to be the only modifiable risk factor consistently associated with an risk for AMD.[82,83] Smoking plays a role as an exogenous trigger that may interact with genetic variations in the pathogenesis of AMD. The underlying mechanism by which smoking increases the incidence and severity of AMD is uncertain, but cigarette smoke is known to contain numerous oxidants. Exposure to cigarette smoke has been shown to result in sub-RPE deposits and diffuse thickening of Bruch's membrane,[83] suggesting that oxidative stress is capable of promoting these phenotypic characteristics of AMD. Oxidative stress has also been implicated in AMD by the Age-Related Eye Disease Study, which showed that antioxidants and zinc reduce the risk of individuals with large drusen progressing to advanced AMD. It has been known that the negative biologic impact of smoking consists of suppression of the release of antioxidants and alteration of choroidal blood flow,[83] as well as suppression of CFH expression.[84] An association between *CFH* polymorphisms and AMD is biologically plausible because this gene is involved with inflammatory and immune pathways.[85] A retrospective cohort study based on the European Genetic Database showed that past smokers and current smokers developed neovascular AMD on average 4.9 and 7.7 years earlier, respectively, than never smokers ($P < .001$ for both). Compared with the reference group, the age at onset was 5.2 years earlier for homozygous carriers of the A69S risk allele in the *ARMD2* gene ($P < .001$). Homozygous carriers of the Y402H risk variant in the *CFH* gene developed neovascular AMD 2.8 years earlier ($P = .02$). Patients carrying four risk alleles in *CFH* and *ARMS2* developed neovascular AMD 12.2 years earlier than patients with zero risk alleles ($P < .001$).[85] Most importantly, the interaction between genetic susceptibility and environmental or modifiable factor such as cigarette smoking confers a significantly higher risk of AMD than either factor alone (Fig. 9.9).[81,87]

A case-control association analysis demonstrated independent effects of smoking and the rs1200638 SNP of *HTRA1* on neovascular AMD risk.[88] There was about a fivefold increased risk of neovascular AMD in patients who were smokers and homozygous for *HTRA1* risk allele than smokers without the risk allele.[88] In contrast, a discordant sib-pairs linkage analysis, which is a powerful method for identifying causal genes, showed the risk from smoking was independent of risk from *CFH* or apolipoprotein E (*ApoE*) genotypes.[81,89] To date, the interaction of risk genes

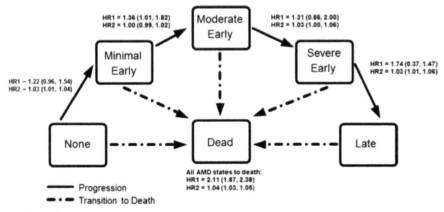

FIGURE 9.9

The impact of cigarette smoking on the 5-step severity scale for AMD recommended by the 3-Continent Consortium. *Arrows* indicate possible transitions along the scale. Hazard ratios (HRs) indicate the hazard of making the transition indicated by the *arrow* for a current smoker compared with a nonsmoker (HR1) and per 5 pack-years smoked (HR2), adjusted for age and sex. The higher HR indicates the smoking population may die at a higher rate per unit time as the control population.

Modified from Myers CE, Klein BEK, Gangnon R, Sivakumaran TA, Iyengar SK, Klein R. Cigarette smoking and the natural history of age-related macular degeneration: the Beaver Dam Eye Study. Ophthalmology. 2014; 121(10):1949–1955. https://doi.org/10.1016/j.ophtha.2014.04.040.

and smoking for late-stage AMD development has not been clearly established. One of the reasons is that one needs very large cohorts to obtain odds ratios or relative risks with small enough confidence intervals. If the combined odds ratios or relative risks are sufficiently different from an additive model, that is, an environmental plus genetic contribution model, an interaction component could be accountable.

Selected potential intrinsic triggers that may interact with genetic variations comprise the regulation of the alternative complement pathway and/or other metabolic pathways such as A2E (N—retinylidene—N—retinylethanolamine), β-amyloid, lipid/oxidized LDL (low-density lipoproteins), and iron metabolism-related molecules. A2E, is formed by cleavage of a precursor A2-phosphatidylethanoloamine deposited in the photoreceptor outer segment in the process of RPE phagocytosis. A2E is considered to be a major source of oxidative products in RPE. These oxidative products are toxic to membranes and inhibit the lysosomal proton pump, resulting in the leakage of the lysosomal membranes and finally apoptosis of RPE cells. The alternative complement pathway is triggered by these processes.[90] Genes that are known to contribute to the production of A2E and lipofuscin accumulation include ABCA4, VMD2, and peripherin/RDS. However, variants in these genes have not been proven to be associated with AMD.

The idea that β-amyloid may play a role in the pathogenesis of AMD arises from several similarities between Alzheimer's disease (AD) and AMD. Both conditions are correlated with aging and the formation of deposits. β-Amyloid accumulation constitutes a critical event in early AD pathogenesis. The amyloid deposits contain a variety of lipids and proteins such as apolipoprotein E that were also found in AMD drusen. HTRA1 may play a role in processing amyloid. The purified HTRA1 can cause proteolytic cleavage of the amyloid precursor protein. On the other hand, HTRA1 inhibitor can cause accumulation of β-amyloid in astrocyte cell culture.[72] Most importantly, HTRA1 protein colocalizes with β-amyloid deposits in human brain samples,[72] thus HTRA1 protein may concur to the individual risk for AD.[91] However, β-amyloid as a possible tissue-specific trigger for AMD has not been reported. In fact, a recent study showed that a HTRA1 inhibitor, FHTR2163, is able to slow the progression of geographic atrophy in a phase 1 clinical trial (see Chapter 11). The possible underlying mechanism is related to a protease function of HTRA1 on extracellular matrix in AMD.[92]

Lipid metabolism has been implicated in extensive studies as a contributing factor for AMD risk. Oxidized LDLs have inhibitory effects on the normal phagocytosis of photoreceptor outer segments by RPE,[93–95] resulting in RPE apoptosis and altered secretion of lysosomal proteases.[95] The association of lipid metabolism with AMD is complicated. One of the first genetic variants associated with AMD was apolipoprotein E (ApoE), a component of low- and high-density lipoproteins (LDL and HDL) in the blood. In a case-control study, the association between *ApoE C112R/R158C* single nucleotide polymorphisms (which determine the E2, E3, and E4 isoforms) and AMD was studied. ApoE112R (E4) distribution differed significantly between AMD patients and controls. *ApoE112R* allele frequency was 10.9% in the AMD group comparing with 16.5% in the younger controls and

18.8% in the clinically screened controls. These results acknowledge the association between *ApoE112R* and a decreased risk of AMD development.[96] These lipoproteins are major carriers of dietary carotenoids such as lutein, zeaxanthin.[62] Evidence exists that HDL metabolism is involved in cholesterol efflux from RPE.[97] Lipid oxidation in PR/RPE/BrM/CC complex may act as a local trigger for AMD. It has been speculated that variants of genes that are responsible for lipid transport and metabolism might be associated with AMD.

Dysregulation of iron homeostasis may also be an etiologic factor in several neurodegenerative disorders such as AMD.[98] Several genetic factors that confer major risk for AMD are polymorphisms within complement component genes as described earlier. As complement dysregulation can lead to inflammatory reactions, both genetic and environmental factors including iron overload may work concurrently to determine the activity of the complement cascade in the outer retinal milieu. In a recent study, by regulating iron-induced *C3* promoter activity, iron-induced *C3* up-regulation was achieved in an animal model. Humans with aceruloplasminemia causing RPE iron overload had increased RPE C3d deposits.[99] However, no variant in the major genes responsible for iron metabolism has yet been shown in association with AMD.

Genetics and response to AMD therapies

As several genetic variants of AMD were identified, the next step is to know whether these high-risk or protective variants would affect the clinical response to therapies. In 2008, AREDS subjects who were considered at high risk for progression to advanced AMD because they had SNPs in *CFH* (Y402H, rs1061170) and *LOC387715/ARMS2* (A69S, rs10490924), received antioxidants plus zinc as a potential therapy.[100] A treatment interaction was observed between the *CFH* Y402H homozygous CC genotype and the supplement with antioxidants plus zinc ($P = .03$). An interaction ($P = .004$) was observed in the AREDS treatment groups taking zinc when compared with that taking no zinc. There was no significant treatment interaction observed with *LOC387715/ARMS2*.[100] These findings indicate that an individual's response to antioxidants plus zinc supplements may be related to *CFH* genotype.

As VEGF is responsible for vascular permeability and neovascularization, anti-VEGF intravitreal injection is the mainstay for the treatment of neovascular AMD, leading to stabilization and quiescence of the choroidal vasculature. Whether the identifiable gene variants interact with the efficacy and outcome of this therapy is a key question for providers. In fact, *VEGF* polymorphisms are associated with the response to an anti-VEGF treatment. *VEGF* SNPs rs3025000 and rs699946 have been associated with improved anti-VEGF treatment.[101,102] For the *VEGF* SNP rs3025000, one T allele appears to be preferable in anti-VEGF treatment with the visual outcome at 6 months.[101] It was also reported that patients with either TT or TC genotypes showed significantly better visual outcome (>7 letter improvement) at 3, 6, and 12 months than did patients with the CC genotype.[101] Evidence exists that patients with the T allele for rs3025000 required less anti-VEGF injections to reach a visual acuity level comparable to other groups.[101] These data indicate the genetic contribution of *VEGF* SNP rs3025000 to the response to anti-VEGF treatment.

Genetic predictive biomarkers of anti-VEGF

In addition to the effects of *VEGF* SNPs, there is some evidence that VEGF receptor (*VEGFR*) SNPs contribute to patient response to anti-VEGF treatment. In two large randomized clinical trials, Comparison of AMD Treatments Trials (CATT) and Alternative Treatment to Inhibitor VEGF in Patients with age-related Macular degeneration (IVAN), the genetic effects of *VEGF* SNPs and *VEGFR* SNPs were studied. These two trials, however, do not support a pharmacogenetics association between *VEGFR* SNPs and change in visual acuity after anti-VEGF treatment.[103] Based on retrospective data collected from patients in replication cohorts in multiple clinics, the mean baseline visual acuity (VA) was 51.3 ETDRS score letters, and the mean change in VA after the loading dose of three monthly injections was a gain of 5.1 letters. Genome-wide single-variant analyses of common variants revealed five independent loci that reached a P-value less than 10×10^{-5}. After replication and meta-analysis of the lead variant among the five loci, rs12138564 located in the *CCT3* gene, remained significantly associated with a better treatment outcome (ETDRS letter gain, 1.7, $P = 1.38 \times 10^{-5}$). On the other hand, genome-wide gene-based optimal unified sequence kernel association test of rare variants showed genome-wide significant associations for the *C10* or *f88* ($P = 4.22 \times 10^{-7}$) and *UNC93B1* ($P = 6.09 \times 10^{-7}$) genes, in both cases leading to a worse treatment outcome. Patients carrying rare variants in the *C10* or *f88* and *UNC93B1* genes lost a mean VA of 30.6 ETDRS score letters and 26.5 ETDRS score letters, respectively, after 3 months of anti-VEGF treatment. These GWAS suggest that rare genetic variants, rather than common variants, may have large effects on treatment outcome after anti-VEGF injections.[104]

From a practical point of view, these differences between the common and rare gene variants are not sufficiently large to predict and modify the therapies for neovascular AMD. However, discovery of additional pharmacogenetic associations with AMD treatment and new genetic and proteomic biomarkers for AMD are needed.

Proteomic biomarkers for AMD risk

Proteomic biomarkers are protein indicators of a biological status of a specific disease. As biochemical species, proteomic biomarkers can be assayed to evaluate the presence of disease and the effect of therapeutic interventions.[105,106] For instance, carboyethylpyrrole (CEP) is a proteomic biomarker for AMD.[107] Modifications of CEP are generated by covalent adduction of primary amino acid groups with 4-hydroxy-7-oxohept-5-enoic acid, an oxidation fragment from docosahexaenoate. Enzyme-linked immunosorbent assay studies showed that mean plasma levels of CEP adducts and their autoantibodies are elevated in AMD patients as compared with the controls.[105] More meaningful, CEP was localized to photoreceptor rod outer segments and RPE cells by immunocytochemical analyses on human retinas.[108] A case-control study showed a 1.6-fold increase in plasma anti-CEP immunoreactivity ($P < .0001$) and a 1.3-fold increase in plasma anti-CEP autoantibody ($P < .0001$) titer in AMD donors as compared with the control donors.[105] Interestingly, proteomic CEP markers alone can differentiate between AMD and normal samples with approximately 76% accuracy and when analyzed together with genomic markers, the discriminatory accuracy increased to about 80%.[105] Donors with *ARMS2, HRTA1, CFH,* or *C3* AMD risk alleles were about 5–10 times more likely to have AMD, whereas when coupled with elevated CEP markers the odds ratios increased an additional 2-to-3-fold.[105] These data are encouraging for the use of CEP plasma biomarkers to predict AMD susceptibility, particularly when analyzed with identified and replicated genomic markers that are associated with AMD. CEP is not the only biomarker available for AMD. Various studies have implicated carboxymethyl lysine (CML), and pentosidine as potential biomarkers for AMD. Oxidatively modified CML and pentosidine were detected in AMD drusen,[108,109] and their plasma levels were higher in AMD patients as compared with control.[106] Further studies should be undertaken to validate proteomic biomarkers for AMD and develop applicable tests for clinical practice.

Finding genetic susceptible loci has provided a framework of genetic architecture of AMD as shown in Fig. 9.10,[86] in which the genetic effect of risk variants ranges from low to high and the frequency of risk variants ranges from very rare to common. Since these variants explain a large proportion of heritability, particularly for late-stage AMD, this has become a paradigm for the genetic examination of complex diseases. By using the genetic association with late-stage AMD, hypothetic pathogenesis pathways may be explored. It highlights inflammatory and lipid metabolic pathways, and also implicates angiogenetic, apoptotic, and extracellular-matrix remodeling processes.[86] Multiple studies, as described earlier, have revealed that the chromosome 1q31-32 and 10q26 regions harbor the major AMD loci. However, our ability to use the variants of these major AMD-related loci to predict the genetic risk of developing AMD for the general population is still inadequate. The current commercially available genetic testing could be useful in selected populations who have a strong family history of AMD or display early AMD phenotypes early in life. For individuals needing a realistic assessment of their future risk of developing AMD, the genetic testing needs to be done in isolation or in conjunction with other measurable external risk factors such as smoking, a modifiable external factor. The predictive value of such testing is also related to the potential interventions that may slow down AMD progression. In future AMD genetics, identification of genetic alleles that contribute more subtly to AMD susceptibility is imperative

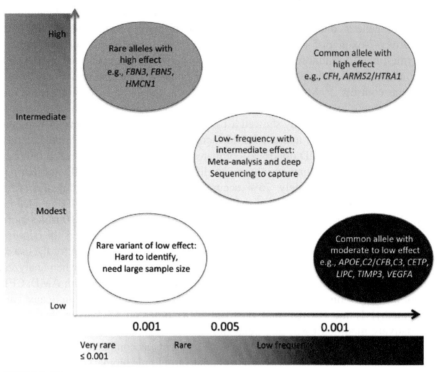

FIGURE 9.10

Genetic architecture of age-related macular degeneration.

Modified from Priya RR, Chew EY, Swaroop A. Genetic studies of age-related macular degeneration. Ophthalmology. 2012;119(12):2526–2536. https://doi.org/10.1016/j.ophtha.2012.06.042.

(Fig. 9.10). Furthermore, functional characterization of genes is also needed, especially when genetic studies cannot clearly pinpoint the susceptibility gene (e.g., *ARMS2* or *HTRA1* at 10q26). Such studies will reveal valuable insights into AMD pathogenesis and suggest new approaches for treatment (see Chapter 12).[86]

References

1. Chong JX, Buckingham KJ, Jhangiani SN, et al. The genetic basis of mendelian phenotypes: discoveries, challenges, and opportunities. *Am J Hum Genet.* 2015;97(2): 199–215. https://doi.org/10.1016/j.ajhg.2015.06.009.
2. Marques SCF, Oliveira CR, Pereira CMF, Outeiro TF. Epigenetics in neurodegeneration: a new layer of complexity. *Prog Neuro-Psychopharmacol Biol Psychiatry.* 2011; 35(2):348–355. https://doi.org/10.1016/j.pnpbp.2010.08.008.
3. Patel N, Adewoyin T, Chong NV. Age-related macular degeneration: a perspective on genetic studies. *Eye.* 2008;22(6):768–776. https://doi.org/10.1038/sj.eye.6702844.

4. Meyers SM, Greene T, Gutman FA. A twin study of age-related macular degeneration. *Am J Ophthalmol*. 1995;120(6):757−766. https://doi.org/10.1016/s0002-9394(14) 72729-1.

5. Hogg RE, Dimitrov PN, Dirani M, et al. Gene-environment interactions and aging visual function: a classical twin study. *Ophthalmology*. 2009;116(2):263−269. https://doi.org/ 10.1016/j.ophtha.2008.09.002.

6. International HapMap Consortium, Frazer KA, Ballinger DG, et al. A second generation human haplotype map of over 3.1 million SNPs. *Nature*. 2007;449(7164):851−861. https://doi.org/10.1038/nature06258.

7. Kruglyak L. The road to genome-wide association studies. *Nat Rev Genet*. 2008;9(4): 314−318. https://doi.org/10.1038/nrg2316.

8. Best S, Wou K, Vora N, Van der Veyver IB, Wapner R, Chitty LS. Promises, pitfalls and practicalities of prenatal whole exome sequencing. *Prenat Diagn*. 2018;38(1):10−19. https://doi.org/10.1002/pd.5102.

9. Tsao H, Florez JC. Introduction to genetic association studies. *J Invest Dermatol*. 2007; 127(10):2283−2287. https://doi.org/10.1038/sj.jid.5701054.

10. Sobrin L, Ripke S, Yu Y, et al. Heritability and genome-wide association study to assess genetic differences between advanced age-related macular degeneration subtypes. *Ophthalmology*. 2012;119(9):1874−1885. https://doi.org/10.1016/j.ophtha.2012.03. 014.

11. Zeggini E, Ioannidis JPA. Meta-analysis in genome-wide association studies. *Pharmacogenomics*. 2009;10(2):191−201. https://doi.org/10.2217/14622416.10.2.191.

12. Seddon JM. The US twin study of age-related macular degeneration: relative roles of genetic and environmental influences. *Arch Ophthalmol*. 2005;123(3):321. https:// doi.org/10.1001/archopht.123.3.321.

13. Hammond CJ, Webster AR, Snieder H, Bird AC, Gilbert CE, Spector TD. Genetic influence on early age-related maculopathy. *Ophthalmology*. 2002;109(4):730−736. https://doi.org/10.1016/S0161-6420(01)01049-1.

14. Barral S, Francis PJ, Schultz DW, et al. Expanded genome scan in extended families with age-related macular degeneration. *Invest Ophthalmol Vis Sci*. 2006;47(12): 5453−5459. https://doi.org/10.1167/iovs.06-0655.

15. Edwards AO, Ritter R, Abel KJ, Manning A, Panhuysen C, Farrer LA. Complement factor H polymorphism and age-related macular degeneration. *Science*. 2005;308(5720): 421−424. https://doi.org/10.1126/science.1110189.

16. Hageman GS, Anderson DH, Johnson LV, et al. A common haplotype in the complement regulatory gene factor H (HF1/CFH) predisposes individuals to age-related macular degeneration. *Proc Natl Acad Sci USA*. 2005;102(20):7227−7232. https://doi.org/ 10.1073/pnas.0501536102.

17. Haines JL, Hauser MA, Schmidt S, et al. Complement factor H variant increases the risk of age-related macular degeneration. *Science*. 2005;308(5720):419−421. https:// doi.org/10.1126/science.1110359.

18. Klein RJ, Zeiss C, Chew EY, et al. Complement factor H polymorphism in age-related macular degeneration. *Science*. 2005;308(5720):385−389. https://doi.org/10.1126/ science.1109557.

19. Jakobsdottir J, Conley YP, Weeks DE, Mah TS, Ferrell RE, Gorin MB. Susceptibility genes for age-related maculopathy on chromosome 10q26. *Am J Hum Genet*. 2005; 77(3):389−407. https://doi.org/10.1086/444437.

20. Spencer KL, Olson LM, Anderson BM, et al. C3 R102G polymorphism increases risk of age-related macular degeneration. *Hum Mol Genet*. 2008;17(12):1821−1824. https://doi.org/10.1093/hmg/ddn075.

21. Fritsche LG, Chen W, Schu M, et al. Seven new loci associated with age-related macular degeneration. *Nat Genet*. 2013;45(4):433−439. https://doi.org/10.1038/ng.2578, 439e1-2.

22. Hodge SE, Greenberg DA. How can we explain very low odds ratios in GWAS? I. Polygenic models. *Hum Hered*. 2016;81(4):173−180. https://doi.org/10.1159/000454804.

23. Holliday EG, Smith AV, Cornes BK, et al. Insights into the genetic architecture of early stage age-related macular degeneration: a genome-wide association study meta-analysis. *PLoS One*. 2013;8(1):e53830. https://doi.org/10.1371/journal.pone.0053830.

24. Grassmann F, Ach T, Brandl C, Heid IM, Weber BHF. What does genetics tell us about age-related macular degeneration? *Annu Rev Vis Sci*. 2015;1:73−96. https://doi.org/10.1146/annurev-vision-082114-035609.

25. American Academy of Ophthalmology. *2019-2020 BCSC: Basic and Clinical Science Course*. 2019.

26. Despriet DDG, Klaver CCW, Witteman JCM, et al. Complement factor H polymorphism, complement activators, and risk of age-related macular degeneration. *J Am Med Assoc*. 2006;296(3):301−309. https://doi.org/10.1001/jama.296.3.301.

27. Boon CJF, van de Kar NC, Klevering BJ, et al. The spectrum of phenotypes caused by variants in the CFH gene. *Mol Immunol*. 2009;46(8−9):1573−1594. https://doi.org/10.1016/j.molimm.2009.02.013.

28. Hughes AE, Orr N, Esfandiary H, Diaz-Torres M, Goodship T, Chakravarthy U. A common CFH haplotype, with deletion of CFHR1 and CFHR3, is associated with lower risk of age-related macular degeneration. *Nat Genet*. 2006;38(10):1173−1177. https://doi.org/10.1038/ng1890.

29. Maller J, George S, Purcell S, et al. Common variation in three genes, including a noncoding variant in CFH, strongly influences risk of age-related macular degeneration. *Nat Genet*. 2006;38(9):1055−1059. https://doi.org/10.1038/ng1873.

30. Harper AR, Nayee S, Topol EJ. Protective alleles and modifier variants in human health and disease. *Nat Rev Genet*. 2015;16(12):689−701. https://doi.org/10.1038/nrg4017.

31. McHarg S, Clark SJ, Day AJ, Bishop PN. Age-related macular degeneration and the role of the complement system. *Mol Immunol*. 2015;67(1):43−50. https://doi.org/10.1016/j.molimm.2015.02.032.

32. Zhang J, Li S, Hu S, Yu J, Xiang Y. Association between genetic variation of complement C3 and the susceptibility to advanced age-related macular degeneration: a meta-analysis. *BMC Ophthalmol*. 2018;18(1):274. https://doi.org/10.1186/s12886-018-0945-5.

33. Chen M, Muckersie E, Robertson M, Forrester JV, Xu H. Up-regulation of complement factor B in retinal pigment epithelial cells is accompanied by complement activation in the aged retina. *Exp Eye Res*. 2008;87(6):543−550. https://doi.org/10.1016/j.exer.2008.09.005.

34. Pickering MC, Cook HT, Warren J, et al. Uncontrolled C3 activation causes membranoproliferative glomerulonephritis in mice deficient in complement factor H. *Nat Genet*. 2002;31(4):424−428. https://doi.org/10.1038/ng912.

35. Chen M, Forrester JV, Xu H. Synthesis of complement factor H by retinal pigment epithelial cells is down-regulated by oxidized photoreceptor outer segments. *Exp Eye Res*. 2007;84(4):635−645. https://doi.org/10.1016/j.exer.2006.11.015.

36. Coffey PJ, Gias C, McDermott CJ, et al. Complement factor H deficiency in aged mice causes retinal abnormalities and visual dysfunction. *Proc Natl Acad Sci USA*. 2007; 104(42):16651−16656. https://doi.org/10.1073/pnas.0705079104.

37. Perkins SJ, Nan R, Li K, Khan S, Miller A. Complement factor H-ligand interactions: self-association, multivalency and dissociation constants. *Immunobiology*. 2012;217(2): 281−297. https://doi.org/10.1016/j.imbio.2011.10.003.

38. Gold B, Merriam JE, Zernant J, et al. Variation in factor B (BF) and complement component 2 (C2) genes is associated with age-related macular degeneration. *Nat Genet*. 2006;38(4):458−462. https://doi.org/10.1038/ng1750.

39. Bora NS, Kaliappan S, Jha P, et al. Complement activation via alternative pathway is critical in the development of laser-induced choroidal neovascularization: role of factor B and factor H. *J Immunol*. 2006;177(3):1872−1878. https://doi.org/10.4049/jimmunol.177.3.1872.

40. Nakata I, Yamashiro K, Yamada R, et al. Significance of C2/CFB variants in age-related macular degeneration and polypoidal choroidal vasculopathy in a Japanese population. *Invest Ophthalmol Vis Sci*. 2012;53(2):794−798. https://doi.org/10.1167/iovs.11-8468.

41. Dinu V, Miller PL, Zhao H. Evidence for association between multiple complement pathway genes and AMD. *Genet Epidemiol*. 2007;31(3):224−237. https://doi.org/10.1002/gepi.20204.

42. Tan PL, Garrett ME, Willer JR, et al. Systematic functional testing of rare variants: contributions of CFI to age-related macular degeneration. *Invest Ophthalmol Vis Sci*. 2017; 58(3):1570−1576. https://doi.org/10.1167/iovs.16-20867.

43. Anderson DH, Talaga KC, Rivest AJ, Barron E, Hageman GS, Johnson LV. Characterization of β amyloid assemblies in drusen: the deposits associated with aging and age-related macular degeneration. *Exp Eye Res*. 2004;78(2):243−256. https://doi.org/10.1016/j.exer.2003.10.011.

44. Akhtar-Schäfer I, Wang L, Krohne TU, Xu H, Langmann T. Modulation of three key innate immune pathways for the most common retinal degenerative diseases. *EMBO Mol Med*. 2018;10(10). https://doi.org/10.15252/emmm.201708259.

45. Lynch AM, Mandava N, Patnaik JL, et al. Systemic activation of the complement system in patients with advanced age-related macular degeneration. *Eur J Ophthalmol*. June 17, 2019. https://doi.org/10.1177/1120672119857896, 1120672119857896.

46. Calippe B, Augustin S, Beguier F, et al. Complement factor H inhibits CD47-mediated resolution of inflammation. *Immunity*. 2017;46(2):261−272. https://doi.org/10.1016/j.immuni.2017.01.006.

47. Loyet KM, DeForge LE, Katschke KJ, et al. Activation of the alternative complement pathway in vitreous is controlled by genetics in age-related macular degeneration. *Invest Ophthalmol Vis Sci*. 2012;53(10):6628. https://doi.org/10.1167/iovs.12-9587.

48. Despriet DDG, Bergen AAB, Merriam JE, et al. Comprehensive analysis of the candidate genes *CCL2* , *CCR2* , and *TLR4* in age-related macular degeneration. *Invest Ophthalmol Vis Sci*. 2008;49(1):364. https://doi.org/10.1167/iovs.07-0656.

49. Blasius AL, Beutler B. Intracellular toll-like receptors. *Immunity*. 2010;32(3):305−315. https://doi.org/10.1016/j.immuni.2010.03.012.

50. Kawai T, Akira S. Pathogen recognition with Toll-like receptors. *Curr Opin Immunol*. 2005;17(4):338−344. https://doi.org/10.1016/j.coi.2005.02.007.

51. McGettrick AF, O'Neill LAJ. Regulators of TLR4 signaling by endotoxins. *Subcell Biochem*. 2010;53:153−171. https://doi.org/10.1007/978-90-481-9078-2_7.

52. Lim K-H, Staudt LM. Toll-like receptor signaling. *Cold Spring Harb Perspect Biol.* 2013;5(1):a011247. https://doi.org/10.1101/cshperspect.a011247.

53. Iyengar SK, Song D, Klein BEK, et al. Dissection of genomewide-scan data in extended families reveals a major locus and oligogenic susceptibility for age-related macular degeneration. *Am J Hum Genet.* 2004;74(1):20−39. https://doi.org/10.1086/380912.

54. Güven M, Batar B, Mutlu T, et al. Toll-like receptors 2 and 4 polymorphisms in age-related macular degeneration. *Curr Eye Res.* 2016;41(6):856−861. https://doi.org/10.3109/02713683.2015.1067326.

55. Yang Z, Stratton C, Francis PJ, et al. Toll-like receptor 3 and geographic atrophy in age-related macular degeneration. *N Engl J Med.* 2008;359(14):1456−1463. https://doi.org/10.1056/NEJMoa0802437.

56. Sharma NK, Sharma K, Gupta A, et al. Does toll-like receptor-3 (TLR-3) have any role in Indian AMD phenotype? *Mol Cell Biochem.* 2014;393(1−2):1−8. https://doi.org/10.1007/s11010-014-2040-4.

57. Edwards AO, Chen D, Fridley BL, et al. Toll-like receptor polymorphisms and age-related macular degeneration. *Invest Ophthalmol Vis Sci.* 2008;49(4):1652−1659. https://doi.org/10.1167/iovs.07-1378.

58. Hageman GS, Luthert PJ, Victor Chong NH, Johnson LV, Anderson DH, Mullins RF. An integrated hypothesis that considers drusen as biomarkers of immune-mediated processes at the RPE-Bruch's membrane interface in aging and age-related macular degeneration. *Prog Retin Eye Res.* 2001;20(6):705−732. https://doi.org/10.1016/s1350-9462(01)00010-6.

59. Saddala MS, Lennikov A, Mukwaya A, Fan L, Hu Z, Huang H. Transcriptome-wide analysis of differentially expressed chemokine receptors, SNPs, and SSRs in the age-related macular degeneration. *Hum Genom.* 2019;13(1):15. https://doi.org/10.1186/s40246-019-0199-1.

60. Goverdhan SV, Ennis S, Hannan SR, et al. Interleukin-8 promoter polymorphism -251A/T is a risk factor for age-related macular degeneration. *Br J Ophthalmol.* 2008;92(4):537−540. https://doi.org/10.1136/bjo.2007.123190.

61. Narayanan R, Butani V, Boyer DS, et al. Complement factor H polymorphism in age-related macular degeneration. *Ophthalmology.* 2007;114(7):1327−1331. https://doi.org/10.1016/j.ophtha.2006.10.035.

62. Kijlstra A, Tian Y, Kelly ER, Berendschot TTJM. Lutein: more than just a filter for blue light. *Prog Retin Eye Res.* 2012;31(4):303−315. https://doi.org/10.1016/j.preteyeres.2012.03.002.

63. Cao S, Ko A, Partanen M, et al. Relationship between systemic cytokines and complement factor H Y402H polymorphism in patients with dry age-related macular degeneration. *Am J Ophthalmol.* 2013;156(6):1176−1183. https://doi.org/10.1016/j.ajo.2013.08.003.

64. Goverdhan SV, Howell MW, Mullins RF, et al. Association of HLA class I and class II polymorphisms with age-related macular degeneration. *Invest Ophthalmol Vis Sci.* 2005;46(5):1726. https://doi.org/10.1167/iovs.04-0928.

65. Rivera A, Fisher SA, Fritsche LG, et al. Hypothetical LOC387715 is a second major susceptibility gene for age-related macular degeneration, contributing independently of complement factor H to disease risk. *Hum Mol Genet.* 2005;14(21):3227−3236. https://doi.org/10.1093/hmg/ddi353.

66. Wang G. Chromosome 10q26 locus and age-related macular degeneration: a progress update. *Exp Eye Res.* 2014;119:1−7. https://doi.org/10.1016/j.exer.2013.11.009.

67. Kanda A, Chen W, Othman M, et al. A variant of mitochondrial protein LOC387715/ ARMS2, not HTRA1, is strongly associated with age-related macular degeneration. *Proc Natl Acad Sci USA.* 2007;104(41):16227−16232. https://doi.org/10.1073/ pnas.0703933104.

68. Yang Z, Camp NJ, Sun H, et al. A variant of the HTRA1 gene increases susceptibility to age-related macular degeneration. *Science.* 2006;314(5801):992−993. https://doi.org/ 10.1126/science.1133811.

69. Dewan A, Liu M, Hartman S, et al. HTRA1 promoter polymorphism in wet age-related macular degeneration. *Science.* 2006;314(5801):989−992. https://doi.org/10.1126/ science.1133807.

70. Tocharus J, Tsuchiya A, Kajikawa M, Ueta Y, Oka C, Kawaichi M. Developmentally regulated expression of mouse HtrA3 and its role as an inhibitor of TGF-beta signaling. *Dev Growth Differ.* 2004;46(3):257−274. https://doi.org/10.1111/j.1440- 169X.2004.00743.x.

71. Sohn EH, Wang K, Thompson S, et al. Comparison of drusen and modifying genes in autosomal dominant radial drusen and age-related macular degeneration. *Retina.* 2015; 35(1):48−57. https://doi.org/10.1097/IAE.0000000000000263.

72. Grau S, Baldi A, Bussani R, et al. Implications of the serine protease HtrA1 in amyloid precursor protein processing. *Proc Natl Acad Sci USA.* 2005;102(17):6021−6026. https://doi.org/10.1073/pnas.0501823102.

73. Liao S-M, Zheng W, Zhu J, et al. Specific correlation between the major chromosome 10q26 haplotype conferring risk for age-related macular degeneration and the expression of HTRA1. *Mol Vis.* 2017;23:318−333.

74. Traboulsi EI, ed. *Genetic Diseases of the Eye.* 2nd ed. Oxford University Press; 2012.

75. Blasiak J, Glowacki S, Kauppinen A, Kaarniranta K. Mitochondrial and nuclear DNA damage and repair in age-related macular degeneration. *Int J Mol Sci.* 2013;14(2): 2996−3010. https://doi.org/10.3390/ijms14022996.

76. Feher J, Kovacs I, Artico M, Cavallotti C, Papale A, Balacco Gabrieli C. Mitochondrial alterations of retinal pigment epithelium in age-related macular degeneration. *Neurobiol Aging.* 2006;27(7):983−993. https://doi.org/10.1016/j.neurobiolaging.2005.05. 012.

77. Jones MM, Manwaring N, Wang JJ, Rochtchina E, Mitchell P, Sue CM. Mitochondrial DNA haplogroups and age-related maculopathy. *Arch Ophthalmol.* 2007;125(9): 1235−1240. https://doi.org/10.1001/archopht.125.9.1235.

78. Udar N, Atilano SR, Memarzadeh M, et al. Mitochondrial DNA haplogroups associated with age-related macular degeneration. *Invest Ophthalmol Vis Sci.* 2009;50(6): 2966−2974. https://doi.org/10.1167/iovs.08-2646.

79. Liu MM, Chan C-C, Tuo J. Genetic mechanisms and age-related macular degeneration: common variants, rare variants, copy number variations, epigenetics, and mitochondrial genetics. *Hum Genom.* 2012;6:13. https://doi.org/10.1186/1479-7364-6-13.

80. Tilleul J, Richard F, Puche N, et al. Genetic association study of mitochondrial polymorphisms in neovascular age-related macular degeneration. *Mol Vis.* 2013;19:1132−1140.

81. Myers CE, Klein BEK, Gangnon R, Sivakumaran TA, Iyengar SK, Klein R. Cigarette smoking and the natural history of age-related macular degeneration: the Beaver Dam Eye Study. *Ophthalmology.* 2014;121(10):1949−1955. https://doi.org/10.1016/ j.ophtha.2014.04.040.

82. Francis PJ, George S, Schultz DW, et al. The *LOC387715* gene, smoking, body mass index, environmental associations with advanced age-related macular degeneration. *Hum Hered.* 2007;63(3−4):212−218. https://doi.org/10.1159/000100046.

83. Espinosa-Heidmann DG, Suner IJ, Catanuto P, Hernandez EP, Marin-Castano ME, Cousins SW. Cigarette smoke−related oxidants and the development of sub-RPE deposits in an experimental animal model of dry AMD. *Invest Ophthalmol Vis Sci.* 2006;47(2):729. https://doi.org/10.1167/iovs.05-0719.

84. Seddon JM, George S, Rosner B, Klein ML. CFH gene variant, Y402H, and smoking, body mass index, environmental associations with advanced age-related macular degeneration. *Hum Hered.* 2006;61(3):157−165. https://doi.org/10.1159/000094141.

85. Lechanteur YTE, van de Camp PL, Smailhodzic D, et al. Association of smoking and CFH and ARMS2 risk variants with younger age at onset of neovascular age-related macular degeneration. *JAMA Ophthalmol.* 2015;133(5):533−541. https://doi.org/10.1001/jamaophthalmol.2015.18.

86. Priya RR, Chew EY, Swaroop A. Genetic studies of age-related macular degeneration. *Ophthalmology.* 2012;119(12):2526−2536. https://doi.org/10.1016/j.ophtha.2012.06.042.

87. Schmidt S, Hauser MA, Scott WK, et al. Cigarette smoking strongly modifies the association of LOC387715 and age-related macular degeneration. *Am J Hum Genet.* 2006;78(5):852−864. https://doi.org/10.1086/503822.

88. Tuo J, Ross RJ, Reed GF, et al. The HtrA1 promoter polymorphism, smoking, and age-related macular degeneration in multiple case-control samples. *Ophthalmology.* 2008;115(11):1891−1898. https://doi.org/10.1016/j.ophtha.2008.05.021.

89. DeAngelis MM, Lane AM, Shah CP, Ott J, Dryja TP, Miller JW. Extremely discordant sib-pair study design to determine risk factors for neovascular age-related macular degeneration. *Arch Ophthalmol.* 2004;122(4):575−580. https://doi.org/10.1001/archopht.122.4.575.

90. Zhou J, Jang YP, Kim SR, Sparrow JR. Complement activation by photooxidation products of A2E, a lipofuscin constituent of the retinal pigment epithelium. *Proc Natl Acad Sci USA.* 2006;103(44):16182−16187. https://doi.org/10.1073/pnas.0604255103.

91. Bai B, Wang X, Li Y, et al. Deep multilayer brain proteomics identifies molecular networks in Alzheimer's disease progression. *Neuron.* 2020;105(6):975−991. https://doi.org/10.1016/j.neuron.2019.12.015. e7.

92. Lin MK, Yang J, Hsu CW, et al. HTRA1, an age-related macular degeneration protease, processes extracellular matrix proteins EFEMP1 and TSP1. *Aging Cell.* 2018;17(4):e12710. https://doi.org/10.1111/acel.12710.

93. Hoppe G, Marmorstein AD, Pennock EA, Hoff HF. Oxidized low density lipoprotein-induced inhibition of processing of photoreceptor outer segments by RPE. *Invest Ophthalmol Vis Sci.* 2001;42(11):2714−2720.

94. Hoppe G, O'Neil J, Hoff HF, Sears J. Products of lipid peroxidation induce missorting of the principal lysosomal protease in retinal pigment epithelium. *Biochim Biophys Acta - Mol Basis Dis.* 2004;1689(1):33−41. https://doi.org/10.1016/j.bbadis.2004.01.004.

95. Rodriguez IR, Alam S, Lee JW. Cytotoxicity of oxidized low-density lipoprotein in cultured RPE cells is dependent on the formation of 7-ketocholesterol. *Invest Ophthalmol Vis Sci.* 2004;45(8):2830. https://doi.org/10.1167/iovs.04-0075.

96. Bojanowski CM, Shen D, Chew EY, et al. An apolipoprotein E variant may protect against age-related macular degeneration through cytokine regulation. *Environ Mol Mutagen.* 2006;47(8):594−602. https://doi.org/10.1002/em.20233.

97. Ishida BY. High density lipoprotein mediated lipid efflux from retinal pigment epithelial cells in culture. *Br J Ophthalmol.* 2006;90(5):616−620. https://doi.org/10.1136/bjo.2005.085076.

98. Dunaief JL. Iron induced oxidative damage as a potential factor in age-related macular degeneration: the cogan lecture. *Invest Ophthalmol Vis Sci.* 2006;47(11):4660. https://doi.org/10.1167/iovs.06-0568.

99. Li Y, Song D, Song Y, et al. Iron-induced local complement component 3 (C3) up-regulation via non-canonical transforming growth factor (TGF)-β signaling in the retinal pigment epithelium. *J Biol Chem.* 2015;290(19):11918−11934. https://doi.org/10.1074/jbc.M115.645903.

100. Klein ML, Francis PJ, Rosner B, et al. CFH and LOC387715/ARMS2 genotypes and treatment with antioxidants and zinc for age-related macular degeneration. *Ophthalmology.* 2008;115(6):1019−1025. https://doi.org/10.1016/j.ophtha.2008.01.036.

101. Abedi F, Wickremasinghe S, Richardson AJ, et al. Variants in the VEGFA gene and treatment outcome after anti-VEGF treatment for neovascular age-related macular degeneration. *Ophthalmology.* 2013;120(1):115−121. https://doi.org/10.1016/j.ophtha.2012.10.006.

102. Fauser S, Lambrou GN. Genetic predictive biomarkers of anti-VEGF treatment response in patients with neovascular age-related macular degeneration. *Surv Ophthalmol.* 2015;60(2):138−152. https://doi.org/10.1016/j.survophthal.2014.11.002.

103. Hagstrom SA, Ying G, Pauer GJT, et al. VEGFA and VEGFR2 gene polymorphisms and response to anti-vascular endothelial growth factor therapy: comparison of age-related macular degeneration treatments trials (CATT). *JAMA Ophthalmol.* 2014;132(5):521−527. https://doi.org/10.1001/jamaophthalmol.2014.109.

104. Lorés-Motta L, Riaz M, Grunin M, et al. Association of genetic variants with response to anti−vascular endothelial growth factor therapy in age-related macular degeneration. *JAMA Ophthalmol.* 2018;136(8):875. https://doi.org/10.1001/jamaophthalmol.2018.2019.

105. Gu J, Pauer GJT, Yue X, et al. Assessing susceptibility to age-related macular degeneration with proteomic and genomic biomarkers. *Mol Cell Proteomics.* 2009;8(6):1338−1349. https://doi.org/10.1074/mcp.M800453-MCP200.

106. Lambert NG, ElShelmani H, Singh MK, et al. Risk factors and biomarkers of age-related macular degeneration. *Prog Retin Eye Res.* 2016;54:64−102. https://doi.org/10.1016/j.preteyeres.2016.04.003.

107. Ardeljan D, Tuo J, Chan C-C. Carboxyethylpyrrole plasma biomarkers in age-related macular degeneration. *Drugs Future.* 2011;36(9):712−718. https://doi.org/10.1358/dof.2011.036.09.1678338.

108. Crabb JW, Miyagi M, Gu X, et al. Drusen proteome analysis: an approach to the etiology of age-related macular degeneration. *Proc Natl Acad Sci USA.* 2002;99(23):14682−14687. https://doi.org/10.1073/pnas.222551899.

109. Ishibashi T, Murata T, Hangai M, et al. Advanced glycation end products in age-related macular degeneration. *Arch Ophthalmol.* 1998;116(12):1629−1632. https://doi.org/10.1001/archopht.116.12.1629.

Management of age-related macular degeneration

10

Age-related macular degeneration (AMD) is a multifactorial disorder with heterogeneous clinical features. Based on clinical and multimodal imaging studies, AMD has been classified with a great extent of consensus into early-stage, that is, from medium- to large-sized drusen and retinal pigmentary abnormalities and late-stage, that is, atrophic and neovascular. At different stages, multiple cell types of retina and choroid, as well as immune cells, interact and participate in pathophysiological events at the macular region. In the macular milieu, dysregulated events in the oxidative stress/ROS generation, bioenergetic homeostasis, complement, inflammation, angiogenesis, and extracellular matrix metabolism contribute to AMD pathogenesis over the disease course. To date, increasing genetic susceptibility loci have been identified, of which the most important ones are in the *CFH* and *ARMS2* genes. The interplay between genetic factors and environmental factors has been gradually elucidated through new findings and the advent of new technologies. Based on the mechanistic understanding, slowing down the dry AMD progression by dietary antioxidants and zinc and preventing vision loss in patients with wet AMD by intravitreal anti-VEGF therapy have been achieved. However, it must be admitted that there is no cure for AMD yet. In this chapter, we are introducing the proven therapies for AMD patients at different stages and discussing some experimental therapies used in the real world clinical practice.

Management of dry AMD
Education on modifiable risk factors

There is no effective treatment for dry AMD to date. Therefore, the management for patients with dry AMD has focused on the prevention of vision loss and maintenance of the remaining visual functions. Smoking and diet habits are considered as important modifiable risk factors for AMD. Evidences exist that patients smoking longer than 40 years are likely to develop AMD two to four times more than nonsmokers of the same age groups.[1] Therefore, for this influential risk factor, patients should be educated at each visit to refrain from smoking to preventing further visual loss. A high intake of certain fats, such as saturated fats, transfats, and omega-6 fatty acids, has been associated with a twofold increase in the prevalence of intermediate AMD, whereas monounsaturated fats were potentially protective.[2] It has been recognized that modifiable factors, such as cigarette smoking and high-fat diet, can convert oxidative stress into a pathological role in AMD development. The negative impact of oxidative stress-related impaired cytoprotective functions of retinal pigment epithelium (RPE) may be the mechanistic bases of these detrimental risk factors.[3]

Self-monitoring by Amsler grid

An Amsler grid should be provided to all AMD patients for self-monitoring purposes at home on a regular basis. Patients should be instructed to seek physicians' advice urgently if any changes on Amsler grid test are noticed such as metamorphopsia and scotoma.

Dietary antioxidants and zinc

Age-related eye disease study (AREDS) and other previous epidemiologic studies pointed out a possible role for antioxidants in reducing the risk of cancer, cardiovascular disease, and eye disease.[4] In addition, a small, randomized clinical trial suggested that pharmacologic doses of zinc provide some protection against vision loss from AMD.[4] In Chapters 7 and 8 of this book, the possible pathogenic role of oxidative stress and ROS generation in AMD development has been discussed. The AREDS now called AREDS1 and the follow-up AREDS2 using high-dose antioxidant vitamins and minerals in dry AMD patients on a regular basis were applied. The results showed that both AREDS1 and AREDS2 formulations can decrease the risk of the development of advanced AMD in patients with dry AMD. Therefore, AREDS2 recommended that the individuals (>55 years old), who have one or more following clinical features, should take the AREDS2 supplements. The indications of AREDS2 are as follows: (1) extensive intermediate drusen (>63−125 μm); (2) at least one large druse (>125 μm); (3) geographic atrophy in one or both eyes; and (4) late stage of AMD in one eye. The formulation used in AREDS1 consisted of vitamin C, vitamin B, the β-carotene form of vitamin A, and 80 mg daily of zinc with copper to prevent zinc-induced copper deficiency. However, a high dose of zinc is potentially associated with genitourinary tract problems.[5] Previous data also showed that 25 mg of zinc may be the maximal level that is absorbed.[6] Additionally, β-carotene could increase the incidence of lung cancer in current and former smokers. Therefore, AREDS2 changed β-carotene and lowered zinc dose (from 80 to 25 mg daily) and tested whether alternative supplementations could enhance the outcome. Based on AREDS2, the carotenoid lutein and zeaxanthin are a safe alternative to β-carotene for peoples who had a smoking history. Comparing AREDS1 and AREDS2 formulations, the result of slowing down AMD progression by AREDS2 is probably superior. The result showed an 18% reduction in risk of advanced AMD above that conferred by the AREDS1 regimen. AREDS2 data demonstrated that lutein and zeaxanthin supplements added to the original AREDS1 formulation were associated with a statistically significant but modestly reduced (26%) risk of AMD.[7] AREDS2 also showed that omega-3 fatty acids added to the formulation did not enhance outcome. The study of AREDS2 formulation with reduced potential side effects of a high dose of zinc showed a statistically significant benefit in AMD progression.

Low vision aids for late-stage AMD

Vision loss due to late stages of AMD can have profound effects on patients' quality of life and psychological well-being. Low-vision rehabilitation is an effective option for coping with AMD-related vision loss when medical or surgical treatments are unsuccessful or are contraindicated. Typical rehabilitative interventions include assessment of residual physical functions including remaining functional vision. Particularly, identification of preferred retinal loci and training in their active use are crucial. Then, the professional providers should prescribe the devices and train patients to use the low-vision aids. It is important to provide training and educational programs (orientation and mobility) and to assist activities of daily living, driving, and lighting adjustments. The success of the low vision aids also depends on counseling or social and financial support.[8]

The implantable miniature telescope

The implantable miniature telescope (IMT) is an optical device that works in conjunction with refractive elements to improve central vision in individuals who have lost bilateral central vision due to both types of end-stage AMD. IMT was approved by FDA in 2010. It is the only implantable telescope commercially available for treatment of end-stage AMD. The IMT is 4.4 mm long and 3.6 mm in diameter. It weighs 115 mg in air and 60 mg in aqueous humor. There are two IMT models, the WA (wide-angle) 2.2X and the WA 3.0X, which are designed to be compatible as routine posterior intraocular lens.[9] The IMT is surgically placed in the posterior chamber after cataract extraction. The FDA determined seven indications of IMT: (1) age 65 years or older with stable, moderate to profound central vision impairment due to end-stage AMD; (2) fovea involved geographic atrophy or disciform scar; (3) unilateral cataract, but no previous cataract surgery; (4) agreement to have training with an external telescope before surgery; (5) improve at least five letters on ETDRS chart with an external telescope; (6) adequate peripheral vision in the fellow eye; (7) willingness to participate in a postoperative visual training program.[9] The studies about the effectiveness and safety of IMT are still cumulating data. Limited cohort studies showed that IMT improves the quality of life and at the same time is cost-effective by conventional standards.[10]

Macular translocation surgery for late-stage AMD

When RPE underlying the fovea is severely damaged in end-stage AMD, it is impossible for any medical treatments to restore the central vision. Surgical treatments aiming translocation of the fovea to an area with relatively healthy RPE become sensible.[11] Macular translocation is performed for this purpose. Two surgical techniques of macular translocation have been used: full macular translocation with 360-degree retinotomy at the periphery, and limited macular translocation (LMT) with the less extensive movement of the retina.[11] Each has advantages and disadvantages in terms of its effectiveness and complications. A long-term follow-up of a cohort study of LMT showed that LMT improves the central vision significantly at 1 year, and the improvement lasted for at least 5 years.[11] These results indicated that the impaired function of the sensory retina at the fovea can recover on the new RPE after the displacement for at least 5 years. Notably, to maintain functional RPE underneath the fovea, the transplantation of RPE cells and/or stem cells might be combined with macular translocation surgery. Overall, because macular translocation surgery has limited success to date, this type of surgery alone is seldom performed.

Visual prostheses for blindness including late-stage AMD

Visual prostheses (VP) are devices using electronic circuitry and electrical impulses to generate vision-compatible stimuli and thus restore lost visual function. Most VP to date focus on how to stimulate different parts of the visual pathway. Currently, the majority of VP has targeted retina. The other nonretinal targets such as lateral geniculate nucleus and visual cortex remain more experimental.[12] In 2013, FDA approved the Second Sight's Argus II Retinal Prosthesis System (Argus II) for patients with rare retinal dystrophy initially. Nowadays, the indications of Argus II have extended to end-stage AMD. The Argus II consists of a small video camera, a transmitter mounted on a pair of eyeglasses, a video processing unit, and a 60-electrode implanted retinal prosthesis.[13] The electrodes send out the electrical impulses to the epi-retina, from which the signals transmit to the optic nerve directly, bypassing the degenerated photoreceptors of the retina. In addition to the Argus II, currently, around two dozen clinical trials for visual prostheses have registered in US National Library of Medicine. The approaches of VP include epiretinal, subretinal, choroidal, and cortical. When each approach was reported with advantages and disadvantages, the epiretinal approach has made substantial progress.[12]

Management of neovascular AMD
VEGF-VEGFR signaling pathway

Neovascular AMD (nAMD) is characterized by the presence of choroidal neovascularization (CNV), a form of pathologic angiogenesis. Vascular endothelial growth factor (VEGF) is a major contributor to CNV formation. The VEGF family comprises seven members including commonly known VEGF-A, VEGF-B, VEGF-C, VEGF-D, and placental growth factor (PlGF) (Fig. 10.1).[14,15] VEGF-A is the best-characterized family member as the most potent stimulator of angiogenic processes (Fig. 10.1).[15] *VEGF-A* gene is alternatively spliced to form multiple isoforms. To date, 16 distinct VEGF-A isoforms have been identified. Most commonly six

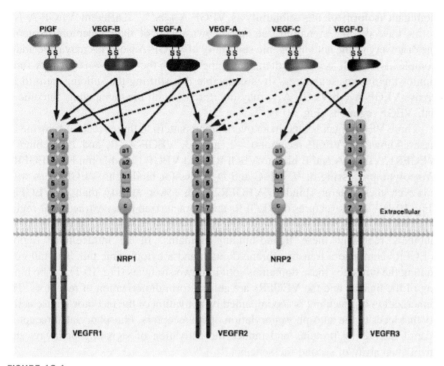

FIGURE 10.1

VEGFR ligands and coreceptors: six different ligands (PlGF, VEGF-B, VEGF-A, VEGF-Axxxb, VEGF-C, and VEGF-D) bind in a partially overlapping manner to VEGFR1–3. The coreceptors NRP1 and NRP2 modulate signal transduction of VEGFRs. PlGF and VEGF-B specifically bind to VEGFR1 and convey their biological function through this receptor. VEGF-A binds to VEGFR1 and VEGFR2. The main biological functions of VEGF-A are transmitted by VEGFR2, while VEGFR1 is thought to serve as a decoy receptor for VEGF-A and thereby limits VEGF-A/VEGFR2 signaling. The antiangiogenic VEGF-Axxxb isoforms bind to VEGFR2 and presumably also VEGFR1. VEGF-C and VEGF-D bind to VEGFR3 that relays their main biological functions. In a proteolytically processed form, VEGF-C and VEGF-D also bind to VEGFR2, albeit with lower affinity. *NRP1*, Neuropilin 1; *NRP2*, Neuropilin 2.

Modified from Álvarez-Aznar A, Muhl L, Gaengel K. VEGF receptor tyrosine kinases: Key Regulators of vascular function. Curr Top Dev Biol. *2017;123:433—482. https://doi.org/10.1016/bs.ctdb.2016.10.001.*

isoforms of VAGF-A are formed as $VEGF_{111}$, $VEGF_{121}$, $VEGF_{145}$, $VEGF_{165}$, $VEGF_{181}$, and $VEGF_{206}$, with different numbers denoting the number of amino acids.[16] A well-studied example of this regulated splicing is that of exon 8 of the *VEGF-A* gene. Within exon 8 of *VEGF-A*, the regulated splice produces proangiogenic family of VEGF-A$_{xxx}$ isoforms (such as VEGF-A$_{165}$, VEGF-A$_{121}$, VEGF-A$_{181}$). Bates et al. characterized a novel splice site in exon 8, which resulted in a new subfamily of antiangiogenic isoforms, termed VEGF-A$_{xxx}$b. The most dominant isoform of this subfamily is VEGF-A$_{165}$b.[17,18] Different VEGF-A isoforms have distinct signaling outcomes downstream of their receptors. Notably, the discovery of the antiangiogenic subfamily of VEGF-A isoforms may have added complexity as well as a novel therapeutic approach to the VEGF-A regulatory function of the microvasculature.[19] It is deducible that shifting the splicing ratio to increase VEGF-A$_{xxx}$b/VEGF-A$_{xxx}$ may interference with the therapeutic outcome of anti-VEGF regimens (Fig. 10.1).[20]

These VEGF ligands bind in an overlapping pattern to three receptor tyrosine kinases, known as VEGF receptor-1, -2, and -3. VEGF-A, B, and PlGF bind to VEGFR1, VEGF-A and E bind to VEGFR2, and VEGF-C and D bind to VEGFR3. Proteolytic processing of VEGF-C and D allows for binding to VEGFR2 as well; however, these factors bind to VEGFR2 with lower affinity than to VEGFR3 (Fig. 10.1).[14] The structures of VEGFRs are characterized by an extracellular region that contains seven immunoglobulin-like ligand-binding domains. In Fig. 10.1, the numbers represent these ligand-binding domains. In an intracellular region, VEGFRs comprise a transmembrane domain and a cytoplasmic tail. The tail containing the tyrosine kinase domain is split into two stretches (Fig. 10.1).[21] The binding of the ligands and the VEGFRs are able to form dimerization of receptors. The dimerization of receptors is accompanied by activation of the receptor-kinase activity that leads to the auto-phosphorylation of the receptors. Phosphorylated receptors recruit interacting proteins and induce the activation of signaling pathways that involve an array of second messengers.

Anti-VEGF agents and tyrosine kinase inhibitors

Anti-VEGF agents block their interaction with receptors on the endothelial cells and so retard or arrest vessel growth. Anti-VEGF regimens are the mainstay of treatment for CNV, which dramatically improve the visual prognosis. Intravitreal injection is the standard method of administration. Anti-VEGF therapy for nAMD and other ocular neovascular diseases is adopted from the research achievement from oncologists. FDA approved the first anti-angiogenic drug, bevacizumab (Avastin), a humanized monoclonal antibody anti-VEGF-A in 2004. Bevacizumab is originally for the treatment of metastatic colorectal cancer, in combination with chemotherapy. The importance of VEGF-A in neovascular AMD was validated by the finding that VEGF-A is localized in the surgically obtained choroidal neovascular membranes of patients with nAMD.[22] These observations and the studies on animal models demonstrated that the VEGF-A blockade is effective to reduce ocular neovascularization. Therefore, the ocular neovascular diseases including nAMD have been defined as VEGF-A-driven disorders.[23] The first anti-VEGF drug for the treatment of nAMD, Pegaptanib (Macugen) was approved by FDA in 2004. Macugen, a PEGylated 28-base ribonucleic aptamer, binds the heparin-binding domain of VEGF-A$_{165}$ isoform. Macugen prevents VEGF-A$_{165}$ activity and slows down the progression of vision loss, but cannot improve visual acuity.[24] Because of the limited effectiveness of Macugen in nAMD patients, a pioneer work of bevacizumab by the off-label intravitreal use was explored by Rosenfeld et al. in 2005. Intravitreal bevacizumab (1 mg) led to dramatically improved optical coherence tomography (OCT) morphology and visual function in a patient with nAMD.[25] In 2006, a recombinant, humanized antibody fragment (Fab) anti-VEGF-A derived from bevacizumab known as ranibizumab (Lucentis) was approved by FDA for nAMD therapy (Fig. 10.2).[26] Compared to bevacizumab, the reduction in molecular size of ranibizumab was theoretically believed to facilitate the penetration of the drugs into the retina. In addition, the smaller ranibizumab molecules are cleared rapidly with a shorter systemic half-life than that of bevacizumab (2.2 h vs. ~21days), implying less systemic side effects. In a multicenter, 2-year, double-blind, sham-controlled study, monthly intravitreal injections of ranibizumab prevented the loss of visual acuity in ~95% of patients. This regimen improved visual acuity in 25%−33% of patients during a 24-month period.[27] However, due to the enormous difference in cost between these two intravitreal anti-VEGF agents, ophthalmologists chose off-label use of bevacizumab instead of ranibizumab to treat nAMD patients worldwide (Fig. 10.2).[26] Therefore, comparison of age-related macular degeneration treatment trials (CATT), a multicenter, randomized clinical trial, was conducted to compare the relative safety and efficacy of ranibizumab with bevacizumab.[28,29] The 1-year CATT data and followed-up for 2 years have been analyzed.[29] Overall, the studies showed that bevacizumab is noninferior to ranibizumab therapy in monthly or as-needed injection regimens over 2 years. Mean letters gained from baseline are 8.8 letters in the ranibizumab-monthly group, 7.8 letters in the bevacizumab-monthly group, 6.7 letters in the ranibizumab as-needed group, and 5.0 letters in the bevacizumab as needed group. Systemic adverse events are significantly greater in the bevacizumab than in the ranibizumab group, but death and arteriothrombotic events are not statistically different between the two drugs. During the second year, participants in the monthly arms were rerandomized to either continue on monthly treatment or switch to pro re nata (PRN) therapy. Participants were released from the study protocol after year 2 and were treated with anti-VEGF therapy (aflibercept, ranibizumab, or bevacizumab) at dosing intervals as determined by the treating physician's best judgment. Associations between visual acuity and morphologic features previously identified in the two groups through year 1 are maintained or strengthened at year 5. At 5 years, 50% of eyes maintain 20/40 or better visual acuity in both CATT groups.[30] In 2011, aflibercept (Eylea) received FDA approval also for the treatment of nAMD and other retinal vascular diseases (Fig. 10.2).[26] Two parallel clinical trials for AMD (VIEW1 and VIEW2),[31] comparing efficacy and safety of aflibercept and ranibizumab, showed that intravitreal injection of aflibercept every 2 months after three consecutive monthly injections is equivalent in efficacy and safety to monthly ranibizumab. Thus, aflibercept offers the advantage to decrease the potential risks associated with intravitreal injections.[32]

For various approaches of angiogenesis inhibition (Fig. 10.2), tyrosine kinase inhibitors can inhibit angiogenesis by directly or indirectly regulating downstream signaling pathways of endothelial cell proliferation, migration, and new vessel

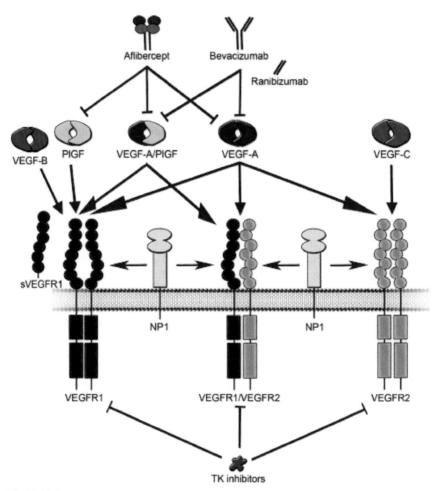

FIGURE 10.2

Anti-VEGF and tyrosine kinase inhibitors for regulation of proangiogenic growth factors and receptors of VEGF family. Anti-VEGF agents are exemplified by bevacizumab, ranibizumab, and aflibercept. They interact with VEGF-A, B, C, PIGF, and VEGF-A/PIGF heterodimer to block VEGFRs including soluble VEGFR1 (sVEGFR1) and their coreceptors such as Neuropilin-1 (NP1 or known NRP1 in Fig. 10.1). Tyrosine kinase (TK) inhibitors suppress phosphorylation of TK.

Modified from Tarallo V, De Falco S. The vascular endothelial growth factors and receptors family: Up to now the only target for anti-angiogenesis therapy. Int J Biochem Cell Biol. *2015;64:185–189. https://doi.org/10.1016/ j.biocel.2015.04.008.*

formation in oncology practice. Tyrosine kinase (TK) is an enzyme that transfers a phosphate group to the amino acid tyrosine on proteins. It can alter the protein's structure and function and thereby facilitate signal transduction between macromolecules. In the eye, both VEGF and platelet-derived growth factor bind to cell surface receptors that rely on a tyrosine kinase to propagate signal transduction. However, the tyrosine kinase inhibitors applied in the treatment of ocular vascular diseases are mostly in the experimental states due to adverse drug events and blood-retina barrier.[33] Some studies on tyrosine kinase inhibitors for nAMD are discussed in Chapter 11.

A bottleneck of nAMD treatment is the requirement of long-term, repeated intravitreal anti-VEGF injections. This regimen has built up the tremendous burden on patients and providers. Therefore, developing anti-VEGF drugs with longer durability and similar or superior efficacy became imperative. Brolucizumab (Beovu), that is, a humanized, single-chain variable fragment (scFv) showed effective inhibition of VEGF-A in the retina at every 12-week interval in clinical studies. Therefore, brolucizumab was approved by FDA in 2019 based on HAWK and HARRIER phase 3 trials.[34] Structurally and pharmacologically, brolucizumab has the smallest molecular weight (26 kDa) among the current anti-VEGF agents and a high affinity to VEGF-A$_{165}$ (Table 10.1), it thus has better molar dosing, better tissue penetration,

Table 10.1 Structural and pharmacokinetic characteristics of the four available anti-VEGF agents.

	Ranibizumab	Bevacizumab	Aflibercept	Brolucizumab
Structure	Recombinant monoclonal antibody fragment (Fab)	Recombinant monoclonal antibody (Mab)	Fusion protein	Single-chain variable fragment (scFv)
Molecular weight (kDa)	48	149	115	26
K$_D$ for VEGF$_{165}$ (pM)	46–192	58–1100	0.5	28.4
Binding targets	VEGF-A	VEGF-A	VEGF-A VEGF-B PlGF	VEGF$_{165, 110, 121}$
Dose (volume)	0.5 mg (0.05 mL)	1.25 mg (0.05 mL)	2 mg (0.05 mL)	6 mg (0.05 mL)
Intravitreal half-life (days)	2.6–2.88 (rabbits) 3–3.2 (monkeys) 7.1 (humans)	4.32–6.61 (rabbits) 3.1 (monkeys) 6.7–10 (humans)	4.5–4.7 (rabbits)	2.37 (monkeys)
Serum half-life humans (days)	0.25	21	18	1.94
Equivalent number of molecules per injection	0.5	0.4	1	11

less systemic exit, and longer VEGF suppression. As a result, it showed better anatomical outcomes in comparison to aflibercept and ranibizumab.[34] Therefore, brolucizumab potentially can achieve better control of neovascular AMD and require fewer injections. Particularly, the reduced systemic exit of brolucizumab can lead to less generation of antidrug antibody, which can play a major role in immunogenicity and treatment failure.[35] The clinical trials showed that brolucizumab (6 mg/0.05 mL) allows for 2.2 to 1.7-fold higher exposure in the retina and RPE/choroid compared to ranibizumab. Importantly, the parallel HAWK and HARRIER phase 3 trials evaluating brolucizumab in nAMD had similar systemic safety results as compared to aflibercept.[34] Increased molar concentration combined with a high binding affinity for VEGF is the advantage of brolucizumab representing a better durability in long-term, repeated treatment of nAMD. However, more and more anecdotal cases of ocular adverse effects after brolucizumab use have been accumulated and reported, even though ocular safety has been assessed in HAWK and HARRIER clinical trials. Fifteen eyes from 12 patients with retinal vasculitis and intraocular inflammation (IOI) after brolucizumab (6 mg/0.05 mL) were reported from 10 practices between December 1, 2019, and March 1, 2020 in the United States. Retinal vasculitis and IOI, unanticipated complications were diagnosed at a mean of 30 days after brolucizumab intravitreal injections.[36] It is important to know that in this case series brolucizumab was used in patients with prior anti-VEGF injections. Unlike the individuals in the clinical trials for FDA approval, they were all treatment-naïve nAMD patients. Whether patients' factors such as prior exposure to proteins with similar peptides as brolucizumab and other immune characteristics merit further study. Therefore, the safety of brolucizumab is under view, although the drug's safety data "continue to support a favorable benefit-risk profile for this drug" (www.AAO.org March 2020).

Switching between anti-VEGF drugs

In various randomized controlled clinical trials and retinal clinics in real world, the major injectable anti-VEGF agents, that is, bevacizumab, ranibizumab, and aflibercept have been used for all CNV subtypes in nAMD.[37] Only the presence of active disease responds to the anti-VEGF therapy. The indications of active CNV consist of fluid or hemorrhage, leakage on multimodal imaging, an enlarging CNV membrane, or deteriorating vision related to CNV activity. The presence of a mature fibrotic disciform scar with little or no fluid makes successful treatment unlikely. However, an eye with almost any level of vision may benefit, although numerous studies showed that the better baseline vision is associated with a better final vision. Patients with very poor vision should be assessed on an individual basis. Generally, four regimens of anti-VEGF therapy are used in nAMD care, namely a fixed regimen using monthly or bimonthly injections, a PRN regimen, a treat-and-extend regimen, and an observe-and-plan regimen. The initial treatment with intravitreal anti-VEGF agents is given at a fixed monthly interval as a loading period. However, once disease stability is achieved, the follow-up and treatment plan are tailored according to clinical status and the judgment of the treating physician, in an attempt to minimize the treatment frequency and achieve the best outcome. The efficacy of current anti-VEGF agents is associated with their structure and pharmacokinetic characteristics (Table 10.1).[38]

Ranibizumab is a humanized monoclonal antibody fragment, which is derived from the same parent mouse antibody as bevacizumab. It nonselectively binds and inhibits all isoforms of VEGF-A. The useful dose for nAMD is 0.5 mg in 0.05 mL (Table 10.1). Three regimens are used in nAMD. The first, a continuously regular monthly injection was the regimen at the initial major clinical trials. Around 95% of patients maintained vision regardless of lesion type, and 35%−40% significantly improved, particularly during the first 3 months. This intensive regimen appears to provide a marginally better visual outcome, but seems to associate with more progression to macular atrophy than that of a less intensive administration.[39] The long-term effects of ranibizumab on RPE degeneration remain undetermined. Because of its small molecular weight (48 KDa) and the resultant fast systemic clearance, the systemic adverse effects may be less than bevacizumab.[29] In the second regimen, three initial monthly injections followed by monthly review with reinjection were conducted if deterioration occurs as assessed by VA, for example, loss of >5 ETDRS letters and/or increase in retinal thickness by OCT, for example, >100 μm. In the third one, a "treat and extend" regimen was used: after three initial monthly injections, the injection intervals were gradually increased until deterioration is evident. A tailored interval increase is determined for each patient.

The use of bevacizumab, a complete antibody against VEGF-A for nAMD is "off label." Clinical trials show that it is approximately comparable to ranibizumab in efficacy and safety, though some assessments suggest a marginally higher systemic side effect than that of ranibizumab.[28] The clinical strategy of bevacizumab use is similar to that used for ranibizumab. The dose of bevacizumab is 1.25 mg/ 0.05 mL (Table 10.1).

Aflibercept is a recombinant fusion protein that binds to VEGF-A, B and placental growth factor (PlGF), showing a multiisoform suppression. After approval by FDA, it was adopted rapidly into clinical practice, because the recommended maintenance regimen consists of one injection every 2 months in contrast to the monthly injections recommended with ranibizumab and bevacizumab. The 2-month regimen is supported by theoretical models showing this molecule with a longer duration of action compared with current treatments.[40] The longer durability is probably related to the feature of multiisoform targets and the strongest binding affinity (0.5 pM K_D) of aflibercept (Table 10.1). The standard dose is 2 mg in 0.05 mL, with three monthly injections as the loading dose.

In various randomized controlled clinical trials, the major injectable anti-VEGF agents, that is, bevacizumab, ranibizumab, and aflibercept represent largely equivalent efficacy and safety in the treatment of nAMD. Based on a systemic review of the literature published before June 2016, bevacizumab and ranibizumab had equivalent efficacy for best correct visual acuity (BCVA), while ranibizumab had a greater reduction in central macular thickness (CMT) and less chance of serious systemic adverse events. Aflibercept and ranibizumab had comparable efficacy for BCVA and CMT.[37] However, in the real world practice, there are always some subgroups of patients with nAMD demonstrating a suboptimal response to any anti-VEGF therapy. Because aflibercept has theoretical advantages over ranibizumab and bevacizumab, including multiple targets on VEGF isoforms, a longer half-life in the eye, and a higher binding affinity to VEGF-A, extensive studies have explored the outcome after switching from bevacizumab or ranibizumab to aflibercept. The majority of studies showed a clear anatomical benefit after the switch in terms of CMT and pigment epithelium detachment characteristics, whereas the functional outcomes were variable.[41] On the other hand, a handful of studies have proposed arguments for and against switching anti-VEGF agents because the majority of the studies supporting switching are lack of control arms and show controversial visual outcomes after switching.[42] How to successfully switch between anti-VEGF agents merits future research.[43]

Other FDA-approved treatments for nAMD

Pegaptanib (Macugen) was the first anti-VEGF agent approved by FDA for ocular use. As the therapeutic effect for nAMD is marginal, its use is now extremely limited.

Thermal argon or diode laser ablation of CNV, which was an FDA-proved treatment of nAMD, is now rarely used. It may be suitable for the treatment of small classic CNV well away from the macular center.

Photodynamic therapy (PDT) utilizes the photosensitive intravenous drug, verteporfin, in combination with a low power, long-duration infrared laser. Verteporfin is a light-activated compound preferentially taken up by dividing cells including new blood vessels. The activated photosensitizer emits high power of energy to cause thrombosis, resulting in new blood vessel closure. The indication of PDT is subfoveal predominantly classic CNV with visual acuity of 20/200 or better. With the advent of anti-VEGF treatment, PDT as monotherapy is rarely used for CNV. Overall, poor response to anti-VEGF treatments requires reevaluation of diagnosis and a possible switch to alternative therapies including other anti-VEGF drugs and/or with PDT. Particularly, idiopathic polypoidal choroidopathy may require treatment with PDT monotherapy or combination with anti-VEGF.[44]

References

1. McCarty CA, Mukesh BN, Fu CL, Mitchell P, Wang JJ, Taylor HR. Risk factors for age-related maculopathy: the visual impairment project. *Arch Ophthalmol.* 2001;119(10): 1455–1462. https://doi.org/10.1001/archopht.119.10.1455.
2. Parekh N, Voland RP, Moeller SM, et al. Association between dietary fat intake and age-related macular degeneration in the Carotenoids in Age-Related Eye Disease Study (CAREDS): an ancillary study of the Women's Health Initiative. *Arch Ophthalmol.* 2009;127(11):1483–1493. https://doi.org/10.1001/archophthalmol.2009.130.

3. Datta S, Cano M, Ebrahimi K, Wang L, Handa JT. The impact of oxidative stress and inflammation on RPE degeneration in non-neovascular AMD. *Prog Retin Eye Res.* 2017;60:201−218. https://doi.org/10.1016/j.preteyeres.2017.03.002.

4. The age-related eye disease study (AREDS). *Contr Clin Trials.* 1999;20(6):573−600. https://doi.org/10.1016/S0197-2456(99)00031-8.

5. Evans J. Antioxidant supplements to prevent or slow down the progression of AMD: a systematic review and meta-analysis. *Eye.* 2008;22(6):751−760. https://doi.org/10.1038/eye.2008.100.

6. Hambidge M. Underwood Memorial Lecture: human zinc homeostasis: good but not perfect. *J Nutr.* 2003;133(5 suppl 1). https://doi.org/10.1093/jn/133.5.1438S, 1438S-42S.

7. Lutein + zeaxanthin and omega-3 fatty acids for age-related macular degeneration: the age-related eye disease study 2 (AREDS2) randomized clinical trial. *J Am Med Assoc.* 2013;309(19):2005. https://doi.org/10.1001/jama.2013.4997.

8. Hooper P, Jutai JW, Strong G, Russell-Minda E. Age-related macular degeneration and low-vision rehabilitation: a systematic review. *Can J Ophthalmol.* 2008;43(2):180−187. https://doi.org/10.3129/i08-001.

9. Gupta A, Lam J, Custis P, Munz S, Fong D, Koster M. Implantable miniature telescope (IMT) for vision loss due to end-stage age-related macular degeneration. Cochrane Eyes and Vision Group. In: *Cochrane Database of Systematic Reviews.* May 30, 2018. https://doi.org/10.1002/14651858.CD011140.pub2.

10. Brown GC, Brown MM, Lieske HB, Lieske PA, Brown KS, Lane SS. Comparative effectiveness and cost-effectiveness of the implantable miniature telescope. *Ophthalmology.* 2011;118(9):1834−1843. https://doi.org/10.1016/j.ophtha.2011.02.012.

11. Oshima H, Iwase T, Ishikawa K, Yamamoto K, Terasaki H. Long-term results after limited macular translocation surgery for wet age-related macular degeneration. Vavvas DG, ed. *PLoS One.* 2017;12(5):e0177241. https://doi.org/10.1371/journal.pone.0177241.

12. Mirochnik RM, Pezaris JS. Contemporary approaches to visual prostheses. *Mil Med Res.* 2019;6(1):19. https://doi.org/10.1186/s40779-019-0206-9.

13. Greenemeier L. FDA approves first retinal implant. *Nature.* February 15, 2013:12439. https://doi.org/10.1038/nature.2013.12439.

14. Álvarez-Aznar A, Muhl L, Gaengel K. VEGF receptor tyrosine kinases: key regulators of vascular function. *Curr Top Dev Biol.* 2017;123:433−482. https://doi.org/10.1016/bs.ctdb.2016.10.001.

15. Ferrara N. Vascular endothelial growth factor: basic science and clinical progress. *Endocr Rev.* 2004;25(4):581−611. https://doi.org/10.1210/er.2003-0027.

16. Peach C, Mignone V, Arruda M, et al. Molecular pharmacology of VEGF-A isoforms: binding and signalling at VEGFR2. *IJMS.* 2018;19(4):1264. https://doi.org/10.3390/ijms19041264.

17. Bates DO, Cui T-G, Doughty JM, et al. VEGF165b, an inhibitory splice variant of vascular endothelial growth factor, is down-regulated in renal cell carcinoma. *Cancer Res.* 2002;62(14):4123−4131.

18. Stevens M, Star E, Lee M, et al. The VEGF-A exon 8 splicing-sensitive fluorescent reporter mouse is a novel tool to assess the effects of splicing regulatory compounds in vivo. *RNA Biol.* 2019;16(12):1672−1681. https://doi.org/10.1080/15476286.2019.1652522.

19. Woolard J, Bevan HS, Harper SJ, Bates DO. Molecular diversity of VEGF-A as a regulator of its biological activity. *Microcirculation.* 2009;16(7):572−592. https://doi.org/10.1080/10739680902997333.

20. Gammons MV, Fedorov O, Ivison D, et al. Topical antiangiogenic SRPK1 inhibitors reduce choroidal neovascularization in rodent models of exudative AMD. *Invest Ophthalmol Vis Sci*. 2013;54(9):6052–6062. https://doi.org/10.1167/iovs.13-12422.

21. Olsson A-K, Dimberg A, Kreuger J, Claesson-Welsh L. VEGF receptor signalling - in control of vascular function. *Nat Rev Mol Cell Biol*. 2006;7(5):359–371. https://doi.org/10.1038/nrm1911.

22. Frank RN, Amin RH, Eliott D, Puklin JE, Abrams GW. Basic fibroblast growth factor and vascular endothelial growth factor are present in epiretinal and choroidal neovascular membranes. *Am J Ophthalmol*. 1996;122(3):393–403. https://doi.org/10.1016/s0002-9394(14)72066-5.

23. Ambati J, Fowler BJ. Mechanisms of age-related macular degeneration. *Neuron*. 2012; 75(1):26–39. https://doi.org/10.1016/j.neuron.2012.06.018.

24. Gragoudas ES, Adamis AP, Cunningham ET, Feinsod M, Guyer DR, VEGF inhibition study in ocular neovascularization clinical trial group. Pegaptanib for neovascular age-related macular degeneration. *N Engl J Med*. 2004;351(27):2805–2816. https://doi.org/10.1056/NEJMoa042760.

25. Rosenfeld PJ, Moshfeghi AA, Puliafito CA. Optical coherence tomography findings after an intravitreal injection of bevacizumab (avastin) for neovascular age-related macular degeneration. *Ophthalmic Surg Lasers Imaging*. 2005;36(4):331–335.

26. Tarallo V, De Falco S. The vascular endothelial growth factors and receptors family: up to now the only target for anti-angiogenesis therapy. *Int J Biochem Cell Biol*. 2015;64: 185–189. https://doi.org/10.1016/j.biocel.2015.04.008.

27. Rosenfeld PJ, Brown DM, Heier JS, et al. Ranibizumab for neovascular age-related macular degeneration. *N Engl J Med*. 2006;355(14):1419–1431. https://doi.org/10.1056/NEJMoa054481.

28. Ranibizumab and bevacizumab for neovascular age-related macular degeneration. *N Engl J Med*. 2011;364(20):1897–1908. https://doi.org/10.1056/NEJMoa1102673.

29. Comparison of Age-related Macular Degeneration Treatments Trials (CATT) Research Group, Martin DF, Maguire MG, et al. Ranibizumab and bevacizumab for treatment of neovascular age-related macular degeneration: two-year results. *Ophthalmology*. 2012;119(7):1388–1398. https://doi.org/10.1016/j.ophtha.2012.03.053.

30. Jaffe GJ, Ying G-S, Toth CA, et al. Macular morphology and visual acuity in year five of the comparison of age-related macular degeneration treatments trials. *Ophthalmology*. 2019;126(2):252–260. https://doi.org/10.1016/j.ophtha.2018.08.035.

31. Heier JS, Brown DM, Chong V, et al. Intravitreal aflibercept (VEGF trap-eye) in wet age-related macular degeneration. *Ophthalmology*. 2012;119(12):2537–2548. https://doi.org/10.1016/j.ophtha.2012.09.006.

32. Schmidt-Erfurth U, Kaiser PK, Korobelnik J-F, et al. Intravitreal aflibercept injection for neovascular age-related macular degeneration: ninety-six-week results of the VIEW studies. *Ophthalmology*. 2014;121(1):193–201. https://doi.org/10.1016/j.ophtha.2013.08.011.

33. Ma J, Waxman DJ. Combination of antiangiogenesis with chemotherapy for more effective cancer treatment. *Mol Cancer Ther*. 2008;7(12):3670–3684. https://doi.org/10.1158/1535-7163.MCT-08-0715.

34. Dugel PU, Koh A, Ogura Y, et al. HAWK and HARRIER: phase 3, multicenter, randomized, double-masked trials of brolucizumab for neovascular age-related macular degeneration. *Ophthalmology*. 2020;127(1):72–84. https://doi.org/10.1016/j.ophtha.2019.04.017.

35. Sharma A, Kumar N, Kuppermann BD, Bandello F, Loewenstein A. Biotherapeutics and immunogenicity: ophthalmic perspective. *Eye*. 2019;33(9):1359−1361. https://doi.org/10.1038/s41433-019-0434-y.

36. Baumal CR, Spaide RF, Vajzovic L, et al. Retinal vasculitis and intraocular inflammation after intravitreal injection of brolucizumab. *Ophthalmology*. April 25, 2020. https://doi.org/10.1016/j.ophtha.2020.04.017.

37. Nguyen CL, Oh LJ, Wong E, Wei J, Chilov M. Anti-vascular endothelial growth factor for neovascular age-related macular degeneration: a meta-analysis of randomized controlled trials. *BMC Ophthalmol*. 2018;18(1):130. https://doi.org/10.1186/s12886-018-0785-3.

38. Stewart MW. Pharmacokinetics, pharmacodynamics and pre-clinical characteristics of ophthalmic drugs that bind VEGF. *Expet Rev Clin Pharmacol*. 2014;7(2):167−180. https://doi.org/10.1586/17512433.2014.884458.

39. Grunwald JE, Daniel E, Huang J, et al. Risk of geographic atrophy in the comparison of age-related macular degeneration treatments trials. *Ophthalmology*. 2014;121(1):150−161. https://doi.org/10.1016/j.ophtha.2013.08.015.

40. Ohr M, Kaiser PK. Aflibercept in wet age-related macular degeneration: a perspective review. *Ther Adv Chronic Dis*. 2012;3(4):153−161. https://doi.org/10.1177/2040622312446007.

41. Empeslidis T, Storey M, Giannopoulos T, et al. How successful is switching from bevacizumab or ranibizumab to aflibercept in age-related macular degeneration? A systematic overview. *Adv Ther*. 2019;36(7):1532−1548. https://doi.org/10.1007/s12325-019-00971-0.

42. Bro T, Hägg S. Worth changing? Clinical effects of switching treatment in neovascular age-related macular degeneration from intravitreal ranibizumab and aflibercept to bevacizumab in a region in southern Sweden. *Eur J Ophthalmol*. October 23, 2019. https://doi.org/10.1177/1120672119883602, 1120672119883602.

43. Mantel I, Gillies MC, Souied EH. Switching between ranibizumab and aflibercept for the treatment of neovascular age-related macular degeneration. *Surv Ophthalmol*. 2018;63(5):638−645. https://doi.org/10.1016/j.survophthal.2018.02.004.

44. Amoaku WM, Chakravarthy U, Gale R, et al. Defining response to anti-VEGF therapies in neovascular AMD. *Eye*. 2015;29(6):721−731. https://doi.org/10.1038/eye.2015.48.

Therapy in pipeline for age-related macular degeneration

11

The therapeutic pipeline for dry AMD

The dry age-related macular degeneration (AMD) affects approximately 85%—90% of individuals with AMD. Geographic atrophy (GA), an advanced form of dry AMD, presents as a discrete area of retinal pigment epithelium (RPE) loss accompanying with the degeneration of overlying photoreceptors. Many of these individuals experience progressive and severe loss of vision when the center of macula is involved. The central GA accounts for approximately 25% of the severe visual impairment attributed to AMD.[1] As GA is a multifactorial disease comprising interplays between causal genetic variants and environmental risk factors, the underlying pathogenesis is still not completely understood. Based on up-to-date clinical findings and research advances, oxidative and metabolic stress, chronic inflammation, complement activation, and uncontrolled programmed cell death all contribute to the development and progression of GA. Although there have been no approved treatments for GA yet, currently numerous therapies in the pipeline to protect the structure and function of the retina have been proposed and explored. In this chapter, the investigating therapies are categorized based on their mechanism of action (MOA) in the ongoing clinical trials. However, the limitation of this chapter is to obtain peer-review published data of these clinical trials in a timely fashion. To overcome this shortcoming, following closely the up-dated news in professional publications and newsletters may be a rapid approach for the readers. This chapter has provided essential information about GA therapy in the pipeline to date, which largely has followed an outline summarized by *Retina Today* in 2019.[2]

Inhibition of inflammation and complement activation
Lampalizumab

Study name: MAHALO phase 2, and CHROMA and SPECTRI phase 3 study.

Objectives: To determine if intravitreal lampalizumab can halt the progression of GA in patients of the late stage of dry AMD.[3,4]

Age-Related Macular Degeneration. https://doi.org/10.1016/B978-0-12-822061-0.00005-0

Sponsors: MAHALO study in the United States and Germany, CHROMA and SPECTRI phase 3 studies in 23 countries.

Study time: MAHALO study 18 months; CHROMA and SPECTRI phase 3 studies 48 weeks.

Patients enrolled; 129 GA patients without CNV in MAHALO study, 906 GA patients without CNV in CHROMA and SPECTRI phase 3 studies.

Treatment regimen: Patients were randomized to receive either lampalizumab 10 mg or sham, administered monthly or every other month in the MAHALO study. Patients were randomized 2:1:2:1 to receive 10 mg of intravitreal lampalizumab every 4 weeks, sham procedure every 4 weeks, 10 mg of lampalizumab every 6 weeks, or sham procedure every 6 weeks in CHROMA and SPECTRI phase 3 studies.

Outcome measures: The primary outcome of MAHALO phase 2 was the mean change in GA lesion area from baseline to month 18.

Results: With an acceptable safety profile, monthly lampalizumab treatment demonstrated a 20% reduction in lesion progression versus sham control. By more substantial monthly treatment, that is,10 mg of lampalizumab every 6 weeks, the benefit of 44% reduction in GA area progression versus sham control was observed in a subgroup of complement factor I (*CFI*) risk-allele carriers.[4] In CHROMA and SPECTRI trials, lampalizumab did not reduce GA enlargement versus sham during 48 weeks of treatment. A mean of GA enlargement was similar in treatment to sham group approximately 2 mm^2 per year.[5]

Present status: Despite the setback with lampalizumab in clinical trial phase 3, complement factor D (CFD) remains a target of interest in the treatment of AMD.

Comments: Lampalizumab is a humanized monoclonal antibody (Fab fragment), which is a selective inhibitor of CFD. MAHALO phase 2 is a proof-of-concept study, indicating the critical role of dysregulation of alternative complement pathway plays a pathogenic role in GA progression. However, the results of CHROMA and SPECTRI trials are disappointing. One of the limitations is that the treatment regimens only apply to 48 weeks. This short application may not be appropriate to all cases of GA, particularly GA cases in extremely chronic process.[5] Another limitation of this study is that the design of the outcome measurement is before the advent of optical coherence tomography (OCT). The high quality of OCT imaging may be able to quantitatively reveal changes of RPE and the interplay of multiple cellular components of the macula.[3]

Eculizumab

Study name: The COMPLETE study (phase 2), namely, systemic complement inhibition with eculizumab for GA in AMD.

Objectives: To determine if the usage of systemic eculizumab can halt GA progression in patients with AMD.

Sponsors: Alexion Pharmaceuticals.

Study time: 6 months.

Patients enrolled: 30 patients with GA but without choroidal neovascularization (CNV).

Treatment regimen: Patients were randomized 2:1 to receive eculizumab or placebo. Patients received eculizumab or placebo for 24 weeks with the primary endpoint at 26 weeks. The treatment was divided into an induction period and a maintenance period. The first 10 patients in the eculizumab group received the low dose of eculizumab (600 mg via intravenous infusion for 4 weeks followed by 900 mg every 2 weeks until week 24), whereas the next 10 patients received the high dose (900 mg eculizumab via intravenous infusion for 4 weeks followed by 1200 mg every 2 weeks until week 24). After 26 weeks, patients were followed up twice without treatment at 3-month intervals.

Outcome measures: The primary outcome was the growth rate measurements of GA area detected by SD OCT sub-RPE slab images. The secondary outcomes were the change in the area of GA measured with autofluorescence and fluorescein angiographic imaging.

Results: In both low- and high-dose treatment groups, there were no significant changes in the GA area. The COMPLETE study found that the progression of GA over 6 months was dependent upon the low luminance deficit at baseline of these patients.

Present status: The COMPLETE study failed to advance to phase 3 trial.

Comments: Eculizumab is an inhibitor of complement component (C5), a humanized monoclonal antibody. Eculizumab inhibits C5 and prevents terminal complement activation and formation of membrane attack complex (C5b-9) with excellent safety profile in systemic utilization.[3] The COMPLETE study utilized accurate parameters currently available monitoring the changes of GA, that is, morphological OCT imaging and functional luminance vision test. However, the sample size of this study was small (30 patients). Most importantly, whether the inhibition of alternative complement pathways via intravenous eculizumab could reach the inhibitory status of C5-mediated cascade in the posterior outer retina may present a concern.[6]

Pegcetacoplan

Study name: The Filly phase 2 study of Pegcetacoplan (APL-2) for GA in AMD.

Objectives: To test the safety and efficacy of intravitreal APL-2 on the reduction of GA growth.

Sponsors: Apellis Pharmaceuticals, Inc.

Study time: 18 months.

Patients enrolled: GA in single eyes of 246 patients without CNV.

Treatment regimen: Patients were assigned randomly in a 2:2:1:1 ratio to receive intravitreal 15 mg pegcetacoplan (APL-2) monthly or every other month or sham intravitreal injections monthly or every other month for 12 months with follow-up at months 15 and 18.

Outcome measures: The primary endpoint was the mean change in the GA area from baseline to month 12 by fundus autofluorescence imaging. The secondary outcome was any change of best-corrected visual acuity (BCVA), low-luminance BCVA, and low-luminance visual acuity deficit.

Results: In APL-2 monthly or every other month groups, the GA growth rate was reduced by 29% and 20% compared with the sham treatment group. However, the eyes treated with both APL-2 regimens developed significantly higher exudative AMD as compared to the sham eyes (8.9%–20.9% in APL-2 groups and 1.2% in the sham group, respectively).

Present status: Completion of phase 2, enrolling for phase 3.

Comments: APL-2 is a pegylated complement C3 inhibitor peptide.[7] The phase 2 results that show significant efficacy of intravitreal APL-2 as compared to the sham treatment on reduction of GA growth are encouraging. This is also a "proof-of concept" study emphasizing the pathogenic role of C3 in the progression of GA. It is of notice that C3 is the central element of the three complement cascades, that is, classical, lectin, and alternative cascades, which is located at the upstream of C5-mediated common pathway. Theoretically, the consequence of C3 inhibition may interfere with the function of whole innate complement systems as described in Chapter 7. Although the current Filly phase 2 study using a local delivery approach (i.e., intravitreal injection) minimized the systemic impact of C3 inhibition, the altered complement defense function in the macular neurovascular complex need to be further monitored. For instance, the APL-2 dose-dependent CNV development in the treated eyes is worrisome in the upcoming phase 3 trial. As this study pointed out, the possible accumulation of active C3 fragments could have continued.[6] In other words, the subretinal macrophage infiltration, which induces an inflammasome activation,[8] can cause the chronic release of inflammatory molecules and tissue damage. Therefore, when the upcoming phase 3 trial is designed, the assembly and activation of inflammasome complex should be monitored.

C5 inhibitor zimura (avacincaptad pegol)

Study name: C5 Inhibitor, Zimura (avacincaptad pegol), for GA in AMD: A phase 2/3 trial (GATHER1 study).[9]

Objectives: To determine the safety and efficacy of intravitreal Zimura on the reduction of GA growth of patients with AMD.

Sponsors: Iveric bio.

Study time: 12 months.

Patients enrolled: 286 patients with GA due to AMD.

Treatment regimen: Patients were assigned randomly in two parts for intravitreal injections: in Part 1, patients were further randomized in a 1:1:1 ratio to receive Zimura 1 mg, Zimura 2 mg, and sham. In Part 2, patients were randomized in a 1:2:2 ratio to receive Zimura 2 mg, Zimura 4 mg, and sham.

Outcome measures: The primary outcome was the mean rate of change in GA over 12 months determined by fundus autofluorescence. Secondary endpoints included the change in best-corrected visual acuity.

Results: Zimura was generally well tolerated. There were no Zimura-related adverse events or serious adverse events. The reduction in the mean GA growth rate over 12 months was 27.4% for the Zimura 2 mg and 27.8% for Zimura 4 mg as compared to their sham-control groups.

Present status: GATHER1 study met its primary efficacy and safety endpoint. GATHER2 study phase 3 trial will compare Zimura 2 mg with a sham-control group.

Comments: There was a higher incidence of CNV or nAMD in study eyes treated with pegcetacoplan (APL-2), a C3 inhibitor as described earlier.[7] In the GATHER1 study, the incidence of CNV for eyes who received Zimura was (9.0%−9.6%) much lower than the incidence of APL-2 (8.9%−20.9%).[7,9] The underlying mechanism of this difference causing CNV formation between C3 and C5 inhibition is not clear. One of the possibilities is that C5 inhibition targets the terminal alternative pathway, which may minimize the disturbance of the C3-mediated complement homeostasis. Larger trials are required to better understand this phenomenon.

CR2-fH

Study name: A preclinical trial of a fusion protein (CR2-fH) consisting of complement receptor 2 fragments (CR2) linked to the inhibitory domain of complement factor H (fH) for both dry and neovascular AMD.[10]

Objectives: To determine the safety and efficacy of AAV-mediated delivery of CR2-fH on anticomplement activation and reduction of laser-induced CNV in a murine model (C57BL/6J mice).

Sponsors: Medical University of South Carolina, USA.

Study time: 1 month.

Treatment regimen: Subretinal AAV5-mediated delivery of CR2-fH to C57BL/6J mice.

Outcome measures: The safety profile of subretinal AAV5-CR2-fH and the efficacy on inhibition of complement activation in animal model.

Results: A safe concentration of AAV5-CR2-fH was identified using ERG, OCT, and RPE morphology. AAV5-mediated CR2-fH expression in the mouse RPE is comparable to that of intravenous injection. CR2-fH expressed in the RPE could reduce the development of laser-induced CNV, attenuate complement activation, as determined by a reduction in C3a production.

Present status: The safety and efficacy profile of CR2-fH to murine with AMD-like retina pathology have met in the preclinical study. Advancing CR2-fH clinical trials for GA and/or CNV is underway.

Comments: The result of this preclinical trial is a "proof-of-concept" work trying to understand the role of complement factor H (FH) in the regulation of alternative complement pathway. Numerous genetic studies have shown strong associations between AMD risk and common variations in genes encoding proteins of the complement system, specifically a variant in FH (Tyr402His). To date, the exact role of complement in AMD pathogenesis remains unclear. However, several structural and functional studies suggest that the 402His form of FH, or its smaller splice product FH-like 1 (FHL1) binds less well than the 402Tyr variant to Bruch's membrane, thus resulting in a reduced inhibitory function of FH, namely, less protection against subretinal chronic inflammation.[11,12] This new product, CR2-fH, may act as a supplement of FH in the regulation of alternative pathways. In addition, the successful delivery of a therapeutic dose of FH to the macular region has validated that the gene delivery is safe and effective for future AMD treatment strategies.[13,14]

ANX007

Study name: Clinical trial phase 1b, intravitreal ANX007 (a C1q inhibitor), for patients affected with GA due to AMD.

Objectives: To determine the safety, tolerability, pharmacokinetics, and targeted endpoints in patients affected with GA.

Sponsors: Annexon bioscience.

Study time: The first evaluation time was 4 weeks after intravitreal ANX007. The designed study time for phase 2 is not available.

Treatment regimen: A single intravitreal ANX007 with varied doses in 17 patients affected with glaucoma was completed. In phase 1b, a single ANX007 injection achieved complete suppression of the C1q for at least 4 weeks, as monitored in aqueous humor samples.[15]

Outcome measures: Primary endpoints are the tolerability of different doses after a single intravitreal injection. Secondary endpoints are the inhibitory effect on C1q.

Results: The primary outcome showed that ANX007 was well tolerated at all dose levels without serious side effects. At the two higher dose levels, a single intravitreal injection of ANX007 achieved complete suppression of the C1q target for at least 4 weeks, as measured in ocular fluid from aqueous humor taps.

Present status: advance to phase 2 clinical trial for GA.

Comments: The role of the alternative complement pathway and its mediation by retinal microglia and macrophages in pathogenesis of AMD has been described in Chapter 7. Recently, a novel approach by using photo-oxidative mice, either $C1q$a knockout ($C1qa^{-/-}$) or mice treated with C1q inhibitor was used. First, this study demonstrated that in addition to alternative pathway, other complement pathway(s) such as classic pathway may contribute to the events of retinal degenerations.[16] Second, for the photo-oxidative damaged mice, $C1qa^{-/-}$ mice showed reduced inflammasome and IL-1β expression in macrophages in the degenerative retina. Neutralization of C1q with intravitreal anti-C1q antibody reduced the progression of retinal degeneration. Third, retinal C1q was found to be expressed by subretinal microglia/ macrophages located in the outer retina of early AMD donor eyes and in mouse photo-oxidative retinas. Fourth, most importantly, systemic delivery of anti-C1q antibody had no such effect in the outer retina, indicating the local regulation of classic complement pathway plays a pathogenic role in retinal degeneration. The regulatory mechanism of the classic complement pathway in the outer retina may be distinct. Although intravitreal ANX007 potently binds to C1q and inhibits activation of all downstream complement cascades, including C3 and C5, it does not interfere with the normal function of C3- and C5-mediated other complement pathways.[15] Therefore, the MOA of ANX007 is via a distinct function of the local classic complement pathway. All these unique findings of ANX007 have met the criteria for the phase 2 trial.

CB2782

Study name: A complement factor C3-inactivating protease (CB2782) and potential long-acting treatment for dry AMD in the preclinical trial.[17]

Objectives: To determine the efficacy of C3 inhibition and pharmacokinetics and pharmacodynamics of intravitreal CB2782 in rabbits.

Sponsors: Catalyst.

Treatment regimen: Intravitreal CB2782 PEG 2 mg, 3–4 times a year in rabbits.

Outcome measures: The inhibitory effect of Pegylated CB-2782 on C3-mediated complement pathway.

Results: Intravitreal CB2782 PEG on C3-mediated complement pathway was documented by using animal models.

Present status: Based on the verified inhibitory effect of intravitreal CB2782 PEG on C3-mediated complement pathway, it will advance to phase 1 clinical trial.

Comments: Despite multiple clinical failures in treating GA by blocking the alternative pathway or the downstream C5 pathways, interest in more completely blocking C3 complement activation in the eye, continues. Pegylated CB-2782 is an enzyme. The pegylated enzyme has indistinguishable enzymatic activity on a C3-mimicking peptide substrate, specifically hydrolyzing C3 at a single site into inactive components, and blocks ex vivo C3-dependent complement-mediated sheep red blood cell hemolysis. Pegylation is an established method to extend the vitreous half-life of macromolecules. The biophysical and biochemical properties of CB2782, which render potential for an extended half-life in the vitreous, may be useful as a long-acting drug for dry AMD treatment.[17]

ALXN1720

ALXN1720 is a novel anti-C5 albumin-binding bispecific antibody that binds and prevents activation of human C5.[18] Bispecific antibodies are antibodies that can simultaneously bind two separate and unique antigens (or different epitopes of the same antigen). Current applications have been explored for cancer immunotherapy and drug delivery. Alexion-developed ALXN1720 bispecific antibody can have an extended half-life.[18] Alexion Pharmaceuticals, Inc., the sponsor company, has completed preclinical study and plans to initiate a phase 1 study of ALXN1720 for treating GA.[15]

HMR59

Study name: Intravitreal HMR59 (AAVCAGsCD59) for the treatment of AMD phase 1 trial.

Objectives: To evaluate the safety of intravitreal HMR59, a transgene product blocking complement at membrane attack complex (MAC).

Sponsors: Hemera Biosciences.

Study time: 24 months.

Patients enrolled: 17 patients affected with GA due to AMD.

Treatment regimen: A phase 1 clinical trial evaluating a single intravitreal injection in patients with advanced dry AMD with 24 months follow-up.

Outcome measures: Primary outcome is to show no severe side effect after a single intravitreal injection. Secondary outcome is to show if HMR59 has the potential to slow down or stop the progression of GA due to AMD with a single intravitreal injection.

Results: HMR59 was delivered intravitreally. The treatment was well tolerated, and there was no dose-dependent toxicity. Four eyes developed mild inflammation. Two of these four patients required pressure-lowering drops as well. While this phase 1 trial was not powered to demonstrate efficacy, the majority of the patients in the high-dose group showed a slower growth rate of GA than the controls.[19]

Present status: Advance to phase 2 for dry AMD clinical trial.

Comments: HMR59 is an AAV2 gene therapy administered as an intravitreal injection. The data of phase 1 showed that a single intravitreal injection with doses up to 1.071×10^{12} vector genomes (vg) has been granted safe to proceed status from the FDA. This AAV-delivered soluble CD59 (sCD59) that inhibits the terminal complement pathway, potentially targets local MAC without disturbance of other defense functions of complement cascades, and appears to be a long-acting drug for dry AMD.[20]

Danicopan (ACH-4471)

Study name: Discovery and development of the oral CFD Inhibitor danicopan.[21]

Objectives: To evaluate if danicopan, a reversible small-molecule inhibitor of CFD is safe, and if oral uptake is feasible for effectiveness on CFD inhibition in preclinical trial and phase 1 clinical trial of healthy volunteers.

Sponsors: Achillion Pharmaceuticals.

Study time: Pharmacokinetic (PK) study of healthy volunteers after single oral dose.

Patients enrolled: 36 healthy volunteers enrolled for safety, tolerability, and PK study after taking single ascending oral doses.

Treatment regimen: In preclinical trial, oral danicopan was administered to cynomolgus monkeys in two oral doses of 200 mg/kg, 12 h apart. In phase 1 study of healthy volunteers, single doses of 200, 600, and 1200 mg, and with two doses of 1200 mg, 12 h apart, as well as placebo group were studied.

Outcome measures: Any side effects and tolerability issue.

Results: At pharmacological levels against CFD in serum of nonhuman primates, a pharmacodynamic study of danicopan on inhibition of alternative pathway (AP) was evaluated.[22] Oral danicopan was well tolerated across all dose groups in healthy volunteers, although posttreatment, two transient, and self-limiting elevations in aspartate transaminase (ALT) were observed.

Present status: Phase 2 clinical trial for dry AMD is ongoing.

Comments: First, the discovery and development of small-molecule reversible CFD inhibitors such as danicopan for AP inhibition is an innovative achievement. This approach has alleviated the potential immunogenicity of irreversible inhibitors that generally are proteins as compared with their reversible counterparts.[23] Second, the oral CFD inhibitors such as danicopan has been modified and identified to make the oral route feasible. Danicopan is the first clinically investigated orally administered small molecule inhibitor of CFD for the treatment of chronic diseases.[21] Third, since CFD inhibitors selectively target the AP and preserve the classical, lectin, and terminal pathways, the antibody-elicited protection should be preserved or rapidly restored after cease of reversible CFD inhibitors.[22]

IONIS-FB-LRX

Study name: Development of IONIS-FB-L$_{Rx}$ to treat GA associated with AMD (phase 1 masked, placebo-controlled single and multiple ascending dose studies).[24]

Objectives: To determine the clinical safety of a novel antisense oligonucleotide (ASO) targeting the human *CFB* gene, and to evaluate if this treatment can inhibit AP activity in the choriocapillaris.

Sponsors: Ionis Pharmaceuticals, Inc.

Study time: 43 days.

Patients enrolled: 54 healthy volunteers.

Treatment regimens: Subcutaneous administrations of 10 and 20 mg of IONIS-FB-L$_{Rx}$.

Outcome measures: Primary outcome is the safety profile after taking IONIS-FB-L$_{Rx}$ by healthy volunteers in 43 days. Secondary outcome is to evaluate the inhibitory effect on reduction of circulating levels of CFB.

Results: There were no safety signals or clinically relevant changes in blood chemistry, hematology, urinalysis, ECGs, or vital signs.

Present status: A placebo-controlled phase 2 trial in patients affected with GA due to AMD in planning.

Comments: The preclinical study demonstrated that a second-generation ASO, that is, IONIS-FB-L$_{Rx}$, targets healthy mouse and monkey CFB mRNA by subcutaneous route.[25] ASO administration reduced CFB mRNA level in the liver. When the plasma level of CFB protein fell by using ASO dramatically, the CFB level in the eye was almost undetectable.[25] In phase 1 study, IONIS-FB-L$_{RX}$ reduced plasma CFB levels of the volunteers in a dose-dependent manner. A larger reduction of CFB levels at the 20 mg dose than that of 10 mg dose was associated with greater suppression of AP activity.[24] Although the mechanistic link between excessive CFB and subretinal/sub-RPE inflammation is still elusive, the upcoming phase 2 and possible phase 3 clinical trial may provide "proof-of-concept" evidence to support this hypothesis.

Neuroprotection

Elamipretide

Study name: The ReCLAIM phase 1 clinical trial of elamipretide for dry AMD.

Objectives: To determine the safety profile of subcutaneous elamipretide in patients affected with dry AMD, and to evaluate if elamipretide administration could improve the visual function and/or reduce the growth rate of GA.[26]

Sponsors: Stealth Biotherapeutics and Duke University.

Study time: 24 weeks.

Patients enrolled: Patients with dry AMD were enrolled into one of two subgroups: (1) noncentral geographic atrophy (NCGA) or (2) high-risk drusen (HRD) without GA.

Treatment regimen: Subcutaneous elamipretide (40 mg) once a day, for 24 weeks.

Outcome measures: Primary outcome is to document any side effect of subcutaneous elamipretide therapy. Secondary outcome measures visual function changes after elamipretide therapy.

Results: Elamipretide therapy was generally safe and well tolerated with no treatment-related serious adverse events. In the NCGA subgroup at week 24, a significant increase both in BCVA and low-luminance visual acuity (LLVA) from baseline was observed. In the NCGA subgroup, the growth rate of the GA area slowed as compared with published data. In the HRD subgroup at week 24, there was a significant increase both in BCVA and LLVA from baseline.

Present status: A phase 2b clinical trial of daily subcutaneous elamipretide in patients with dry AMD and NCGA is underway.

Comments: Elamipretide is a novel tetrapeptide drug that binds to cardiolipin, resulting in the restoration of defects in mitochondrial function including improved ATP production, restoration of mitochondrial membrane potential, normal calcium flux, and the reduced superoxide generation.[27] Cardiolipin is a key component of the inner mitochondrial membrane, where it constitutes about 20% of the total lipid composition.[28] Based on ReCLAIM study, elamipretide is the first drug that can improve the visual function of patients with dry AMD including noncentral GA. The proposed mechanism of elamipretide is to keep bioenergetic homeostasis of RPE mitochondria, because the impaired energy metabolism of RPE mitochondria drives overall retinal damage (see Chapter 7).[29]

Risuteganib

Study name: Intravitreal risuteganib for intermediate dry AMD phase 2a study[30]

Objectives: To determine if intravitreal risuteganib is safe; to evaluate if the primary endpoint can be reached, that is, a gain of BCVA in early treatment of diabetic retinopathy study (ETDRS) vision of >8 letters.

Sponsors: Allegro Ophthalmics.

Study time: 28 weeks.

Patients enrolled: 39 eyes with intermediate AMD.

Treatment regimen: 25 eyes received two intravitreal risuteganib (1 mg) at week 1 and week 16, and 14 eyes received one sham injection. At week 16, the injecting investigator was then unmasked and participants in the sham group were crossed over to receive a single injection of risuteganib (1.0 mg).

Outcome measures: The primary endpoint in this study is a gain in ETDRS vision of ≥8 letters. The safety profile is documented.

Results: Risuteganib has a good safety profile based on more than 1200 injections.[31] When the BCVA of risuteganib treatment group at week 28 was compared to the sham group at week 12, 48% patients in risuteganib group versus 7.1% in the sham group achieved this endpoint.

Present status: A larger trial to confirm these results is underway.

Comments: Risuteganib is a synthetic RGD (arginyl-glycyl-aspartic acid)-class peptide that regulates the functions of multiple integrin isoforms. Integrins are cell adhesion and signaling receptors that interact with the extracellular matrix. They located on cell surfaces throughout the body, play a major role in cell-to-cell interactions. Risuteganib is a novel antiintegrin peptide that targets the multiple integrin heterodimers involved in the pathophysiology of dry AMD. Preclinical investigations of risuteganib suggest that the MOA of this drug is antiinflammation, mitochondrial stabilization, and antiapoptosis.[32]

Photobiomodulation

Study name: Photobiomodulation (PBM) for dry AMD (LIGHTSITE 1 study), a double-masked, randomized, sham-controlled, parallel group format.

Objectives: To determine if PBM therapy can improve visual function such as visual acuity and contrast sensitivity and reduce druse volume and thickness structurally.[33]

Sponsors: LumiThera.

Study time: 1 year.

Patients enrolled: 30 subjects for a total of 46 qualifying eyes with dry AMD.

Treatment regimen: PBM versus sham treatment randomized at a 1:1 ratio, PBM with LumiThera Valeda Light Delivery System, two series of treatments (3 per week for 3–4 weeks) over 1 year.

Outcome measures: Outcome measures included best-corrected visual acuity, contrast sensitivity, microperimetry, central drusen volume and drusen thickness, and quality-of-life assessments.

Results: Overall, 50% and 46% of the patients after PBM showed >5 ETEDS letters improvement after the first and second series of treatment, respectively. PBM benefited the patients with dry AMD functionally as determined by improved contrast sensitivity and microperimetry results, also structurally as reduced druse volume and thickness. This clinical study showed a good safety profile of PBM without serious adverse events.[34]

Present status: Further LIGHTSITE 2 and 3 study are underway.

Comments: PBM is a light-based technology that stimulates bioenergetic output in targeted tissues.[33] The Valeda light delivery system (LumiThera) was designed as a multiwavelength platform for PBM. PBM using low-level light between 500 and 1000 nm can be applied to selected tissues.[35] Although the MOA remains poorly understood, preclinical data demonstrated that the light at the therapeutic window, which is accepted by mitochondrial enzyme cytochrome C oxidase, may improve mitochondrial energy generation, RNA and protein synthesis.[36] In the LIGHTSITE 1 study, the visual function of patients treated with PBM improved significantly from month 1 to 4. From month 4 to 6, the visual benefits of PBM started fading out. The similar therapeutic effect was observed in the second series of PBM. These data indicate that PBM needs to be repeated after 4–6 months for maintenance of continuous benefits. However, whether the long-term, repeated PBM is safe for human retinal cells, for instance what is the capacity of mitochondrial energy generation, merits to be answered in the future studies.

Brimonidine tartrate

Study name: Brimonidine delivery system (Brimo DDS) phase 2 study in patients with GA due to AMD.[37]

Objectives: To evaluate the safety and efficacy of Brimo DDS, a biodegradable intravitreal implant, in the treatment of GA secondary to AMD.

Sponsors: Allergan Inc.

Study time: 24 months.

Patients enrolled: 113 patients were randomized in a 2:2:1 ratio to receive Brimo DDS 132 µg, Brimo DDS 264 µg, or sham treatment.

Treatment regimen: Intravitreal implants with different doses of brimonidine (132 µg, 264 µg, or sham) at Day 1 and Month 6; follow-up visits extended to Month 24.

Outcome measures: The outcome measures were based on stereoscopic fundus photography and fluorescein angiography.

Results: Brimo DDS showed a favorable safety profile. The efficacy of Brimo DDS on the reduction of GA growth demonstrated a dose-dependent fashion at Month 3. The Brimo DDS treatment groups could reduce GA growth, particularly in patients with GA lesions 6 mm^2 or larger at baseline.[37]

Present status: Consider to advance this study to phase 3

Comments: Numerous in vitro and in vivo studies showed that brimonidine, an alpha2-adrenergic agonist utilizing as an antiglaucoma medicine, has cytoprotective and neuroprotective functions. Brimonidine protected human RPE and Muller cell lines from the detrimental effects of reactive oxygen species.[38] In multiple animal models, topical or systemic administration of brimonidine promoted the survival of retinal neurons such as retinal ganglion cells and experimentally injured optic nerve.[39,40] In the study of a rat spinal cord injury model, the neuroprotective mechanism of alpha2-adrenergic agonist appears to be associated with modulation of neuroinflammation, which is partially mediated via α2-adrenergic receptor signaling.[41]

Based on the phase 2 study of brimo DDS, the efficacy of brimonidine on the reduction of GA growth rate is brimonidine-dose dependent.[37] These findings suggest that a high intraocular brimonidine concentration needs to be kept for maintaining efficacy. The level should be at least above 2 nM, because this is the concentration required for alpha2-receptor activation within the target tissues.[40] For this purpose, a new polymer as a platform for an ocular drug delivery system was developed for bromonidine application.[42] The brimonidine implant, brimo DDS, was applied to maintain a therapeutic level for 90 days in the posterior segment.[43]

The limitation of this study is a small sample size. Thus, this study was not powered for statistical comparisons between treatment groups.[37] However, the proof-of-concept result that shows a significantly reduced GA growth in brimo DDS group as compared to the sham group at Month 3 has made the study advance to phase 3.

GAL-101 (MRZ-99030)

Study name: Neuroprotective effect of β-amyloid (Aβ) aggregation modulator GAL-101 in dry AMD (preclinical and phase 1 studies).[44]

Objectives: To determine the safety profile of a novel topical Aβ aggregation modulator (GAL-101), to evaluate if topical GAL-101 can reduce amyloid-beta oligomers.

Sponsors: Galimedix Therapeutics, Inc.

Study time: Not available.

Patients enrolled: 70 patients in phase 1

Treatment regimen: Topical GAL-101.

Outcome measures: Any side effect and drop-out due to intolerability.

Results: GAL-101 eye drops are safe and tolerable without serious side effects in phase 1 study. All 70 randomized subjects completed the study and adverse events occurred at low frequencies across the treatment and control groups. The drops in monkeys have demonstrated that therapeutic levels are quickly reached in the retina. Single eye drops in monkeys sustained GAL-101 concentrations >100 nM in the retina for >2 h. Compelling data from GAL-101 eye drops in animal models have demonstrated more than 90% neuroprotection. In vitro studies of neuronal cells that have lost function have shown reversal neural function by GAL-101.[44]

Present status: Based on preclinical and phase 1 study, planning to advance to phase 2/3.

Comments: GAL-101 is a novel small molecule and blocks the formation of all forms of toxic Aβ oligomers, in which it binds with high affinity to the misfolded amyloid-β monomers before they can form toxic soluble oligomers.[44] GAL-101 prevents synaptotoxic effects of $A\beta_{1-42}$ oligomers on synaptic plasticity and cognition, thus showing a promising applicability in Alzheimer's disease. Moreover, long-lasting in vivo effects indicate that GA-101 seeds a beneficial self-replication of nontoxic Aβ aggregates.[45] In animal models of Alzheimer's disease and dry AMD, both systemic and topical administration of CAL-101 demonstrate the neuroprotective effects.

RT011

Study name: Second deuterated polyunsaturated fatty acid (D-PUFA) drug (RT011), targeting the treatment of AMD phase 1 study.

Objectives: To determine if oral D-PUFA is safe; to evaluate if long-term oral D-PUFA can reduce PUFA peroxidation, because oxidative PUFA is associated with neurodegenerative diseases including AMD.[46]

Sponsors: Retrotope.

Study time: 36 months.

Patients enrolled: 59 participants.

Treatment regimen: Oral dosing at 1.8 g/d and 9.0 g/d.

Outcome measures: The safety profile of a long-term treatment, the accumulation in the percentage of D-PUFA in plasma and red blood cell membrane, and pharmacokinetics of RT001 were studied.

Results: RT011 has a good safety profile and a clear MOA.

Present status: Because of the good safety profile and a clear MOA of RT001, the phases of the clinical trial will be advanced.

Comments: RT001 is a bis-allylic-di-deuterated analog of linoleic acid.[47] RT001 has a novel MOA. When the concentrations of tissue deuterium-stabilized PUFA (D-PUFA) reach a certain level, deuterium stabilization confers oxidation-resistance and maintains PUFA's essential functional properties. Evidence suggests that toxic byproducts from PUFA oxidation are major drivers of AMD and multiple other retinal atrophies.[47]

Visual cycle modulation
ALK-001

Study name: Study of C20-D3-vitamin A molecule (ALK-001) in GA (phase 1).[48]

Objectives: To determine if oral ALK-001 is safe; to evaluate if it could slow the progression of GA.

Sponsors: Alkeus Pharmaceuticals, Inc.

Study time: 24 months.

Patients enrolled: 300 participants.

Treatment regimen: 300 participants randomized in a 2:1 ratio to receive oral daily capsule ALK-001 or placebo.

Outcome measures: Growth rate of GA lesions, as assessed by fundus autofluorescence (FAF); Secondary outcome measures include safety and tolerability, pharmacokinetics, plasma concentrations of ALK-001 and metabolites, incidence of choroidal neovascularization, visual acuity, and reading speed changes from baseline to 24 months.[48]

Results: C20-D3-vitamin A molecule began human clinical trials in Stargardt macular dystrophy. A phase 1 trial, an assessment of the safety and pharmacokinetics in healthy volunteers, has been completed.

Present status: The clinical trial phase 2/3 is ongoing.

Comments: The visual cycle is a series of biochemical events in outer retina photoreceptors and RPE, in which light is converted to an electric signal transmitting to the brain. The fundamental goal of the visual cycle is to convert all-trans-retinal back to 11-cis-retinal and to shuttle them between RPE and photoreceptors.[49] Several promising visual cycle modulators have been tested to maintain and restore this function in retinal diseases. It has been known that the rate-determining step in vitamin A dimerization is at the C20 carbon—hydrogen bond of the retinaldehyde—PE Schiff base.[50] Replacing the C20 hydrogen of vitamin A with deuterium (i.e., ALK-001) makes this bond resistant to cleave and retards vitamin A dimerization. Whether retardation of vitamin A dimerization could slow lipofuscin formation in RPE of dry AMD patients requires further study.

Inflammasome inhibition

Kamuvudine

Study name: Preclinical study of kamuvudine, an inhibitor of inflammasome activation, for AMD associated inflammatory events.

Objectives: To determine if kamuvudine is safe and effective for inhibition of inflammasome activation.

Sponsors: Inflammasome Therapeutics.

Comments: Kamuvudine is derived from nucleoside reverse-transcriptase inhibitors (NRTIs). It showed robust inhibition on inflammasome activation in cell culture and animal models. In multiple preclinical tests, it showed over 1000-times less toxic than its parent molecules and highly effective in models of AMD. The pathogenic role of the activated inflammasome in dry AMD has been introduced in Chapter 7.[51]

Xiflam

Study name: Xiflam (Tonabersat), an inhibitor of inflammasome, for the potential treatment of dry AMD (preclinical and phase 1 trial).

Objectives: To determine the safety and antiinfalmmatory efficacy of oral Xiflam via inhibition of inflammasome on in vitro and in vivo models of AMD.

Sponsors: OcuNexus.

Present status: Based on preclinical data and over 1000 humans in clinical trials (for prophylactic treatment of migraine, oral Xiflam showed a good safety profile and inhibitory effects on connexin hemichannel opening.[52,53] Therefore, Xiflam for treatment of dry AMD (phase 2 trial) is ongoing.

Comments: Xiflam is a novel small molecule, known as a hemichannel blocker. Connexins are gap junction proteins. Each connexin molecule is composed of two hemichannels. Under physiological conditions, hemichannels at the cell surface confer low membrane permeability. When hemichannels responding to insults such as ischemia and inflammation, a large nonselective membrane channel opens, which has been termed "pathologic membrane pore."[54] Mugisho et al. recently demonstrated in animal models that connexin43 is upregulated with inflammation. The upregulated connexin43 protein correlates with NLRP3 inflammasome complex assembly. These findings indicate that the inhibition of connexin hemichannels, resulting suppressed inflammasome assembly, is a rational approach mitigating inflammatory events in AMD.[53]

Matrix modulation

Doxycycline

Study name: Clinical study to evaluate treatment with ORACEA (doxycycline) for geographic atrophy (TOGA).[55]

Objectives: To evaluate the inhibitory effect of oral doxycycline on GA growth.

Sponsors: Oracea.

Study time: 30 months.

Patients enrolled: 286 patients with GA.

Treatment regimen: Patients randomized in a 1:1 ratio to either ORACEA (40 mg doxycycline) or placebo capsule once daily for 24 months, extending to 30-month.

Outcome measures: Primary outcome measures the rate of enlargement in the area of geographic atrophy in the study eye during the treatment period. Secondary outcome measures changes in best corrected visual acuity.

Results: ORACEA(doxycycline) has a good safety profile in long-term clinical observation. Numerous experiments demonstrated the doxycycline functions of matrix modulation and antiinflammation.

Present status: Advancing to phase2/3 clinical trial for GA.

Comments: Doxycycline was FDA-approved an antibiotic in 1967, which was labeled with same side-effects as that of tetracycline.[56] Notably, recent studies reported that little or no effects of doxycycline on tooth staining or dental enamel hypoplasia in children under 8 years old. In the United States, the Centers for Disease Control and Prevention confirmed the antibiotic properties, antiinflammatory properties, and good safety profile of doxycycline.[57] In addition, the effect of doxycycline on matrix remodeling has been proposed to play a regulatory role in the extracellular matrix (ECM) pathology of AMD patients.[58] For instance, the formation of drusen is due to the malfunction of the RPE cells and the dysregulation of the remodeling of the ECM in specific regions of Bruch's membrane.[59] The ECM remodeling is closely regulated by matrix metalloproteinases (MMPs) and the tissue inhibitors of metalloproteinases (TIMPs). AMD is characterized by the reduced function of the photoreceptor and RPE cells, including pathological matrix remodeling, cell degradation, cell proliferation, neovascularization, and chronic inflammation. The modulation of ECM turnover by changing the RPE secretion of MMPs and TIMPs may play a central role in the pathogenesis of AMD. One of the molecular targets of doxycycline is MMPs.[57] Doxycycline is a derivative and the most potent MMP inhibitor among tetracyclines. Similarly to doxycycline, another second-generation product of tetracycline, minocycline, has been shown to slow the growth rate of GA associated with dry AMD.[60]

HtrA1 inhibitor
FHTR2163

Study name: A Study Assessing the Safety, Tolerability, and Efficacy of RO7171009 (FHTR2163) in Participants affected with GA due to AMD (GALLEGO).

Objectives: To determine the safety, tolerability, and efficacy of FHTR2163.

Sponsors: Genentech, Inc.

Study time: 72 weeks.

Patients enrolled: 285 participants.

Treatment regimen: Participants receive intravitreal FHTR2163 either every four or 8 weeks compared with sham at Q4W or Q8W.

Outcome measures: Primary outcome measures change from baseline in GA Area by FAF at week 72; secondary outcome measures ocular and systemic adverse events.

Results: In the phase 1 study, FHTR2163 demonstrated a good safety profile.

Present status: Enrolling for phase 2 trial.

Comments: Genome-wide association studies (GWAS) identified three mutations of AMD-associated genetic locus at 10q26 (see Chapter 9). These mutations are inseparable because of high linkage disequilibrium.[61] Among them, the SNP, rs11200638, in the promoter of High-Temperature Requirement A Serine Peptidase 1 (*HTRA1*) is linked to AMD.[62] HtrA1 protein is expressed in the RPE of the human retina.[63] It contains a protease domain, catalytic domain, and several functional domains. The change of HtrA1 activity is thought to be linked to AMD pathology. Therefore, inhibition of HtrA1 became a strategy to treat AMD. Based on preclinical and phase 1 study, FHTR2163, a HtrA1 inhibitor with a good safety profile, has been designed to test the therapeutic hypothesis that inhibition of HtrA1 leads to a slow progression of GA.

Stem cell-based treatment

Although there are numerous advances in the therapeutic pipeline for dry AMD, the late stage of dry AMD, that is, geographic atrophy, is still an incurable blinding condition. Therefore, cell-based treatment replacing or rejuvenating the diseased cells of the outer retina in GA is an attractive approach. As we have assumed, the primary GA pathology originates from the RPE layer. In AMD, the capacity of RPE for maintaining the normal function of the overlying photoreceptor and the integrity of the underlying Bruch's membrane is gradually lost. As the comprehensive introduction of stem cell-based transplantation strategies for GA is beyond the scope of this chapter, only a few sources of stem cells for derived-RPE in the pipeline are listed as follows:

(1). Induced pluripotent stem cells (iPSC) are from autologous tissue sources. The major advantage of iPSC-RPE is the prevention of immune rejection. However, this kind of advantage of iPSC-RPEs may be lost because during the reprogramming from somatic cells they turn to be immunogenic.[64] Recent studies reported that successfully differentiated the iPSCs toward an iPSC-RPEs are able to possess specific characteristics of healthy RPE.[65] This preclinical achievement may lead to the application of iPSC-RPE as a cell-based treatment to GA.

(2). Human embryonic stem cells (hESC) are promising allogenic source for cell-based replacement therapies due to their availability and pluripotency. da Cruz et al. reported a phase 1 clinical study using engineered hESC-RPE patch for transplantation to subretinal space for two end-stage exudative AMD patients, although the authors actually aimed to study the RPE patch in dry AMD in the future.[66] This study showed an encouraging safety profile including well-controlled immunogenicity and tumorigenicity. After 12-month postoperative period, the transplanted hESC survived and the patients' vision gained substantially. The successful phase 1/2 transplantation of hESC-derived RPE for advanced Stargardt disease was also reported recently.[67] All of these studies have laid down the foundation for further hESC-RPE clinical trials of GA. Currently, hESC-RPE replacement therapy sponsored by Lineage Cell Therapeutics is in a phase 1/2a, multicenter, clinical trial.[68]

The studies on other stem cell-derived RPE such as umbilical stem cells and human retinal progenitor cells are underway.[69]

By using cellular and gene-based therapies to date, the aim for the regeneration of the degenerated cells and/or the continuous secretion of cell-protecting agents has been explored in different clinical trials. These trials include cell-based drug delivery systems, stem cells of different origins, as well as virus-mediated gene therapy approaches.

Therapies for neovascular AMD in pipeline

Neovascular AMD (nAMD) is characterized by the pathologic CNV beneath the macula. CNV causes exudation of blood and/or fluid into the outer retina. Progressively, neovascular tissue, exudates, and associated inflammation develop into a destructive macular scar, resulting in central blindness. Scientific evidences showed that VEGF is one of the main drivers of angiogenesis in CNV development.[70] The application of intravitreal anti-VEGF agents has revolutionized the treatment of nAMD. However, to improve visual outcomes and overcome the bottle-necks in anti-VEGF therapy, the ongoing nAMD treatments in the pipeline focus on targets of VEGF-related angiogenetic pathways, combination strategies, long-acting/sustained release agents, and gene therapies. In this chapter, only pharmaceutical pipelines involved in selected angiogenetic pathways, that is, extracellular VEGF, tyrosine kinase, angiopoietin-Tie2, and integrin are introduced.

Extracellular VEGF pathways
KSI-301

Study name: KSI-301phase 1 study.[71]

Objectives: To determine the safety and tolerability of intravitreal KSI-301, and to evaluate if it can impact the improvement of vision.

Sponsors: Kodiak Sciences.

Study time: 12 weeks.

Patients enrolled: 9 patients with severe diabetic macular edema.

Treatment regimen: Up to 5 mg of each dose.

Outcome measures: Primary outcome measures any side effect after intravitreal KSI-301. Secondary outcome measures BCVA changes from baseline.

Results: At 12-week postinjection follow-up, no serious side effects were documented. The median of 9 ETDRS letter vision improvement across all dose groups was achieved.

Present status: Phase 1b study in patients with treatment-naïve nAMD is recruiting. The efficacy of KSI-301 will be compared with 8-week dosing of aflibercept.[71]

Comments: The antibody biopolymer conjugate technique is used to synthesize KSI-301 with high molecular weight.[72] It has two components, that is, a specific anti-VEGF IgG1 antibody and an inert immune effector that is covalently and stably linked to a high molecular weight phosphorycholine biopolymer.[73] When the molecular weight is compared among the following compounds, it shows 950 kDa for KSI-301, 48 kDa for ranibizumab, 115 kDa for aflibercept, and 149 kDa for bevacizumab, respectively. If a 3.5-fold greater molar dose than aflibercept is used, the estimated intraocular anti-VEGF effect at 3 months could be 1000-fold greater than aflibercept.[73] Therefore, a high intraocular durability is expected for intravitreal KSI-301.

OPT-302

Study name: OPT-302 combination therapy for neovascular AMD phase 2b study.[71]

Objectives: To evaluate the efficacy of intravitreal OPT-302 on the improvement of visual acuity and reduction of macular thickness as compared with the control.

Sponsors: Opthea.

Study time: 24 weeks.

Patients enrolled: 366 wet AMD patients.

Treatment regimen: This is a randomized, double-masked, sham-controlled clinical trial.

The patients are randomized in a 1:1:1 ratio to receive one of the following treatment regimens: every 4 weeks for 24 weeks: OPT-302 (0.5 mg) in combination with ranibizumab (0.5 mg); OPT-302 (2.0 mg) in combination with ranibizumab (0.5 mg); or sham in combination with ranibizumab (0.5 mg).

Outcome measures: Primary endpoint was mean visual acuity gain and macular thickness by OCT at 24 weeks compared to ranibizumab monotherapy in treatment-naïve patients with nAMD.

Results: Based on phase 1/2a study for treatment-naïve patients, intravitreal OPT-302 has been proven to be a safe procedure for nAMD. Phase 2b study met the primary endpoints, showing the superiority of efficacy over ranibizumab alone for nAMD.

Present status: Primary endpoint in phase 2b study has met.

Comments: OPT-302 specifically targets VEGF-C and VEGF-D, which may play a complementary role in nAMD pathogenesis (see Chapter 10). The phase 2b trial entry criteria allowed for randomization of patients with a broad range of CNV that is divided into type 1 (occult) and type 2 (classic) membranes as well as more distinct subtypes of polypoidal choroidal vasculopathy (PCV) and retinal angiomatous proliferation.[74] The expanded indication of OPT-302 for different types of CNV may potentially overcome some limitations of therapies that only target VEGF-A in neovascular eye diseases.

Tyrosine kinase inhibitor pathways
PAN-90806

Study name: PAN-90806 phase 1/2 trial: Once-daily topical anti-VEGF biologics eye drop for nAMD.[75]

Objectives: To determine the safety and tolerability of topical PAN-90806 eye drop; to evaluate anti-VEGF response through tyrosine kinase inhibition.

Sponsors: Panoptica.

Study time: 28 weeks.

Patients enrolled: 51 patients.

Treatment regimen: Patients were randomized to three dose groups (10 mg/mL, 6 mg/mL, and 2 mg/mL) as 1:1:1 ratio; once a day monotherapy for 12 weeks and follow up to 16 weeks.

Outcome measures: Primary endpoints were safety and tolerability; secondary endpoints were anti-VEGF biological response.

Results: 88% patients who followed the treatment regimen without any rescued treatment showed clinical improvement or stability.

Present status: Advancing to phase 2 and phase 3 trials.

Comments: PAN-90806 (PanOptica) is a tyrosine kinase inhibitor (TKi) eye drop. It is able to produce an anti-VEGF-A response comparable to currently available anti-VEGF-A therapies in half of 51 treatment naïve nAMD patients.[75] The newer eye drop (suspension) is designed to reduce the incidence of punctate keratopathy as a side effect.

Tie2 activation pathways

Faricimab

Study name: Phase 2 studies in nAMD for bispecific molecule, Faricimab.[76]

Objectives: To determine faricimab is a safe and well-tolerated agent; to evaluate if faricimab could provide sustainable vision improvement of nAMD patients who received the treatment.

Sponsors: Genentech/Roche.

Study time: 52 weeks.

Patients enrolled: 76 nAMD patients.

Treatment regimen: Faricimab (6.0 mg) was given in four weekly loading doses followed by two different dosing schedules of q16w (6 mg) and q12w (1.5 mg) dosing and compared to 0.5 mg of ranibizumab in q4w dosing.

Outcome measures: The primary endpoint is the change in BCVA at week 48 from baseline.

Results: Overall, 65% patients treated with faricimab were free of disease activity at week 24. Measurements of the BCVA showed that the gains in vision achieved with the every-16-week flex dosing and every-12-week dosing were maintained at week 52 and were comparable to those seen with monthly ranibizumab (+11.42, +10.08, and +9.59 letters, respectively).[77]

Present status: Advancing to phase 3 trial.

Comments: The bottle-necks in anti-VEGF therapy for nAMD include resistance, nonresponse, and recurrences of pathology in many cases. Faricimab was developed on CrossMAB platform by Genentech/Roche to produce biologically engineered bispecific molecules. In other words, faricimab is able to block both angiopoietin 2 (Ang-2) and VEGF. Both of them synergistically drive vascular instability, neovascularization, and inflammation in nAMD (see Chapter 8). Therefore, faricimab discovery, known as bsAb, is conceptually beyond the horizon of VEGF in the treatment of nAMD.[78]

AXT107

Study name: AXT107 for treatment of neovascular AMD.

Objectives: In preclinical study on AXT107, a collagen IV-derived peptide, AXT107 was tested if it has antiangiogenic effect via regulation of the integrin pathway.

Sponsors: Asclepix Therapeutics.

Treatment regimen: By using mouse models with laser-induced CNV, ischemia-induced CNV, sub-retinal NV in *rho/VEGF* mice, and VEGF-induced leakage, intraocular injection of 0.1 or 1 μg of AXT107 was performed.[79]

Outcome measures: Suppression of CNV, subretinal NV and VEGF-induced leakage and binding AXT107 to α5β1 and αvβ3 integrin.

Results: The primary outcome are met (see Comments below).

Present status: Phase 1 clinical trial is underway.

Comments: The interaction between integrin and extracellular matrix is pivotally important to keep optimal ligand-induced phosphorylation of multiple receptors such as VEGFR2, c-Met (a receptor tyrosine kinase), and PDGFRβ. The complex formation with β3 integrin was reduced by AXT107 binding to αvβ3. AXT107 also reduced total VEGFR2 levels by increasing internalization, ubiquitination, and degradation.[79] In a separated study, AXT107 potentiated Tie2 phosphorylation and stabilizes retinal vasculature in vivo. When AXT107 disrupts α5β1, it stimulates the relocation of Tie2 and α5 to cell junctions, leading to a reduction of permeability.[80] In a uveitis model, intravitreal AXT107 substantially suppressed inflammation-induced vascular leakage via disruption of integrin.[81] AXT107, a biomimetic peptide appears to be a sustained, multitargeted therapy that may be proved to have advantages over routine intraocular injections of specific VEGF-neutralizing proteins in future clinical trials.

Integrin pathways

Integrins are cell-adhesion molecules involved in angiogenesis signaling pathways and are overexpressed in many angiogenic processes including nAMD.[80,82] Therefore, integrin-targeted molecules have been designed to control the balance between proangiogenic and antiangiogenic proteins for exploring the new treatment of nAMD. In the pipeline of nAMD therapies, integrin-targeted agents, risuteganib and AXT107, have been exemplified in this chapter (vide supra).

This chapter has briefly discussed the ongoing investigative treatment in the pipeline. At the end of the discussion, we must admit that this summary is neither comprehensive nor detailed enough, because following the new development in AMD treatment is difficult. It is best to cite Dr. Peter Kaiser's comments that "Therapeutic options move from one phase to the next at different times and at different rates, and drugs may start their path in one disease only to find success treating another."[2]

References

1. Fisher DE, Klein BEK, Wong TY, et al. Incidence of age-related macular degeneration in a multi-ethnic United States population. *Ophthalmology*. 2016;123(6):1297—1308. https://doi.org/10.1016/j.ophtha.2015.12.026.

2. Kaiser P. Retina pipeline A view into ongoing innovation. *Retina Today.* November/December 2019.

3. Gil-Martínez M, Santos-Ramos P, Fernández-Rodríguez M, et al. Pharmacological advances in the treatment of age-related macular degeneration. *Comput Mater Continua.* 2020;27(4):583–598. https://doi.org/10.2174/0929867326666190726121711.

4. Yaspan BL, Williams DF, Holz FG, et al. Targeting factor D of the alternative complement pathway reduces geographic atrophy progression secondary to age-related macular degeneration. *Sci Transl Med.* 2017;9(395). https://doi.org/10.1126/scitranslmed.aaf1443.

5. Holz FG, Sadda SR, Busbee B, et al. Efficacy and safety of lampalizumab for geographic atrophy due to age-related macular degeneration: chroma and spectri phase 3 randomized clinical trials. *JAMA Ophthalmol.* 2018;136(6):666–677. https://doi.org/10.1001/jamaophthalmol.2018.1544.

6. Yehoshua Z, de Amorim Garcia Filho CA, Nunes RP, et al. Systemic complement inhibition with eculizumab for geographic atrophy in age-related macular degeneration: the COMPLETE study. *Ophthalmology.* 2014;121(3):693–701. https://doi.org/10.1016/j.ophtha.2013.09.044.

7. Liao DS, Grossi FV, El Mehdi D, et al. Complement C3 inhibitor pegcetacoplan for geographic atrophy secondary to age-related macular degeneration: a randomized phase 2 trial. *Ophthalmology.* 2020;127(2):186–195. https://doi.org/10.1016/j.ophtha.2019.07.011.

8. He Y, Hara H, Núñez G. Mechanism and regulation of NLRP3 inflammasome activation. *Trends Biochem Sci.* 2016;41(12):1012–1021. https://doi.org/10.1016/j.tibs.2016.09.002.

9. Jaffe GJ, Westby K, Csaky KG, et al. *C5 Inhibitor Avacincaptad Pegol for Geographic Atrophy Due to Age-Related Macular Degeneration: A Randomized Pivotal Phase 2/3 Trial. Ophthalmology.* 2020. https://doi.org/10.1016/j.ophtha.2020.08.027. Published online August 31.

10. Harris CL, Pouw RB, Kavanagh D, Sun R, Ricklin D. Developments in anti-complement therapy; from disease to clinical trial. *Mol Immunol.* 2018;102:89–119. https://doi.org/10.1016/j.molimm.2018.06.008.

11. Clark SJ, Perveen R, Hakobyan S, et al. Impaired binding of the age-related macular degeneration-associated complement factor H 402H allotype to Bruch's membrane in human retina. *J Biol Chem.* 2010;285(39):30192–30202. https://doi.org/10.1074/jbc.M110.103986.

12. Prosser BE, Johnson S, Roversi P, et al. Structural basis for complement factor H–linked age-related macular degeneration. *J Exp Med.* 2007;204(10):2277–2283. https://doi.org/10.1084/jem.20071069.

13. Schnabolk G, Parsons N, Obert E, et al. Delivery of CR2-fH using AAV vector therapy as treatment strategy in the mouse model of choroidal neovascularization. *Mol Ther - Meth Clin Develop.* 2018;9:1–11. https://doi.org/10.1016/j.omtm.2017.11.003.

14. Tomlinson S, Thurman JM. Tissue-targeted complement therapeutics. *Mol Immunol.* 2018;102:120–128. https://doi.org/10.1016/j.molimm.2018.06.005.

15. Johnson G. *Annexon Biosciences Reports Top-Line Phase 1b Results for Novel C1q Inhibitor ANX007 in Glaucoma.* October 9, 2019.

16. Jiao H, Rutar M, Fernando N, et al. Subretinal macrophages produce classical complement activator C1q leading to the progression of focal retinal degeneration. *Mol Neurodegener.* 2018;13(1):45. https://doi.org/10.1186/s13024-018-0278-0.

17. Furfine E, Rao A, Baker S, et al. Pegylated CB2782: a complement factor C3-inactivating protease and potential long-acting treatment for dry AMD. In: *Investigative Ophthalmology & Visual Science July 2019.* Vol. 60. 2019:374.

18. Nie S, Wang Z, Moscoso-Castro M, et al. Biology drives the discovery of bispecific antibodies as innovative therapeutics. *Antibody Therap.* 2020;3(1):18−62. https://doi.org/10.1093/abt/tbaa003.

19. Dugel PU. Clinical trial download: data on a gene therapy for dry and wet AMD. *Retin Physician.* 2020;17(April 1, 2010):16, 17.

20. Biosciences H. Preventing progression of dry age-related macular degeneration (AMD). *June.* 2020;16.

21. Wiles JA, Galvan MD, Podos SD, Geffner M, Huang M. Discovery and development of the oral complement factor D inhibitor danicopan (ACH-4471). *Comput Mater Continua.* 2020;27(25):4165−4180. https://doi.org/10.2174/0929867326666191001130342.

22. Yuan X, Gavriilaki E, Thanassi JA, et al. Small-molecule factor D inhibitors selectively block the alternative pathway of complement in paroxysmal nocturnal hemoglobinuria and atypical hemolytic uremic syndrome. *Haematologica.* 2017;102(3):466−475. https://doi.org/10.3324/haematol.2016.153312.

23. Johnson DS, Weerapana E, Cravatt BF. Strategies for discovering and derisking covalent, irreversible enzyme inhibitors. *Future Med Chem.* 2010;2(6):949−964. https://doi.org/10.4155/fmc.10.21.

24. J Jaffe G, Sahni J, Fauser S, Geary RS, Schneider E, McCaleb M. Development of IONIS-FB-LRx to treat geographic atrophy associated with AMD. In: *Investigative Ophthalmology & Visual Science July 2019.* Vol. 61. 2020:4305.

25. Grossman TR, Carrer M, Shen L, et al. Reduction in ocular complement factor B protein in mice and monkeys by systemic administration of factor B antisense oligonucleotide. *Mol Vis.* 2017;23:561−571.

26. Priyatham (prithu) mettu, scott cousins. The ReCLAIM phase 1 clinical trial of elamipretide for dry AMD. *Retin Physic.* November/December 2019;16(Issue).

27. Petcherski A, Trudeau KM, Wolf DM, et al. Elamipretide promotes mitophagosome formation and prevents its reduction induced by nutrient excess in INS1 β-cells. *J Mol Biol.* 2018;430(24):4823−4833. https://doi.org/10.1016/j.jmb.2018.10.020.

28. Liu S, Soong Y, Seshan SV, Szeto HH. Novel cardiolipin therapeutic protects endothelial mitochondria during renal ischemia and mitigates microvascular rarefaction, inflammation, and fibrosis. *Am J Physiol Renal Physiol.* 2014;306(9):F970−F980. https://doi.org/10.1152/ajprenal.00697.2013.

29. Bartel K, Pein H, Popper B, et al. Connecting lysosomes and mitochondria - a novel role for lipid metabolism in cancer cell death. *Cell Commun Signal.* 2019;17(1):87. https://doi.org/10.1186/s12964-019-0399-2.

30. Shaw LT, Mackin A, Shah R, et al. Risuteganib-a novel integrin inhibitor for the treatment of non-exudative (dry) age-related macular degeneration and diabetic macular edema. *Expert Opin Investig Drugs.* 2020;29(6):547−554. https://doi.org/10.1080/13543784.2020.1763953.

31. BARUCH D. KUPPERMANN. Risuteganib for intermediate dry AMD. *Retin Physic.* November/December, 2019;16:28, 30, 31.

32. Bhatwadekar AD, Kansara V, Luo Q, Ciulla T. Anti-integrin therapy for retinovascular diseases. *Expert Opin Investig Drug.* 2020:1−11. https://doi.org/10.1080/13543784.2020.1795639. Published online September 9.

33. Hakan K, Hartmut S. *Photobiomodulation as a Treatment in Dry AMD. Retina Today.* May/June 2020.

34. Markowitz SN, Devenyi RG, Munk MR, et al. A double-masked, randomized, sham-controlled, single-center study with photobiomodulation for the treatment OF dry age-

related macular degeneration. *Retina*. 2020;40(8):1471–1482. https://doi.org/10.1097/IAE.0000000000002632.

35. Chung H, Dai T, Sharma SK, Huang Y-Y, Carroll JD, Hamblin MR. The nuts and bolts of low-level laser (light) therapy. *Ann Biomed Eng*. 2012;40(2):516–533. https://doi.org/10.1007/s10439-011-0454-7.

36. Wong-Riley MTT, Liang HL, Eells JT, et al. Photobiomodulation directly benefits primary neurons functionally inactivated by toxins: role of cytochrome *c* oxidase. *J Biol Chem*. 2005;280(6):4761–4771. https://doi.org/10.1074/jbc.M409650200.

37. Kuppermann BD, Patel SS, Boyer DS, et al. *Phase 2 Study of the Safety and Efficacy of Brimonidine Drug Delivery System (BRIMO DDS) Generation 1 in Patients with Geographic Atrophy Secondary to Age-Related Macular Degeneration. Retina (Philadelphia, Pa)*. 2020. https://doi.org/10.1097/IAE.0000000000002789. Published online March 3.

38. Ramírez C, Cáceres-del-Carpio J, Chu J, et al. Brimonidine can prevent in vitro hydroquinone damage on retinal pigment epithelium cells and retinal müller cells. *J Ocul Pharmacol Ther*. 2016;32(2):102–108. https://doi.org/10.1089/jop.2015.0083.

39. Ortín-Martínez A, Valiente-Soriano FJ, García-Ayuso D, et al. A novel in vivo model of focal light emitting diode-induced cone-photoreceptor phototoxicity: neuroprotection afforded by brimonidine, BDNF, PEDF or bFGF. *PloS One*. 2014;9(12):e113798. https://doi.org/10.1371/journal.pone.0113798.

40. Saylor M, McLoon LK, Harrison AR, Lee MS. Experimental and clinical evidence for brimonidine as an optic nerve and retinal neuroprotective agent: an evidence-based review. *Arch Ophthalmol*. 2009;127(4):402–406. https://doi.org/10.1001/archophthalmol.2009.9.

41. Gao J, Sun Z, Xiao Z, et al. Dexmedetomidine modulates neuroinflammation and improves outcome via alpha2-adrenergic receptor signaling after rat spinal cord injury. *Br J Anaesth*. 2019;123(6):827–838. https://doi.org/10.1016/j.bja.2019.08.026.

42. Manickavasagam D, Wehrung D, Chamsaz EA, et al. Assessment of alkoxylphenacyl-based polycarbonates as a potential platform for controlled delivery of a model anti-glaucoma drug. *Eur J Pharm Biopharm*. 2016;107:56–66. https://doi.org/10.1016/j.ejpb.2016.06.012.

43. Shinno K, Kurokawa K, Kozai S, Kawamura A, Inada K, Tokushige H. The relationship of brimonidine concentration in vitreous body to the free concentration in retina/choroid following topical administration in pigmented rabbits. *Curr Eye Res*. 2017;42(5):748–753. https://doi.org/10.1080/02713683.2016.1238941.

44. Abraham J. *Galimedix Therapeutics, Inc.'s GAL-101 Gains from Target Validation by Positive Phase 3 Results of Biogen's Aducanumab*. Galimedix Therapeutics, Inc.; 2019.

45. Rammes G, Parsons CG. The Aβ aggregation modulator MRZ-99030 prevents and even reverses synaptotoxic effects of Aβ1-42 on LTP even following serial dilution to a 500:1 stoichiometric excess of Aβ1-42, suggesting a beneficial prion-like seeding mechanism. *Neuropharmacology*. 2020;179:108267. https://doi.org/10.1016/j.neuropharm.2020.108267.

46. Molinari RJ. A novel class ofDrugs to fighta multitude of degenerative diseases. *Retrotope Newslett*. July 21, 2020.

47. Brenna JT, James G, Midei M, et al. Plasma and red blood cell membrane accretion and pharmacokinetics of RT001 (bis-Allylic 11,11-D2-linoleic acid ethyl ester) during long term dosing in patients. J Pharmaceut Sci. Published online August 2020: S0022354920304895. doi:10.1016/j.xphs.2020.08.019.

48. Saad L. *Phase 3 Study of ALK-001 in Geographic Atrophy (SAGA)*. Alkeus Pharmaceuticals, Inc; 2019.

49. Hussain RM, Gregori NZ, Ciulla TA, Lam BL. Pharmacotherapy of retinal disease with visual cycle modulators. *Expert Opin Pharmacother.* 2018;19(5):471−481. https://doi.org/10.1080/14656566.2018.1448060.

50. Kaufman Y, Ma L, Washington I. Deuterium enrichment of vitamin A at the C20 position slows the formation of detrimental vitamin A dimers in wild-type rodents. *J Biol Chem.* 2011;286(10):7958−7965. https://doi.org/10.1074/jbc.M110.178640.

51. Jedynak B. Boehringer ingelheim partners with inflammasome therapeutics to develop novel therapies for patients with retinal diseases. *Inflammasome Therap.* 2019;20. September.

52. Kim Y, Griffin JM, Nor MNM, et al. Tonabersat prevents inflammatory damage in the central nervous system by blocking Connexin43 hemichannels. *Neurotherap: J Am Soci Experiment NeuroTherap.* 2017;14(4):1148−1165. https://doi.org/10.1007/s13311-017-0536-9.

53. Mugisho OO, Rupenthal ID, Paquet-Durand F, Acosta ML, Green CR. Targeting connexin hemichannels to control the inflammasome: the correlation between connexin43 and NLRP3 expression in chronic eye disease. *Expert Opin Ther Targets.* 2019; 23(10):855−863. https://doi.org/10.1080/14728222.2019.1673368.

54. Decrock E, Vinken M, De Vuyst E, et al. Connexin-related signaling in cell death: to live or let die? *Cell Death Differ.* 2009;16(4):524−536. https://doi.org/10.1038/cdd.2008.196.

55. P.A Yates. Clinical Study to Evaluate Treatment with ORACEA® for Geographic Atrophy (TOGA). Published online December 2020.

56. Gaillard T, Briolant S, Madamet M, Pradines B. The end of a dogma: the safety of doxycycline use in young children for malaria treatment. *Malar J.* 2017;16(1):148. https://doi.org/10.1186/s12936-017-1797-9.

57. Henehan M, Montuno M, De Benedetto A. Doxycycline as an anti-inflammatory agent: updates in dermatology. *J Eur Acad Dermatol Venereol.* 2017;31(11):1800−1808. https://doi.org/10.1111/jdv.14345.

58. García-Onrubia L, Valentín-Bravo FJ, Coco-Martin RM, et al. Matrix metalloproteinases in age-related macular degeneration (AMD). *IJMS.* 2020;21(16):5934. https://doi.org/10.3390/ijms21165934.

59. Luibl V, Isas JM, Kayed R, Glabe CG, Langen R, Chen J. Drusen deposits associated with aging and age-related macular degeneration contain nonfibrillar amyloid oligomers. *J Clin Invest.* 2006;116(2):378−385. https://doi.org/10.1172/JCI25843.

60. Wright C, Mazzucco AE, Becker SM, Sieving PA, Tumminia SJ. NEI-supported age-related macular degeneration research: past, present, and future. *Trans Vision Sci Technol.* 2020;9(7):49. https://doi.org/10.1167/tvst.9.7.49.

61. Tom I, Pham VC, Katschke KJ, et al. Development of a therapeutic anti-HtrA1 antibody and the identification of DKK3 as a pharmacodynamic biomarker in geographic atrophy. *Proc Nat Academy Sci U S A.* 2020;117(18):9952−9963. https://doi.org/10.1073/pnas.1917608117.

62. Yang Z, Camp NJ, Sun H, et al. A variant of the HTRA1 gene increases susceptibility to age-related macular degeneration. *Science.* 2006;314(5801):992−993. https://doi.org/10.1126/science.1133811.

63. Melo E, Oertle P, Trepp C, et al. HtrA1 mediated intracellular effects on tubulin using a polarized RPE disease model. *EBioMedicine.* 2018;27:258−274. https://doi.org/10.1016/j.ebiom.2017.12.011.

64. Zhao T, Zhang Z-N, Rong Z, Xu Y. Immunogenicity of induced pluripotent stem cells. *Nature*. 2011;474(7350):212−215. https://doi.org/10.1038/nature10135.

65. Hazim RA, Karumbayaram S, Jiang M, et al. Differentiation of RPE cells from integration-free iPS cells and their cell biological characterization. *Stem Cell Res Ther*. 2017;8(1):217. https://doi.org/10.1186/s13287-017-0652-9.

66. da Cruz L, Fynes K, Georgiadis O, et al. Phase 1 clinical study of an embryonic stem cell-derived retinal pigment epithelium patch in age-related macular degeneration. *Nat Biotechnol*. 2018;36(4):328−337. https://doi.org/10.1038/nbt.4114.

67. Mehat MS, Sundaram V, Ripamonti C, et al. Transplantation of human embryonic stem cell-derived retinal pigment epithelial cells in macular degeneration. *Ophthalmology*. 2018;125(11):1765−1775. https://doi.org/10.1016/j.ophtha.2018.04.037.

68. Hone IC. *Lineage Cell Therapeutics Reports Regeneration of Retinal Tissue in Patient Treated with OpRegen RPE Cells for Dry AMD with Geographic Atrophy*. Lineage Cell Therapeutics, Inc; June 1, 2020.

69. Kvanta A, Grudzinska MK. Stem cell-based treatment in geographic atrophy: promises and pitfalls. *Acta Ophthalmol*. 2014;92(1):21−26. https://doi.org/10.1111/aos.12185.

70. Marneros AG. Increased VEGF -A promotes multiple distinct aging diseases of the eye through shared pathomechanisms. *EMBO Mol Med*. 2016;8(3):208−231. https://doi.org/10.15252/emmm.201505613.

71. Al-Khersan H, Hussain RM, Ciulla TA, Dugel PU. Innovative therapies for neovascular age-related macular degeneration. *Expert Opin Pharmacother*. 2019;20(15):1879−1891. https://doi.org/10.1080/14656566.2019.1636031.

72. Samanta A, Aziz AA, Jhingan M, Singh SR, Khanani A, Chhablani J. Emerging therapies in neovascular age-related macular degeneration in 2020. *Asia Pac J Ophthalmol*. 2020;9(3):250−259. https://doi.org/10.1097/APO.0000000000000291.

73. Cunningham Jr ET. *Potential of KSI-301 to Extend Treatment*. 2019.

74. Baldwin M. Opthea presents additional data from OPT-302 phase 2b wet AMD trial. *BioSpace*. 2019;14. October.

75. Paul GC. *PAN-90806: Once-Daily Topical Anti-VEGF Eye Drop for Wet AMD*. 2019.

76. Khanani AM, Patel SS, Ferrone PJ, et al. Efficacy of every four monthly and quarterly dosing of faricimab vs ranibizumab in neovascular age-related macular degeneration: the STAIRWAY phase 2 randomized clinical trial. *JAMA Ophthalmol*. 2020;138(9):964. https://doi.org/10.1001/jamaophthalmol.2020.2699.

77. Danzig C. *ASRS 2020: Trial Shows Faricimab Blocks Ang-2 and VEGF-A*. Uly: Ophthalmology times; 2020.

78. Sharma A, Kumar N, Kuppermann BD, Bandello F, Loewenstein A. Faricimab: expanding horizon beyond VEGF. *Eye*. 2020;34(5):802−804. https://doi.org/10.1038/s41433-019-0670-1.

79. Lima e Silva R, Kanan Y, Mirando AC, et al. Tyrosine kinase blocking collagen IV−derived peptide suppresses ocular neovascularization and vascular leakage. *Sci Transl Med*. 2017;9(373):eaai8030. https://doi.org/10.1126/scitranslmed.aai8030.

80. Mirando AC, Shen J, Silva RLE, et al. A collagen IV-derived peptide disrupts α5β1 integrin and potentiates Ang2/Tie2 signaling. *JCI insight*. 2019;4(4). https://doi.org/10.1172/jci.insight.122043.

81. R. Formica. AXT107, a peptide that disrupts integrins, suppresses vascular leakage in the setting of ocular inflammation. In: ARVO Meeting Abstract. Vol Vol. 60. Investigative Ophthalmology & Visual Science July 2019,; 2019:4073.

82. Fang I-M, Yang C-H, Yang C-M, Chen M-S. Overexpression of integrin alpha6 and beta4 enhances adhesion and proliferation of human retinal pigment epithelial cells on layers of porcine Bruch's membrane. *Exp Eye Res*. 2009;88(1):12–21. https://doi.org/10.1016/j.exer.2008.09.019.

Basic and clinical studies of AMD in future: questions more than answers

Epidemiology models herald a challenging future

According to various forecasting models, life expectancy is projected to increase worldwide. There is a more than a 50% probability that by 2030 in 35 industrialized countries studied, national female life expectancy will break the 90-year barrier. In several countries on the top of this list, there is a roughly 27% probability that by 2030, male life expectancy will surpass 85 years.[1] As a consequence, by 2050 approximately a quarter of the world population will be the elderly.[2] Longer life actually is an incredibly valuable resource, not a socioeconomic burden.[3] However, aging that is defined as an age-specific decline in physiological function leads to an increase in age-specific diseases and mortality.[4] A systematic literature review identified all population-based studies of age-related macular degeneration (AMD) published before May 2013. By using the standard classification and severity scale as described in Chapters 3 and 4, the prevalence of different ethnicity subgroups was also measured. Overall, it has shown that the projected number of people with AMD is around 196 million in 2020, increasing to 288 million in 2040.[5] AMD affects central vision that significantly impairs patients' life of quality. Despite such a high disease burden, to date there is no proven treatment for advanced dry AMD, and current treatment for wet AMD is incompletely efficacious. Both the patients and physicians are facing great challenges ahead.

Molecular genetics-based strategies for AMD prevention and treatment

Molecular genetics-based GWAS have identified numerous loci coding for rare and common variants for AMD risk (see Chapter 9). However, translation of these loci into biological insights remains a challenge, because it is difficult to pinpoint very small effects of common disease-associated variants.[6] In addition, based on AMD-associated common variants, the genetics of AMD can only account for about

Age-Related Macular Degeneration. https://doi.org/10.1016/B978-0-12-822061-0.00008-6

70% of the predicted risk.[7] Future efforts will continue to identify rare and potentially highly penetrant variants in the genes already implicated from common loci, and discover other genes that may have been overlooked by traditional GWAS.[8]

The goals of molecular genetics in future research are to better understand AMD pathogenesis and to identify potentially preventive and therapeutic targets, as outlined in the following. The first aim is how to predict AMD initiation. To date, the study of genetic risk of AMD is based on the primary endpoint of advanced stages of disease, that is, neovascular AMD (nAMD) or geographic atrophy (GA). It has been realized that the genetic risks for AMD initiation are not necessarily the same as those for AMD progression. The latter is anticipated to develop into advanced AMD.[9] Because the presence of certain types of drusen can be defined as incident AMD, that is, the initiation of AMD pathology, the current genetic risk models are actually predicting disease progression beyond drusen formation. In other words, these models are not helpful for predicting incident AMD. Since the majority of the population has intermediate AMD risk, the predictive genetics for AMD progression would not be appropriate for predicting and preventing AMD initiation. Therefore, predictive genetic testing for incident AMD needs to be established.

The second aim is how to identify predictive genetics for AMD progression. The signaling pathways affected by functions of responsible genes will surely vary according to the gene involved. For instance, vascular endothelial growth factor receptor (VEGFR) gene variants may alter the risk of nAMD, but not play an important role in the initiation of AMD.[10] One way to obtain risk models for AMD progression is to use a longitudinal approach, in which combined genetic, environmental, and retinal feature risk are included.[11] Longitudinal risk models may be able to improve the prediction for AMD progression. The third aim is to correlate the genetic profiles of patients with the success or failure of their AMD treatment. The treatments for AMD are limited to date, comprising only nutritional supplements for certain types of dry AMD and anti-VEGF therapy for nAMD. The molecular genetic studies on the differential effect of the AREDS supplements among genotype groups have been inconclusive. A subgroup that could benefit from zinc supplementation in reducing progression to advanced AMD has been identified with risk allele for *CFH* or *ARMS2*.[12] In contrast, some reports have suggested that AREDS supplements are in fact harmful to a subset of patients.[13] Thus, the effectiveness of AREDS supplement appears to differ by genotype. Further study is needed to determine the biological basis for the interplay between genetic risk in specific subgroups and AREDS supplement intervention. In terms of anti-VEGF strategy for nAMD, clinicians have been eager to identify the anti-VEGF treatment responsive patients, hopefully by genetic testing. Numerous epidemiological and clinical studies showed that the degree of differential response among current anti-VEGF agents is relatively small.[14] Still, molecular genetic testing should be able to guide patients toward more effective prevention strategies, when considered in the context of environmental exposures, retinal or systemic biomarkers, and therapeutic options. At present, no genetic test can clearly establish if a patient is going to fail or succeed with a particular treatment protocol. In future research, genetics-based selection of therapies will only be relevant when there are multiple options. In the future, genetic testing may offer treatment choices for patients who are at the same stage of AMD.

Future translational research of AMD: learning from oncology

In 1963 Judah Folkman found a new way to think about cancer. He provided the first evidence that in the absence of a blood supply, tumors cannot grow more than 1–2 mm diameter.[15] In 1971, Folkman raised a hypothesis that tumor growth is angiogenesis-dependent and that antiangiogenesis could be therapeutic.[16] Based on the pioneering work of Folkman et al., antiangiogenesis has become one of the key strategies for treating angiogenesis-dependent tumors as well as other angiogenic disorders. The discovery of vascular endothelial growth factor (VEGF) and the identification of its role in angiogenesis in health and disease have conceptually elucidated the underlying process of physiological and pathological angiogenesis.[17,18] Pathological angiogenesis, that is, neovascularization, tends to occur at a relatively late stage in the course of many angiogenic disorders, such as neovascular AMD. However, as it represents a final common pathway with multifactorial etiologies, the upstream players of angiogenesis become attractive targets in different disease stages. For instance, upstream players like hypoxia, oxidative stress, or inflammation need to be considered at different stages of AMD. Rosenfeld et al. set up the best example learning from oncology, which is an intravitreal injection of bevacizumab, an anti-VEGF monoclonal antibody, for neovascular ocular diseases. The anti-VEGF therapy that is one of the essential therapies for cancer has been transplanted into the armamentarium for neovascular AMD.[19] Most importantly, the multifactorial mechanistic pathways leading to late-stage AMD share incredible similarity with pathogenic events of cancer. Therefore, it may be proposed that since multiple pathogenic targets of cancer have been investigated in preclinical and clinical trials, whether the harvested pharmacological fruits in the cancer research can prompt us to modify them for treating AMD to halt the disease progression and to improve the vision of patients?

Antiangiogenesis in cancer and AMD

Antiangiogenesis therapies are the best example of ophthalmologists learning from oncology. Judah Folkman initiated antitumor angiogenesis, which is much complex than that of nontumor conditions. Tumor cells persistently generate proangiogenic factors. Antitumor angiogenesis therapy can only achieve temporarily neovascular suppression. This is due to the characteristics of human cancer cells. Tumor cells possess sustained proliferation capacity, the capability of escaping apoptosis, and pervasive genomic instability, as a result of mutations in oncogenes and tumor suppressor genes.[20] Therefore, antitumor angiogenesis must combine with other therapies such as radiotherapy, chemotherapy, immune checkpoint blockers, and surgeries.[21] Currently, in the field of antitumor angiogenesis, the focus has been on developing VEGF and VEGFR inhibitors. Meanwhile, other antiangiogenic agents are in development for a variety of targets, such as the Ang-1/2 and Tie2 receptor axis, the $\alpha v\beta 3$, $\alpha v\beta 5$ and $\alpha 5\beta 1$ integrins, and the receptors FGFR-1-4, PDGFRβ, and VEGFR-1-3.[22,23]

Neovascular AMD is a nontumor, angiogenic disorder. Since the introduction of bevacizumab from oncology, anti-VEGF therapy has revolutionized nAMD treatment. In Chapter 11, we briefly described the antiangiogenesis drugs for nAMD currently in the pipeline, which essentially follows the rationale and ideas raised by oncology (Figure 10.2, in Chapter 10). However, the requirements for antiangiogenesis therapy in ophthalmology are different from that in oncology. First, the routes of local application such as intravitreal, suprachoroidal, and topical utilization are specific for ocular use. Second, as antiangiogenesis therapy is a long-term regimen, options of extended duration include an increase in half-life in the posterior segment, sustained delivery system, and polymer-extended release. Third, developing drugs with a minimal systemic exit is critical for reducing immunogenicity and treatment failure.[24] Based on these requirements, new antiangiogenic drugs including some previously antitumor angiogenesis agents will undergo clinical trials.[25]

Antioxidant supplements in cancer and AMD

Reactive species, mainly reactive oxygen species (ROS), are products generated by metabolic reactions of cells. In normal cells, low-level concentrations of these compounds are required for signal transduction. However, under pathological conditions such as cancer, cardiovascular diseases, and AMD, the ROS concentration is high. This happens by means of a feed-forward ROS-induced ROS-release loop coordinated by the endogenous NADPH oxidase/mtROS axis as described in Chapter 8. Oxidative stress, an imbalance between oxidative and antioxidative systems in cells and tissues, is a result of overproduction of ROS, causing damage to many intracellular molecules, including DNA, RNA, lipids, and proteins.[26] Specifically, antioxidant supplementation in cancer therapy is much more complicated than in AMD management. The antioxidant therapy may be a double-edged sword in cancer treatment. Radiotherapy and some chemotherapy regimens generate free radicals for cytotoxic functions, whereas, exogenous antioxidants such as vitamins, minerals, and polyphenols may quench ROS activity. Therefore, whether antioxidants could alter antitumor effects during radiotherapy and some types of chemotherapy remains unclear.[27] Meanwhile, the AREDS study demonstrated that dietary antioxidant supplementation has modest efficacy in slowing down AMD progression. However, the question remains whether the AREDS findings are generalizable to the population as a whole? As described earlier, whether subgroups with specific genetic risk factors may have different responses to the AREDS formula is still unclear. Clearly, antioxidant supplement therapy is complex and must be considered in the context of different diseases. Evidence-based clinical trials with the appropriate design are needed to answer the unmet questions in AMD.

Targeting the NADPH oxidase complex in cancer and AMD

Oxidative stress is a consequence of high levels of ROS generated in mitochondria by several enzymes, including NADPH oxidase (NOX) as described in Chapter 7. Numerous studies pointed out the pathogenic role of oxidative stress in the development and progression of AMD. Therefore, suppression of oxidative stress by inhibition of NOX is a rational therapeutic strategy in AMD and other oxidative-stress driven diseases, including cancer. In fact, the research on NOX inhibition therapy for both cancer and AMD is ongoing.[28] Increasing evidence shows that ROS generated by NOX systems plays a crucial role in the invasive potential of certain types of cancer.[29] Specific isoforms of NOX such as NOX2, in combination with the inflammatory activity of endothelial cells within the tumor, can facilitate tumor growth. Thus, inhibition of NOX2 may block the proangiogenic survival signals that are responsible for tumor cell proliferation. Isoform-specific NOX inhibitors are currently being developed. Evidence has shown that NOX inhibition by small molecules appears to effectively decrease tumor growth in vivo.[30,31] For instance, when Setanaxib (GKT137831), a selective NADPH oxidase inhibitor, was used in isolated cancer-associated fibroblasts (CAFs) from human cancers, more normal fibroblast-phenotype is restored, and CAF-dependent increase in cell migration is rescued.[30] In future research, it remains to be determined whether selective NADPH oxidase inhibitors can be developed to control ROS generation in the outer retina in AMD?

NLRP3 inflammasome inhibitor in cancer and AMD

The NLRP3 inflammasome is characterized as a cytosolic complex, which belongs to the nucleotide-binding and oligomerization domain-like receptor (NLR) family, as described in Chapter 7. This inflammasome complex comprises NLRP3 protein, ASC (apoptosis-associated speck-like protein containing a caspase recruitment domain), and procaspase 1. Activated NLRP3 inflammasome is associated with numerous age-related disorders such as Alzheimer's disease and AMD. In addition, the NLRP3 inflammasome is also linked with various cancers, such as colon cancer, breast cancer, melanoma, and gastrointestinal cancers.[32] Because assembly of NLRP3 inflammasome involves in multiple signaling pathways, diverse targets of these pathways can be used to inhibit this activation. In recent years, clinical interest in exploring potential inhibitors of the NLRP3 inflammasome has grown. For instance, as NLRP3 inflammasome activation in RPE is observed in atrophic AMD, NLRP3 inhibitors have been studied in preclinical models of AMD, showing a reduction of photooxidative damage in RPE cells.[33] Meanwhile, a variety of pharmacological NLRP3 inflammasome inhibitors that regulate the link between innate immunity and cancer immunosurveillance may lead to an increase in tumoricidal function of immune cells in tumor tissues.[34–36] For example, MCC950, an inhibitor of NLRP3 inflammasome, suppressed the NLRP3 inflammasome activation and increased the number of effective CD4[+] and CD8[+] T cells in a mouse model of head and neck squamous cell carcinoma.[37] It is likely that more effective NLRP3 inflammasome inhibitors will emerge for clinical trials in cancer and AMD.

Future translational research of AMD by multidisplinary approach

The neurons of the CNS form a complex network to perform CNS functions. Because intrinsic regenerative capacity of CNS is limited, damage to the neuronal network is difficult to repair or reconstruct. The optic nerve and retina are components of the CNS. Their regenerative capacity is limited as well. GA in AMD is characterized by retinal pigmented epithelium (RPE) death and resultant photoreceptor degeneration. Therefore, protecting neurons and minimizing neuronal damage is a logical approach for the treatment of injuries and nerve disorders such as the GA happening in late dry AMD. Numerous endogenous and exogenous protectants have been investigated; however, the exact biological effects of each neuroprotectant are complex and in most cases remain unclear. In addition to small-molecule neuroprotectants, the following endogenous neuroprotectants have been extensively studied: pituitary adenylate cyclase-activating polypeptide, hepatocyte growth factor, neurotrophic factors, apolipoprotein E-containing lipoprotein, prothymosin α, erythropoietin, and tissue inhibitor of metalloproteinase.[38] Notably, one of the essential mechanisms of neuroprotectants is the attenuation of neuronal apoptosis, blocking the final common pathways of cell death.[38,39] For example, ciliary neurotrophic factor, an endogenous factor that combats amyloid beta (Aβ)-induced cytotoxicity, oxidative injury, and cell apoptosis,[40] underwent a phase 2 clinical trial for macular telangiectasia.[41] Another endogenous neuroprotectant, erythropoietin (EPO), has been proposed for the treatment of atrophic AMD, because of its antiapoptotic, antiinflammatory, and antioxidative functions.[42] EPO is a glycoprotein expressed in the fetal liver and is then predominantly produced in the kidney after birth.[38] EPO is characterized as a humoral regulator of erythropoiesis. EPO and its receptor are expressed in various tissues including brain and retina. Evidence exists that exogenous EPO acts as a potent neuroprotectant for retinal vascular and neuronal cells against apoptosis.[43] By using in vitro oxidative models of retinal neurons, our laboratory documented that EPO is able to enhance BAD phosphorylation and Bcl-xL expression while downregulating Bax. The neuroprotective effect of EPO in the regulation of the apoptosis-related proteins is mediated through the ERK and Akt pathways.[44] Recently, we used a rat model of retinal degeneration to explore the efficacy of EPO administered via subretinal transplantation of *EPO* gene-modified rat mesenchymal stem cells (rMSCs).[45] The results demonstrated the ability of rMSCs to differentiate into RPE cells in the niche of the host subretinal space and showed improved therapeutic effect of *EPO* gene-modified rMSCs on retinal morphology and visual functions, as compared to unmodified rMSCs alone.[45] This study may not only show the efficacy of neuroprotectants such as EPO on the rescue of retinal degeneration but also suggest a novel delivery system combining gene therapy with cell-based therapy for long-acting treatment. To develop novel and effective treatments for AMD, valid clinical trials demonstrating cytoprotection of RPE and photoreceptors in AMD patients are needed.

As the comprehensive discussion of the future studies needed on AMD is beyond the scope of this chapter, we intend to emphasize some anatomically and functionally unique aspects of the eye, which could offer opportunities accelerating AMD research in the future. First, the optic nerve (ON) and retina are the only directly visible components of the CNS. It has been realized that structural and functional features of the retina and ON such as optical coherence tomography (OCT)-measured retinal thickness and electrophysiological tests, for example, VEP and PERG, can be used as biomarkers for specific disorders of CNS.[46,47] Future studies may discover and develop retinal and/or ON specific biomarkers, by which AMD can be differentiated from other CNS disorders, and vice versa.

Second, the anterograde transmission of visual signals begins from outer to inner retina, that is, from photoreceptors to bipolar cells to ganglion cells. When the outer retina is destroyed in late AMD, engineered devices such as Argus II can bypass the outer retina and send signals directly to the brain. There is evidence that retrospective trans-synaptic activity from ON to retina exists and exerts special neurological function.[48,49] For instance, persistent strengthening or weakening of synapses, so-called long-term potentiation (LTP) or long-term depression (LTD), is induced by retrograde spread from the optic tectum to the retina. The retrograde spread of LTP and LTD. is initiated by brain-derived neurotrophic factor, resulting in potentiation and depression of bipolar cells.[50] A future study may use bidirectional regulation of the strength of input synapses between bipolar cells and photoreceptors, to direct whether the degenerative process in cones and rods can be halted and degenerative neurons and glia "trained" or rejuvenated?

Third, the transparency of ocular media and the neuroretina provides a unique opportunity to visualize and surgically manipulate the retina directly. The multimodal imaging system of OCT has helped gain visualization of the subretinal and sub-RPE structures at the posterior pole. Future clinical trials may use standard and new imaging techniques, for example, choroidal blood flow, choriocapillaris density by optical coherence tomographic angiography (OCTA) and others, for categorizing subgroups of AMD and evaluating the efficacy of new drugs for AMD treatment.

Fourth, the subretinal space is a special location for pathogenic events in AMD. The subretinal space is devoid of immune cells, due to the potent immunosuppressive factors produced by the RPE, which eliminate infiltrating leukocytes. It has been discussed in Chapter 7 that AMD causes macrophage infiltration into this space, resulting in a chronic inflammatory microenvironment. The by-products of inflammation form drusen, the hallmark of AMD. Future studies should target keeping the subretinal space in an antiinflammatory condition. If antiinflammatory therapy is used, the focus should be on monitoring druse formation and development in the subretinal space.

Fifth, the subretinal space has attracted special attention because it is an ideal location for gene therapy and cell-based therapy. The subretinal space is nonvascular and protected from systemic circulation by the outer blood-retinal barrier, that is, tight junction of RPE cells. Additionally, the RPE produces a variety of immunosuppressive molecules. Therefore, the classical immune responses are limited in the subretinal space. In other words, the subretinal space possesses the so-called immune privilege. This condition is amenable to for gene therapy because studies have shown that adaptive humoral and cellular responses to the transgene, as well as to the AAV2 capsid, are negative.[51] However, gene augmentation clinical trials via subretinal injections showed limited success in the real-world practice.[52,53] The high rate of complication such as disturbance of remaining photoreceptors, damage to underlying Bruch's membrane, and iatrogenic retinal detachment has become the bottleneck for this technique. In future clinical studies, the technique of subretinal manipulation needs to be improved. Meanwhile, other routes for delivering gene-based materials should be investigated? In fact, the intravitreal route has gained popularity. Jacobson and Aguirre et al. pointed out that not only is the intravitreal technique simpler and safer, but also it has proven to be effective.[52] Supportive evidence showed that in primates the intravitreal vectors penetrate large areas of the retina, particularly photoreceptors in the macula.[54−56] The improved technique for the subretinal space delivery and the enlarged applicability of intravitreal injection for gene-vectors will promote future clinical trials with various gene therapies.[57] Further, stem cell-based therapies are showing progress as discussed in Chapter 11. Schwartz et al. have reported phase 1 and 2 studies using subretinal transplantation of human embryonic stem cell-derived RPE to treat AMD patients with GA.[58−60] Ten of 18 (56%) patients showed visual improvement. The main adverse events were associated with para-operative immune suppression. Overall, the results of this pilot study are encouraging. On the other hand, it is recognized that although the subretinal space is considered as a unique and promising target for cell-based therapy, it cannot provide a complete immune-privileged environment. There is much to learn about cell-based therapy, as there is with other treatment modalities for AMD.

References

1. Kontis V, Bennett JE, Mathers CD, Li G, Foreman K, Ezzati M. Future life expectancy in 35 industrialised countries: projections with a Bayesian model ensemble. *Lancet.* 2017; 389(10076):1323−1335. https://doi.org/10.1016/S0140-6736(16)32381-9.
2. Guest PC, ed. *Reviews on Biomarker Studies in Aging and Anti-aging Research.* Adv. Exp. Med. Biol. 1st; Vol. 1178. Springer International Publishing; 2019.

3. Beard JR, Officer A, de Carvalho IA, et al. The World report on ageing and health: a policy framework for healthy ageing. *Lancet.* 2016;387(10033):2145−2154. https://doi.org/10.1016/S0140-6736(15)00516-4.

4. Flatt T. A new definition of aging? *Front Genet.* 2012;3. https://doi.org/10.3389/fgene.2012.00148.

5. Wong WL, Su X, Li X, et al. Global prevalence of age-related macular degeneration and disease burden projection for 2020 and 2040: a systematic review and meta-analysis. *Lancet Glob Health.* 2014;2(2):e106−116. https://doi.org/10.1016/S2214-109X(13)70145-1.

6. Gibson G. Rare and common variants: twenty arguments. *Nat Rev Genet.* 2012;13(2):135−145. https://doi.org/10.1038/nrg3118.

7. Fritsche LG, Igl W, Bailey JNC, et al. A large genome-wide association study of age-related macular degeneration highlights contributions of rare and common variants. *Nat Genet.* 2016;48(2):134−143. https://doi.org/10.1038/ng.3448.

8. Gorin MB, daSilva MJ. Predictive genetics for AMD: hype and hopes for genetics-based strategies for treatment and prevention. *Exp Eye Res.* 2020;191:107894. https://doi.org/10.1016/j.exer.2019.107894.

9. Heesterbeek TJ, de Jong EK, Acar IE, et al. Genetic risk score has added value over initial clinical grading stage in predicting disease progression in age-related macular degeneration. *Sci Rep.* 2019;9(1):6611. https://doi.org/10.1038/s41598-019-43144-3.

10. Lazzeri S, Orlandi P, Figus M, et al. The rs2071559 AA VEGFR-2 genotype frequency is significantly lower in neovascular age-related macular degeneration patients. *Sci World J.* 2012:420190. https://doi.org/10.1100/2012/420190.

11. Seddon JM, Reynolds R, Yu Y, Daly MJ, Rosner B. Risk models for progression to advanced age-related macular degeneration using demographic, environmental, genetic, and ocular factors. *Ophthalmology.* 2011;118(11):2203−2211. https://doi.org/10.1016/j.ophtha.2011.04.029.

12. Awh CC, Lane A-M, Hawken S, Zanke B, Kim IK. CFH and ARMS2 genetic polymorphisms predict response to antioxidants and zinc in patients with age-related macular degeneration. *Ophthalmology.* 2013;120(11):2317−2323. https://doi.org/10.1016/j.ophtha.2013.07.039.

13. Seddon JM, Silver RE, Rosner B. Response to AREDS supplements according to genetic factors: survival analysis approach using the eye as the unit of analysis. *Br J Ophthalmol.* 2016;100(12):1731−1737. https://doi.org/10.1136/bjophthalmol-2016-308624.

14. Park DH, Sun HJ, Lee SJ. A comparison of responses to intravitreal bevacizumab, ranibizumab, or aflibercept injections for neovascular age-related macular degeneration. *Int Ophthalmol.* 2017;37(5):1205−1214. https://doi.org/10.1007/s10792-016-0391-4.

15. Ribatti D. Judah Folkman, a pioneer in the study of angiogenesis. *Angiogenesis.* 2008;11(1):3−10. https://doi.org/10.1007/s10456-008-9092-6.

16. Folkman J. Tumor angiogenesis: therapeutic implications. *N Engl J Med.* 1971;285(21):1182−1186. https://doi.org/10.1056/NEJM197111182852108.

17. Ferrara N, Henzel WJ. Pituitary follicular cells secrete a novel heparin-binding growth factor specific for vascular endothelial cells. *Biochem Biophys Res Commun.* 1989;161(2):851−858. https://doi.org/10.1016/0006-291x(89)92678-8.

18. Carmeliet P, Ferreira V, Breier G, et al. Abnormal blood vessel development and lethality in embryos lacking a single VEGF allele. *Nature.* 1996;380(6573):435−439. https://doi.org/10.1038/380435a0.

19. Rosenfeld PJ, Brown DM, Heier JS, et al. Ranibizumab for neovascular age-related macular degeneration. *N Engl J Med*. 2006;355(14):1419−1431. https://doi.org/10.1056/NEJMoa054481.

20. Macheret M, Halazonetis TD. DNA replication stress as a hallmark of cancer. *Annu Rev Pathol*. 2015;10:425−448. https://doi.org/10.1146/annurev-pathol-012414-040424.

21. Russo M, Giavazzi R. Anti-angiogenesis for cancer: current status and prospects. *Thromb Res*. 2018;164(Suppl 1):S3−S6. https://doi.org/10.1016/j.thromres.2018.01.030.

22. Ramjiawan RR, Griffioen AW, Duda DG. Anti-angiogenesis for cancer revisited: is there a role for combinations with immunotherapy? *Angiogenesis*. 2017;20(2):185−204. https://doi.org/10.1007/s10456-017-9552-y.

23. Qin S, Li A, Yi M, Yu S, Zhang M, Wu K. Recent advances on anti-angiogenesis receptor tyrosine kinase inhibitors in cancer therapy. *J Hematol Oncol*. 2019;12(1):27. https://doi.org/10.1186/s13045-019-0718-5.

24. Sharma A, Kumar N, Kuppermann BD, Bandello F, Loewenstein A. Biotherapeutics and immunogenicity: ophthalmic perspective. *Eye*. 2019;33(9):1359−1361. https://doi.org/10.1038/s41433-019-0434-y.

25. Al-Khersan H, Hussain RM, Ciulla TA, Dugel PU. Innovative therapies for neovascular age-related macular degeneration. *Expet Opin Pharmacother*. 2019;20(15):1879−1891. https://doi.org/10.1080/14656566.2019.1636031.

26. Veskoukis AS, Tsatsakis AM, Kouretas D. Dietary oxidative stress and antioxidant defense with an emphasis on plant extract administration. *Cell Stress Chaperones*. 2012;17(1):11−21. https://doi.org/10.1007/s12192-011-0293-3.

27. Yasueda A, Urushima H, Ito T. Efficacy and interaction of antioxidant supplements as adjuvant therapy in cancer treatment: a systematic review. *Integr Canc Ther*. 2016;15(1):17−39. https://doi.org/10.1177/1534735415610427.

28. Terluk MR, Ebeling MC, Fisher CR, et al. N-Acetyl-L-cysteine protects human retinal pigment epithelial cells from oxidative damage: implications for age-related macular degeneration. *Oxid Med Cell Longev*. 2019;2019:5174957. https://doi.org/10.1155/2019/5174957.

29. Roy K, Wu Y, Meitzler JL, et al. NADPH oxidases and cancer. *Clin Sci*. 2015;128(12):863−875. https://doi.org/10.1042/CS20140542.

30. Hanley CJ, Mellone M, Ford K, et al. Targeting the myofibroblastic cancer-associated fibroblast phenotype through inhibition of NOX4. *J Natl Cancer Inst*. 2018;110(1). https://doi.org/10.1093/jnci/djx121.

31. Doroshow JH, Gaur S, Markel S, et al. Effects of iodonium-class flavin dehydrogenase inhibitors on growth, reactive oxygen production, cell cycle progression, NADPH oxidase 1 levels, and gene expression in human colon cancer cells and xenografts. *Free Radic Biol Med*. 2013;57:162−175. https://doi.org/10.1016/j.freeradbiomed.2013.01.002.

32. Zahid A, Li B, Kombe AJK, Jin T, Tao J. Pharmacological inhibitors of the NLRP3 inflammasome. *Front Immunol*. 2019;10:2538. https://doi.org/10.3389/fimmu.2019.02538.

33. Wang L, Schmidt S, Larsen PP, et al. Efficacy of novel selective NLRP3 inhibitors in human and murine retinal pigment epithelial cells. *J Mol Med*. 2019;97(4):523−532. https://doi.org/10.1007/s00109-019-01753-5.

34. Moossavi M, Parsamanesh N, Bahrami A, Atkin SL, Sahebkar A. Role of the NLRP3 inflammasome in cancer. *Mol Canc*. 2018;17(1):158. https://doi.org/10.1186/s12943-018-0900-3.

35. Swanson KV, Deng M, Ting JP-Y. The NLRP3 inflammasome: molecular activation and regulation to therapeutics. *Nat Rev Immunol*. 2019;19(8):477−489. https://doi.org/10.1038/s41577-019-0165-0.

36. Dupaul-Chicoine J, Arabzadeh A, Dagenais M, et al. The Nlrp3 inflammasome suppresses colorectal cancer metastatic growth in the liver by promoting natural killer cell tumoricidal activity. *Immunity*. 2015;43(4):751–763. https://doi.org/10.1016/j.immuni.2015.08.013.

37. Chen L, Huang C-F, Li Y-C, et al. Blockage of the NLRP3 inflammasome by MCC950 improves anti-tumor immune responses in head and neck squamous cell carcinoma. *Cell Mol Life Sci*. 2018;75(11):2045–2058. https://doi.org/10.1007/s00018-017-2720-9.

38. Hayashi H, Takagi N. Endogenous neuroprotective molecules and their mechanisms in the central nervous system. *Biol Pharm Bull*. 2015;38(8):1104–1108. https://doi.org/10.1248/bpb.b15-00361.

39. Sun X, Dai L, Zhang H, et al. Neuritin attenuates neuronal apoptosis mediated by endoplasmic reticulum stress in vitro. *Neurochem Res*. 2018;43(7):1383–1391. https://doi.org/10.1007/s11064-018-2553-4.

40. Wang K, Xie M, Zhu L, Zhu X, Zhang K, Zhou F. Ciliary neurotrophic factor protects SH-SY5Y neuroblastoma cells against Aβ1-42-induced neurotoxicity via activating the JAK2/STAT3 axis. *Folia Neuropathol*. 2015;53(3):226–235. https://doi.org/10.5114/fn.2015.54423.

41. Small R. Neurotech pharmaceuticals, inc. and lowy medical research institute announce publication of NT-501 phase 2 results. Cision PR Newswire. January 16, 2019 09:34 ET.

42. Wang Z-Y, Zhao K-K, Song Z-M, Shen L-J, Qu J. Erythropoietin as a novel therapeutic agent for atrophic age-related macular degeneration. *Med Hypotheses*. 2009;72(4):448–450. https://doi.org/10.1016/j.mehy.2008.09.055.

43. Zhang J, Wu Y, Jin Y, et al. Intravitreal injection of erythropoietin protects both retinal vascular and neuronal cells in early diabetes. *Invest Ophthalmol Vis Sci*. 2008;49(2):732–742. https://doi.org/10.1167/iovs.07-0721.

44. Shen J, Wu Y, Xu J-Y, et al. ERK- and Akt-dependent neuroprotection by erythropoietin (EPO) against glyoxal-AGEs via modulation of Bcl-xL, Bax, and BAD. *Invest Ophthalmol Vis Sci*. 2010;51(1):35–46. https://doi.org/10.1167/iovs.09-3544.

45. Guan Y, Cui L, Qu Z, et al. Subretinal transplantation of rat MSCs and erythropoietin gene modified rat MSCs for protecting and rescuing degenerative retina in rats. *Curr Mol Med*. 2013;13(9):1419–1431. https://doi.org/10.2174/15665240113139990071.

46. den Haan J, Csinscik L, Parker T, et al. Retinal thickness as potential biomarker in posterior cortical atrophy and typical Alzheimer's disease. *Alzheimer's Res Ther*. 2019;11(1):62. https://doi.org/10.1186/s13195-019-0516-x.

47. Janáky M, Jánossy Á, Horváth G, Benedek G, Braunitzer G. VEP and PERG in patients with multiple sclerosis, with and without a history of optic neuritis. *Doc Ophthalmol*. 2017;134(3):185–193. https://doi.org/10.1007/s10633-017-9589-7.

48. Munteanu T, Noronha KJ, Leung AC, Pan S, Lucas JA, Schmidt TM. Light-dependent pathways for dopaminergic amacrine cell development and function. *Elife*. 2018;7. https://doi.org/10.7554/eLife.39866.

49. Zhang D-Q, Belenky MA, Sollars PJ, Pickard GE, McMahon DG. Melanopsin mediates retrograde visual signaling in the retina. *PloS One*. 2012;7(8):e42647. https://doi.org/10.1371/journal.pone.0042647.

50. Du J, Wei H, Wang Z, Wong ST, Poo M. Long-range retrograde spread of LTP and LTD from optic tectum to retina. *Proc Natl Acad Sci U S A*. 2009;106(45):18890–18896. https://doi.org/10.1073/pnas.0910659106.

51. Bainbridge JWB, Smith AJ, Barker SS, et al. Effect of gene therapy on visual function in Leber's congenital amaurosis. *N Engl J Med*. 2008;358(21):2231–2239. https://doi.org/10.1056/NEJMoa0802268.

52. Garafalo AV, Cideciyan AV, Héon E, et al. Progress in treating inherited retinal diseases: early subretinal gene therapy clinical trials and candidates for future initiatives. *Prog Retin Eye Res*. 2020;77:100827. https://doi.org/10.1016/j.preteyeres.2019.100827.

53. Davis JL. The blunt end: surgical challenges of gene therapy for inherited retinal diseases. *Am J Ophthalmol*. 2018;196:xxv–xxix. https://doi.org/10.1016/j.ajo.2018.08.038.

54. Dalkara D, Byrne LC, Klimczak RR, et al. In vivo-directed evolution of a new adeno-associated virus for therapeutic outer retinal gene delivery from the vitreous. *Sci Transl Med*. 2013;5(189). https://doi.org/10.1126/scitranslmed.3005708, 189ra76-189ra76.

55. Boye SE, Alexander JJ, Witherspoon CD, et al. Highly efficient delivery of adeno-associated viral vectors to the primate retina. *Hum Gene Ther*. 2016;27(8):580–597. https://doi.org/10.1089/hum.2016.085.

56. Khabou H, Garita-Hernandez M, Chaffiol A, et al. Noninvasive gene delivery to foveal cones for vision restoration. *JCI Insight*. 2018;3(2). https://doi.org/10.1172/jci.insight.96029.

57. Ammar MJ, Hsu J, Chiang A, Ho AC, Regillo CD. Age-related macular degeneration therapy: a review. *Curr Opin Ophthalmol*. 2020;31(3):215–221. https://doi.org/10.1097/ICU.0000000000000657.

58. Schwartz SD, Regillo CD, Lam BL, et al. Human embryonic stem cell-derived retinal pigment epithelium in patients with age-related macular degeneration and Stargardt's macular dystrophy: follow-up of two open-label phase 1/2 studies. *Lancet*. 2015;385(9967):509–516. https://doi.org/10.1016/S0140-6736(14)61376-3.

59. Schwartz SD, Hubschman J-P, Heilwell G, et al. Embryonic stem cell trials for macular degeneration: a preliminary report. *Lancet*. 2012;379(9817):713–720. https://doi.org/10.1016/S0140-6736(12)60028-2.

60. Schwartz SD, Tan G, Hosseini H, Nagiel A. Subretinal transplantation of embryonic stem cell-derived retinal pigment epithelium for the treatment of macular degeneration: an assessment at 4 years. *Invest Ophthalmol Vis Sci*. 2016;57(5). https://doi.org/10.1167/iovs.15-18681. ORSFc1-9.

Index

'*Note*: Page numbers followed by "f" indicate figures and "t" indicate tables.'

Printed and bound by CPI Group (UK) Ltd, Croydon, CR0 4YY

03/10/2024

01040373-0002